NEURODEVELOPMENTAL DISEASES - LABORATORY AND CLINICAL RESEARCH

HANDBOOK ON CEREBRAL PALSY

RISK FACTORS, THERAPEUTIC MANAGEMENT AND LONG-TERM PROGNOSIS

NEURODEVELOPMENTAL DISEASES - LABORATORY AND CLINICAL RESEARCH

Additional books in this series can be found on Nova's website under the Series tab.

Additional e-books in this series can be found on Nova's website under the e-book tab.

NEURODEVELOPMENTAL DISEASES - LABORATORY AND CLINICAL RESEARCH

HANDBOOK ON CEREBRAL PALSY

RISK FACTORS, THERAPEUTIC MANAGEMENT AND LONG-TERM PROGNOSIS

HAROLD YATES
EDITOR

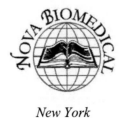

New York

Copyright © 2014 by Nova Science Publishers, Inc.

All rights reserved. No part of this book may be reproduced, stored in a retrieval system or transmitted in any form or by any means: electronic, electrostatic, magnetic, tape, mechanical photocopying, recording or otherwise without the written permission of the Publisher.

For permission to use material from this book please contact us:
Telephone 631-231-7269; Fax 631-231-8175
Web Site: http://www.novapublishers.com

NOTICE TO THE READER

The Publisher has taken reasonable care in the preparation of this book, but makes no expressed or implied warranty of any kind and assumes no responsibility for any errors or omissions. No liability is assumed for incidental or consequential damages in connection with or arising out of information contained in this book. The Publisher shall not be liable for any special, consequential, or exemplary damages resulting, in whole or in part, from the readers' use of, or reliance upon, this material. Any parts of this book based on government reports are so indicated and copyright is claimed for those parts to the extent applicable to compilations of such works.

Independent verification should be sought for any data, advice or recommendations contained in this book. In addition, no responsibility is assumed by the publisher for any injury and/or damage to persons or property arising from any methods, products, instructions, ideas or otherwise contained in this publication.

This publication is designed to provide accurate and authoritative information with regard to the subject matter covered herein. It is sold with the clear understanding that the Publisher is not engaged in rendering legal or any other professional services. If legal or any other expert assistance is required, the services of a competent person should be sought. FROM A DECLARATION OF PARTICIPANTS JOINTLY ADOPTED BY A COMMITTEE OF THE AMERICAN BAR ASSOCIATION AND A COMMITTEE OF PUBLISHERS.

Additional color graphics may be available in the e-book version of this book.

Library of Congress Cataloging-in-Publication Data

ISBN: 978-1-63321-852-9
Library of Congress Control Number: 2014948645

Published by Nova Science Publishers, Inc. † New York

Contents

Preface		**vii**
Chapter 1	Cerebral Palsy in an Era of Neuroprotection and Evidence Based Interventions: Risk Factors, Therapeutic Management, and Prognoses for Long Term Functioning and Participation *Petra Karlsson, Sarah McIntyre Ph.D. and Michael E. Msall M.D.*	**1**
Chapter 2	Integration of Exergames and Virtual Reality in the Treatment of Cerebral Palsy Children *Bruno Bonnechère, Bart Jansen, Lubos Omelina and Serge Van Sint Jan*	**25**
Chapter 3	Unilateral Cerebral Palsy: Epidemiology, Etiology, Imaging and Treatment of Hand Function Problems *Lucianne Speth M.D. and Hans Vles M.D., Ph.D.*	**41**
Chapter 4	The Problem Patella of Crouch Gait in Adolescents with Cerebral Palsy *Tim O'Brien, Damien Kiernan and Rory O'Sullivan*	**53**
Chapter 5	Infant Cerebral Palsy in Hemiplegic Children: Treatment Options and Outcome *Melissa Rosa-Rizzotto, M.D., Ph.D., Cristina Ranzato, Ph.D. and Paola Facchin, M.D., Ph.D.*	**63**
Chapter 6	Assessment of Postural Control and Functionality in Children with Cerebral Palsy: Possibilities and Relevance *Cristina dos Santos Cardoso de Sá and Raquel de Paula Carvalho*	**97**
Chapter 7	Improving Gait in Individuals with Cerebral Palsy: Novel Treatment Options *Luanda André Collange Grecco, Natália de Almeida Carvalho Duarte and Alejandra Malavera*	**115**

Contents

Chapter 8   Fine Motor Performance of Children with Ataxic Cerebral Palsy
during Tracing Activity: A Case Report   **127**
*Maraísa Fonseca Machado, Rita de Cássia Tibério Araújo
and Lígia Maria Presumido Braccialli*

Chapter 9   The Value of Providing Cerebral Palsy Children and Caregivers
an Oral Health Program   **141**
*Renata Oliveira Guaré, Ph.D.,
Daniel Cividanis Gomes Nogueira Fernandes, M.D.,
Ana Lídia Ciamponi, Ph.D.
and Maria Teresa Botti Rodrigues Santos, Ph.D.*

Chapter 10   The Use of Weight Bracelet in Individuals with Encephalopathy   **151**
*Mauro Audi, Andréia Naomi Sankako
and Lígia Maria Presumido Braccialli*

Chapter 11   Is Cerebral Palsy Associated with Cardiac Changes?   **161**
*Maria Cristina Duarte Ferreira, Jaqueline Wagenfuhr,
Renata de Oliveira Guaré, Sergio Tufik, Dalva Poyares,
Wercules Oliveira, Carlos Alberto Pastore
and Maria Teresa Botti Rodrigues Santos*

Chapter 12   Cerebral Palsy, Which Risk Factors Could Be Important:
Are They the Same for All Populations?   **169**
María de la Luz Arenas-Sordo, M.D., Ph.D.

Chapter 13   Management of Postural Abnormalities in Children
with Cerebral Palsy   **177**
*Michiyuki Kawakami, M.D., Ph.D.
and Meigen Liu, M.D., Ph.D.*

Chapter 14   Shock Wave Therapy for Reduction of Muscle Spasticity
in Children with Cerebral Palsy   **193**
*Elena Milkova Ilieva M.D., Ph.D.
and Maria Ilieva Gonkova, M.D.*

Chapter 15   Latest Trends in Neurorehabilitation of Patients with Cerebral Palsy   **205**
Stanislava Klobucká, Elena Žiaková and Robert Klobucký

Chapter 16   Improvement of Gross Motor Functions in Patients with Cerebral
Palsy After Robotic Assisted Treadmill Training (RATT)
Depending on Age   **231**
Stanislava Klobucká, Elena Žiaková and Robert Klobucký

Chapter 17   Effect of Social Support on Parenting Stress of Mothers of Children
with Cerebral Palsy   **249**
*Yeon-Gyu Jeong, Jeong-A Bang, Yeon-Jae Jeong,
and Hyun-Sook Kim, Ph.D.*

Index   **259**

Preface

Cerebral palsy (CP) is an extremely heterogeneous condition. There is any number of aetiological pathways possible for causing brain damage to the developing fetus and into early childhood, and these are morphing and changing over time. There are also numerous clinical manifestations of CP encompassing: different motor types, topographies, gross motor function levels, manual abilities, intellectual, communication, behavioral, sensory, abilities and impairments. Understanding the risk factors and complex causal pathways to CP has been a slow and protracted process. This handbook discusses the risk factors of cerebral palsy, as well as the therapeutic management options, and long-term prognosis of the condition.

Chapter 1 – The purpose of this chapter is to examine current knowledge of risk factors among term and preterm infants for developing cerebral palsy. The authors will highlight advances in understanding the changing epidemiology and the contribution of registries and case-control studies with respect to our knowledge of causal pathways. The authorswill also highlight advances in neuroprotection with a focus on optimizing early identification and introducing evidence based interventions to optimize gross motor, fine motor, communicative and developmental functioning. Among adults with cerebral palsy without intellectual disability, the majority are completing high school, living independently, and participating in community activities. However, challenges in health, social skills, and executive function can lead to suboptimal adult outcomes. To improve health and developmental trajectories for individuals with cerebral palsy it will require clinical and translational community networks that emphasize prevention, neuroprotection, and neurorehabilitation. The authors propose one such model for the research community to debate and consider.

Chapter 2 – How to motivate children (patients) to perform their exercises during rehabilitation or at home? This is the challenge met by physical therapists in their daily professional practice with disabled patients. Indeed, a lack of motivation is one of the most frequent reasons for patients to drop out. Commercial video games have significantly evolved over the last decade. Today computer performance and play experience allow new perspectives for rehabilitation. Thanks to new gaming controllers (Nintendo Wii Fit™, Microsoft Xbox Kinect™, etc.) video game playing has changed from a passive (i.e., the player is seated on a sofa) to an active experience: players have to move in order to interact with games. Clinicians are now prospecting the new potential use of these games in rehabilitation mainly through testing available commercial games with patients suffering from various pathologies (e.g., cerebral palsy, brain stroke, Parkinson disease, elderly…). Physical rehabilitation must be based on active exercises, and new gaming strategy allows it. Furthermore, the game environment is obviously a major advantage to increase patient motivation to perform their rehabilitation schemes. Today challenge is to use games as rehabilitation. However, results of these first clinical tests using commercial video games are not as good as first expected. Several limitations appeared when using commercial video games in rehabilitation. Such games are designed for entertainment purpose and obviously do not include any therapeutically know-how and strategies. Further, the architecture of the games (i.e., tasks to achieve, visual background, etc) is not adapted for patients showing various kinds of disabilities like motor or visual disorders. For example, most games are based on scenario fast movements to succeed while such quick execution is often contraindicated during many physical rehabilitation schemes related to neurological disorders. Also, player motion accuracy requested by the player during the games is low while most therapists will aim to improve patient joint control and coordination. In short, commercial video games are not adapted for rehabilitation; contrariwise the different gaming controllers used offer interesting new perspectives for rehabilitation. The current challenge for therapists is to help the game industry to develop specific games well-adapted for specific pathologies. Since a few years specific solutions have been developed and tested with cerebral palsy children. This chapter presents an overview of the different works that have been done in the field both using commercial games as well as games specifically developed for the target group. Advantages and limits of each approach will be then discussed. Finally, the last part of this chapter will focus on global trends for future work and perspectives will be provided on how to integrate rehabilitation aspects (physiotherapy, occupational therapy) in game scenarios.

Chapter 3 – Cerebral Palsy (CP) describes a group of permanent disorders of development of movement and posture, causing activity limitation, that are attributed to non-progressive disturbances that occurred in the developing fetal or infant brain. The prevalence of CP remains constant over the last years at 2.11 per 1000 live births. Unilateral spastic CP (uCP), also called hemiplegic CP, has a prevalence of 0.6 per 1,000 live births, and amounts to about 30% of the CP subtype proportion. In children with a birth weight of 2,500g or more, there is an increase of the uCP subtype. The definition of CP gives no etiological explanation. However, with the introduction of modern neuro-imaging, the authors are more informed in detail about the different etiological and risk factors. Different etiology will have different consequences with concern to cortical and sub-cortical re-organization. In this review chapter the authors will focus on a vascular event (hypoxic ischemic, HI or stroke) as a cause for uCP, using definitions related to gestational age. Ultrasound (US) and Magnetic Resonance Imaging (MRI) are not only of importance in studying etiology but also can be of help to determine the time the insult took place. The clinical presentation of uCP is variable due to the severity and localization of the lesion, associated pathology and the aspect of the incident: chronic HI versus acute asphyxia. With the introduction of new neuro-imaging techniques, such as functional MRI (fMRI) and Diffusion Tensor Imaging (DTI), we are more informed about the relation of structure and function and the possibilities of neuronal adaptation. This is of utmost clinical importance, because the way the re-organization of neuronal networks (ipsi or contra lateral) takes place and the severity and localization of the lesion correlates with hand function and bimanual performance and even influences therapy outcome. Developmental disuse is a problem typically occurring in uCP and also influencing therapy outcome. Evidence of several treatment modalities of unilateral hand function problems in children with unilateral CP, i.e., bimanual intensive goal directed treatment, constraint induced movement therapy and botulinum toxin A treatment, will be discussed.

Chapter 4 – The purpose of this review is to demonstrate the etiology and effects of patellar fractures in adolescents with crouch gait. The authors describe the correlation between these fractures and Gait Laboratory kinematic and kinetic data. These fractures are not incidental findings as they are always associated with a significant deterioration in gait. The kinematic and kinetic data that accompanies displaced fractures are typical of knee extensor disruption. The more common oblique fracture through the distal pole of the patella is caused by an increased bending force on the patella while the increased traction of crouch can also result in a sleeve fracture. The authors outline the surgical options for treatment of knee extensor disruption.

Chapter 5 – Cerebral palsy (CP) describes a group of disorders of the development of movement and posture, causing activity limitation, that are attributed to non progressive disturbances that occurred in the developing fetal or infant brain. CP is the leading cause of childhood disability affecting function and development. This disorder affects the development of movement and is believed to arise from nonprogressive disturbances in the developing fetal or infant brain. In addition to the motor disorders that characterize cerebral palsy, which may limit a patient's activities, individuals with cerebral palsy often display epilepsy, secondary musculoskeletal problems, and disturbances of sensation, perception, cognition, communication, and behavior. CP is characterized by sensorimotor dysfunction as manifested by atypical muscle tone, posture and movement. Severity of impairment varies widely, depending on the site and severity of brain damage. Hemiplegia is a unilateral physical impairment, is a common type of CP accounting for 36-40% of all CP. Typically, the upper limb is more involved than the lower, with impairments of spasticity, sensation and reduced strength. One of the most disabling symptoms of hemiplegia is unilaterally impaired hand and arm function, which affects self-care activities such as feeding, dressing, and grooming. The impairment of the hand is often the result of damage to the motor cortex and corticospinal pathways responsible for the fine motor control of the fingers and hand. Thus, skilled independent finger movements do not develop typically in children with hemiplegia. During tasks that require fine manipulation, such children often use several fingers, and often show abnormal hand posturing as well as reduction in distal strength and dexterity.

Sensory disturbances can occur as well, further complicating any motor impairment. Furthermore, children with hemiplegia due to cerebral palsy (CP, the most motorically studied subtype of hemiplegia) have difficulty with the timing and coordination of reaching movements, grasping, movement planning, and a deficient capacity to modulate postural adjustments during reaching. The resulting sensory and motor impairments in children with hemiplegia compromise movement efficiency. Such children often tend not to use the affected extremity, resulting in a developmentally learned non-use of the involved upper extremity that can be termed 'developmental disuse. Typically, rehabilitation techniques have focused on teaching and reinforcing compensatory strategies that encourage use of the non-involved upper extremity to decrease functional limitations. Strong evidence for the successful application of any therapeutic approach is lacking. Recent evidence suggests that children with hemiplegic CP can improve motor performance if provided sufficient practice. This finding indicates that intensive practice may improve function in the involved upper extremity that could lead to increased use in daily life. In the last decades, several treatment approaches have been employed to improve upper limb function in hemiplegic CP.

The chapter provides a review of current efficacy of the most recent treatment approaches, including a focus on Constraint Induced Movement Therapy and bimanual intensive rehabilitation approach.

Chapter 6 – Cerebral palsy (CP) is one of the most common causes of chronic disability in childhood, with an incidence of 2 to 2.5 in 1000 live births in developed countries. In Brazil, 24.5 million people have some kind of disability, including CP. Cerebral palsy is group of permanent disorders related to mobility and postural development due to a non-progressive disturbance in immature brain during fetal period or childhood. Brain abnormalities associated with CP may also contribute to sensory, cognitive, communication and behavioral disorders including motor disabilities and spasticity. Children and adolescents with CP have lower level of physical activity than those with typical development. Problems in motor control can reduce the amount of movements performed by children resulting in a lack of experience with motor activities, which would delay concept formation about sensation and motor activity, sociality. The capability of maintaining postural control is essential for performing Activities of Daily Living (ADL's). In accordance with the level of motor function, children with CP have different degrees of trunk control and level of functionality that affect their performance in ADL's mainly when the upper limbs are affected. Therefore, CP can impose many limitations on social activity and participation. There is an ongoing effort to develop assessment methods that are suitable for people with CP to provide relevant information about their postural control and level of functionality to clinical and research proposes. The proposal of this chapter is to introduce the relevant aspects and evaluation protocols about postural control and functionality in children with CP.

Chapter 7 – Independently of the size of the brain lesion in individuals with cerebral palsy (CP), a global reduction occurs in the activation of the central nervous system during the execution of movements[1] with changes in the excitability of the primary motor cortex and a reduction in the processing of corticospinal and somatosensory circuits. Thus, approximately 90% of individuals with CP have some degree of gait impairment stemming from neurological abnormalities that result in muscle weakness, reductions in selective motor control and postural reactions as well as changes in joint kinematics.[5] Gait pattern and independent locomotion are closely associated with the topography of the motor impairment (hemiparesis, diparesis or quadriparesis) and the level of gross motor function determined by the Gross Motor Function Classification System (GMFCS, Levels I to V).

A number of methods and resources are currently employed in the rehabilitation process of children and adults with CP, such as stretching and muscle strengthening exercises, spasticity control through muscle relaxant drugs (e.g., botulinum toxin) and gait training methods (treadmill training with or without body weight support). More recently, encouraging preliminary results have been achieved with noninvasive cerebral stimulation, specifically transcranial direct current stimulation, which has been used to facilitate the excitability of the primary motor cortex during gait and balance training.

In the last five years, a large number of studies have demonstrated and discussed the effects of treadmill training with body weight support. Despite the divergences, the findings suggest benefits mainly in gait velocity and gross motor function in children classified on Levels II to IV of the GMFCS. The most important results are achieved with training protocols that involve a gradual reduction in body weight support and sessions with a frequency of two or three times a week. Papers published in the last two years report positive results with treadmill training without body weight support and training velocity performed at the aerobic threshold in children classified on Levels I to III of the GMFCS. Besides an increase in gait velocity, these studies also report important improvements in balance and cardiopulmonary fitness, which favors the independence of the child.

Chapter 8 – The aim of this study was to test the effect of weight bracelet and adapted pen on fine motor graphic activity performance. Two patients with a diagnosis of ataxic cerebral palsy from the Occupational Therapy service participated in the study. The effect of these adaptations was tested during tracing activities on a tablet, with records related to time, jerk, pressure and strokes. The data represent four experimental situations: a) without adaptation, b) with weight bracelet, c) with weight bracelet and weight on an adapted pen, and d) with weight on an adapted pen. Participant P1 showed less tremor and execution time in situation "d", and less stroke and pressure in situation "c". Participant P2 had a shorter execution time, tremor and pen force in situation "d", and less stroke incidence in situation "c". This study suggests that the prescription of weight using weight bracelet in addition to weight on an adapted a pen to cerebral palsy patients would be suitable to perform graphic tasks with higher quality

Chapter 9 – Purpose: The purpose was to evaluate the effect of an education program on the oral health of individuals with cerebral palsy (CP) and their caregivers. Methods: 67 individuals with CP (8.87±3.91) of both sexes were evaluated, together with their caregivers (38.43±9.78) by a single examiner (kappa=0.88). Oral hygiene was evaluated using the Simplified Oral Hygiene Index (OHI-S) and the Gingival Index (GI). The general linear model for repeated measures was used to compare the effect of the intervention. Multivariate linear regression models were used to identify predictor variables. Results: The intervention achieved through the oral health program managed to reduce the OHI-S and GI in both the individuals with CP and their caregivers. The study also revealed that the only significant predictor for periodontal disease in individuals with CP was age. Conclusion: This research highlights the importance of early preventive guidelines through an oral health program that is also directed toward the caregivers.

Chapter 10 – This study aimed to analyze the function of upper limbs, in the reach movement to a target, with and without a weight bracelet, in individuals with encephalopathy who had involuntary movements of upper limbs. 7 individuals with diagnosis of encephalopathy who had involuntary movements, 2 females, 5 males, aged 21 to 38 years (mean = 26) participated in this study. Significant statistical differences were found (p = 0.03) to the obtained results of the distance gone through upper limb and to straightness index values (p = 0.03), comparing the obtained results with and without weight bracelet. The use of weight bracelet on the wrist influenced the values of the traveled distance and the straightness index during the reach movement to a target, which were lesser when compared to the movement without weight bracelet. Results demonstrated a better motor performance of upper limbs from participants of this study with weight bracelet.

Chapter 11 – Background: Some studies have suggested that an autonomic abnormality is associated with cerebral palsy. The modulation effects on autonomic function might be disturbed resulting in unbalanced sympathovagal activity. Aim: To investigate whether children with cerebral palsy (CP) present any cardiac abnormalities compared with healthy controls. Methods: Thirty-three CP children aged 5-14 years and 22 sibling controls underwent echocardiography and heart rate variability evaluations. Snoring and body mass index were also assessed. Results: The CP children presented lower values of body mass index (p=0.02), left ventricular mass index (p=0.03) and E/A ratio (p=0.01), as well as higher cardiac output (p=0.05), heart rate and blood pressure (p=0.01, both) compared with controls. With regard to heart rate variability, CP children presented higher values of High-frequency and Low-frequency and lower Low-frequency/High-frequency ratios (p=0.04, all) than controls. Conclusion: Children with CP present with chronic autonomic imbalance and some degree of diastolic impairment. The present results suggest that a cardiac investigation of these patients is warranted.

Chapter 12 – The concept of cerebral palsy (CP) has been created to include different neurological sequels that affect our motor sphere. In 1958, the first accepted definition was published by Mac-Keith and Polani: ''CP is a persistent motor disorder appearing before the age of 3 due to a non-progressive interference in the development of the brain taking place before the growth of the central nervous system is complete'' Cerebral palsy has remained unchanged over the past 50 years; its incidence is approximately 2.5 per 1000 live births, almost the same in different countries. Usually and in the classical form, CP has its origin in three important moments: Prenatal, perinatal and postnatal. In all of these, one same situation: hypoxic events, could appear. Of course there are other many possibilities in each one, for example, infections, malformations and accidents. The prenatal and perinatal causes are responsible for 70 to 80% of the cases; the rest corresponds to postnatal ones. There are many risk factors that cause CP in pre, peri or postnatal stages; they depend on the type of country, genetic characteristics of the populations and environment, all of which we know are different. To conclude, up to date, it is a fact that the important risk factors are preterm birth, pre or perinatal infections, hypoxia in the partum and thrombophilia and they can be more important or not, depending on the population. It is important to remember that the predisposition or protection afforded by our genes may allow or not that a determined condition presents itself depending on the rest of the genome and the environment that interacts with it.

Chapter 13 – Postural problems play a central role in the motor dysfunction of children with cerebral palsy. The performance of everyday activities is noticeably influenced by such postural deficits. In this chapter, the authors will review the epidemiology of postural deformities such as scoliosis, pelvic obliquity and hip subluxation/dislocation in these children. The authors then relate these deformities with secondary problems like pain, loss of ability, increased care burden, pressure problems, cardio-pulmonary dysfunctions, swallowing difficulties and sleep disturbance, which can all adversely affect the quality of life of the children as well as that of their caregivers. Many factors are involved in the development and aggravation of postural deformities, such as tone abnormalities, persistent primary reflexes, handedness, habitual posture, pain and inappropriate postural management. Among these factors, recent studies suggest that asymmetrical skull deformity (ASD) is frequently observed in cerebral palsy and closely related with asymmetric postural deformities. ASD is thought to be brought about by a predominantly one-sided facial direction during early childhood when the skull is softer, and once ASD becomes established, it aggravates the asymmetrical posture further. An asymmetrical tonic neck reflex caused by a one-sided face direction could contribute to the development and aggravation of postural abnormalities and limb and spinal deformities. A recent consensus statement by an expert multidisciplinary group defined a postural management program for children with cerebral palsy as "a planned approach encompassing all activities and interventions which impact on an individual's posture and function". In this comprehensive approach, postural management focused on

ASD and facial direction appears to be necessary to prevent deformities in children with cerebral palsy.

Chapter 14 – Extracorporeal shock wave therapy has been used for the treatment of chronic musculo-skeletal disorders in the last decades. Recently a new field of its application has been studied - for reduction of muscle spasticity as a result of central motor neuron disease. The authors present the knowledge about extracorporeal shock wave therapy: physical characteristics, types, evidence based mechanisms of its effect and indications for its use. The results of the studies about the efficacy of SWT in the treatment of muscle spasticity in adults after stroke and in children with cerebral palsy are presented and discussed.

The authors discuss also the results of their original study about the effect of radial shock wave therapy for reduction of muscle hypertonus of plantar flexor muscles of children with spastic diplegia and hemiplegia. One placebo session was applied followed four weeks later by one active treatment session. The authors used passive range of motion, Modified Aschworth Scale and pedobarometric measurements (static and dynamic) for outcome assessment. After RSWT, a significant increase in passive range of motion and decrease of the score of the Modified Ashworth Scale were observed, which persisted at fourth week follow-up. Pedobarometric measurement showed a significant increase in the contact plantar surface area and in heel pressure. Conclusion: Shock wave therapy could be considered as a treatment of choice for reduction of muscle spasticity in children with cerebral palsy.

Chapter 15 – Cerebral palsy (CP) still represents a live medical as well as social issue. It is one of the most common neurodevelopmental disorders in the childhood. The aim of this paper is to highlight the need for early diagnosis and adequate rehabilitation therapy of cerebral palsy. The early start of rehabilitation is the fundamental and crucial therapeutic procedure. Ever increasing emphasis has currently been placed on active approach in the therapy, including intensive repetitive task-specific training in support of neuroplasticity. A good understanding of the maturity of gait for normal children and for each individual child with CP is decisive in planning the treatment. Locomotor functions training has become an effective means to improve walking performance in patients with gait impairment. In the past decade there was increase in the use of robotic therapy, especially in patients with strokes, cerebrospinal trauma, and last but not least, in children with cerebral palsy. In this paper the authors present some of new trends in neurorehabilitation - robotic-assisted treadmill training in virtual reality environment, functional therapy of upper extremity and coordination dynamic therapy. The authors report here the results of robotic–assisted treadmill therapy of patient suffering from ataxic form of cerebral palsy.

Chapter 16 – Introduction: Robotic-assisted body-weight-supported treadmill therapy (RATT) enabled by driven gait orthosis can improve motor functions in patients with movement disorders. The aim of the study was to assess the impact of patient´s age on improvement of motor functions in patients with cerebral palsy (CP). Methods: 78 patients (44 males) with bilateral spastic CP, aged 4 – 25 years underwent 20 therapeutic units (T.U.) of RATT using driven gait orthosis with a frequency of 3 to 5 times a week. The patients participating in the study were divided into groups according to age and severity of motor impairment determined by the Gross Motor Function Classification System (GMFCS). Outcome measures were dimension A (lying,rolling), B (sitting), C (crawling, kneeling), D (standing) and E (walking, running, jumping) of the Gross Motor Function Measure (GMFM-88). Results: After completing 20 therapeutic units patients demonstrated highly statistically significant improvement (p<0,001) in all dimensions of the GMFM. Comparing the average improvement (%) in outcome parameters in all groups after 20 T.U., the authors didn't recorded the difference in any of the subgroups. Conclusion: The authors study indicates, that RATT can improve the gross motor functions. Effect of the age on improvement in this study has not been demonstrated. RATT can be suitable for patients with cerebral palsy of all ages. Thus, RATT is a promising treatment option in ambulatory and nonambulatory patients with CP of all ages.

Chapter 17 – Background: This study investigated the effect of perceived social support on the parenting stress of mothers who have children with cerebral palsy (CP). [Method] This study was conducted using surveys, literature review, and interviews. Survey data were collected from 181 mothers of children (under 18 years of age) with CP. Results: Level of disability, mother's health status and social support were significant predictors of the parenting stress of mothers. Conclusion: The authors have to comprehend and share the psychological and physical affliction of mothers having much difficulty nurturing children with CP. Also, the government should take social responsibility for the upbringing of their children, developing back-up programs for mothers and making them comprehensively available to support the psychological and physical health of mothers of children with CP.

In: Handbook on Cerebral Palsy
Editor: Harold Yates

ISBN: 978-1-63321-852-9
© 2014 Nova Science Publishers, Inc.

Chapter 1

Cerebral Palsy in an Era of Neuroprotection and Evidence Based Interventions: Risk Factors, Therapeutic Management, and Prognoses for Long Term Functioning and Participation

Petra Karlsson M.Sc. (O.T.), Sarah McIntyre Ph.D. and Michael E. Msall[*] M.D.

[1]Research Institute, Cerebral Palsy Alliance School of Medicine,
University of Notre Dame Australia, Darlinghurst NSW, Australia
[2]Cerebral Palsy Alliance, Sydney
University of Notre Dame Australia, Darlinghurst NSW, Australia
[3]Pediatrics/University of Chicago
Comer Children's Hospital, Kennedy Research Center on Intellectual
and Neurodevelopmental Disabilities, Chicago, Illinois, US

Abstract

The purpose of this chapter is to examine current knowledge of risk factors among term and preterm infants for developing cerebral palsy. We will highlight advances in understanding the changing epidemiology and the contribution of registries and case-control studies with respect to our knowledge of causal pathways. We will also highlight advances in neuroprotection with a focus on optimizing early identification and introducing evidence based interventions to optimize gross motor, fine motor, communicative and developmental functioning. Among adults with cerebral palsy

---

[*] Email: mmsall@peds.bsd.uchicago.edu.

without intellectual disability, the majority are completing high school, living independently, and participating in community activities. However, challenges in health, social skills, and executive function can lead to suboptimal adult outcomes. To improve health and developmental trajectories for individuals with cerebral palsy it will require clinical and translational community networks that emphasize prevention, neuroprotection, and neurorehabilitation. We propose one such model for the research community to debate and consider.

Introduction

Cerebral palsy (CP) is an extremely heterogeneous condition. There are a myriad of known aetiological pathways that can interfere with brain development throughout prenatal, perinatal, and postnatal life. Importantly, our knowledge is far from complete in fully understanding these factors and being able to intervene to prevent or ameliorate their consequences on neuromotor and neurodevelopmental processes. There are also numerous clinical manifestations of cerebral palsy involving different motor types (spastic, extrapyramidal, ataxic), topographies (diplegia, hemiplegia, quadriplegia) and functioning in gross motor, manual, intellectual, communication, behavioural, and sensory activities. Understanding the risk factors/aetiology and complex causal pathways underlying cerebral palsy has evolved slowly over the past 75 years. Because of its relative rarity in the population (and low absolute numbers i.e., 2 per 1000 live births) for many years "all CP" was used as one total outcome of interest. Inadvertently, this practical decision may have held back research findings.

In the only population based prospective study, the National Collaborative Perinatal Project (NCPP), over 50,000 pregnant women and their babies were followed for seven years to identify almost 200 children with cerebral palsy [1]. This study helped the field expand rapidly and is still being used today. Even though lessons learned from this study were many, 200 children with cerebral palsy are not nearly enough once stratifications take place to look into detailed aetiological subtypes. Since this prospective population study, a number of population based retrospective case control studies from total population CP Registers have taken place, enabling up to four times as many children with cerebral palsy to be included, although with the inherent biases associated with retrospective designs [2-4]. Similarly, population cohort studies [5] predominantly linking large data sets, have also allowed more children with cerebral palsy to be included in the outcome group but nowhere near the level of detail obtainable by case control studies.

Aetiology researchers searching to identify causal pathways with the ultimate aim of prevention, are now moving away from studies that have "all CP" as the outcome group, trying to identify more homogenous outcome groups to study in cerebral palsy. Some are focussing on subtypes as an outcome e.g., hemiplegia [6, 7], others are suggesting that magnetic resonance imaging (MRI) findings should be the outcome of interest e.g., focal vascular insults [8], and others again are looking at working alongside neuoprotective trials for a particular pathway, for example, working with cooling trials for infants with hypoxic ischemic encephalopathy (HIE).

The advent of neonatal intensive care units has enabled many more premature infants to survive, some free of neurological impairment, others with neurodevelopmental disabilities including cerebral palsy. Today, 35% of all cerebral palsy arises from premature infants, which is quite a contrast to the NCPP where 90% were born at term equivalent weight. At a minimum, we recommend that singletons and multiples should be studied separately and that term and preterm infants have (some overlapping but) many different aetiologies and should also be studied separately.

Premature Infants

The purpose of this section is to describe our current understanding of the relationship of cerebral palsy to prematurity and the role of neonatal morbidities in increasing the risks for adverse neurodevelopmental outcomes. This section will emphasize the current epidemiology of prematurity, relationship between gestational age and concurrent antecedent risk factors and cerebral palsy, the predictors of cerebral palsy in very and extremely preterm birth, and the current status of neonatal and postnatal neuroprotection interventions.

Over the past 30 years, major advances in maternal fetal medicine, neonatology, and translational developmental biology have resulted in unprecedented survival rates for extremely preterm (<28 weeks gestation) or extremely low birth-weight (<1000 g) infants who received neonatal intensive care. Currently the survival rates exceed 98% for those born between 33 and 36 weeks gestation, are 90% at 28-32 weeks gestation, and are 80% for <28 weeks [9].

Prematurity is a significant public health problem in both developing and developed economies. World-wide, preterm births defined by the World Health Organization as: a delivery that occurs prior to 37 weeks gestation occurs in 1 of 9 births. To date, effective interventions for preventing preterm birth include the use of progestins and cerclage in appropriate high-risk mothers, smoking cessation, limiting embryo transfer in assisted reproduction, and reduction of elective preterm birth in uncomplicated pregnancies [10, 11]. Since the major causal pathways of preterm birth are unknown, the widespread adoption of these interventions would only result in a slight reduction and not total elimination of preterm birth. This epidemiological data further highlight the critical need for evidence based prenatal and postnatal interventions, especially in order to reduce known complications of prematurity that increase the risk of cerebral palsy.

Prematurity, Short Term Outcomes and Neurodevelopmental Disabilities

The majority (84%) of all preterm births occur after 32 weeks gestation [10]. However, 1-2 per 1000 children are born before 28 weeks and previously, the majority of these extremely preterm children died. Over the last past two decades we have seen an increased survival as noted in the EPICURE cohort [12]. In Epicure 2006, survival of live born babies was 2% (n=3) for those born at 22 weeks' gestation, 19% (n=66) at 23 weeks, 40% (n=178) at 24 weeks, 66% (n=346) at 25 weeks, and 77% (n=448) at 26 weeks (P<0.001). At discharge from hospital, 68% (n=705) of survivors had bronchopulmonary dysplasia (receiving supplemental oxygen at 36 weeks postmenstrual age), 13% (n=135) had evidence of serious abnormality on cerebral ultrasonography, and 16% (n=166) had laser treatment for retinopathy of prematurity. Overall rates of severe neurodevelopmental disabilities at age 2 were approximately 1 in 5 for both cohorts [12].)

It must be emphasized that there is a wide spectrum of neurodevelopmental consequences after prematurity. These not only include neuromotor and neurosensory disabilities, such as cerebral palsy, sensory-neural hearing loss, visual disability (i.e., cortical or optic blindness), epilepsy, and significant intellectual disability (IQ <55 with concurrent adaptive delays), but also more subtle neurobehavioral and learning impairments. The current epidemiology of cerebral palsy reflects as many as 2 in 5 children with cerebral palsy have had preterm birth and, among those who are very preterm or extremely preterm, there are high rates (50%) of needing special education supports to address difficulties in perception, coordination, attention, phonological processing, memory, learning, handwriting, and mathematics.

Prematurity and Cerebral Palsy

Himpens and colleagues [13] examined the relationship between gestational age and prevalence, type, distribution, and severity of functional challenges in individuals with cerebral palsy. This was a comprehensive medical meta-analysis and targeted 4 gestational age categories: gestational age (GA) less than 28 weeks, GA 28-31 weeks, GA 32-36 weeks, and GA > 37 weeks. The classification guidelines operationalized by the Surveillance of Cerebral Palsy in Europe (SCPE) [14] was used [15]. The prevalence of cerebral palsy decreased significantly with increasing GA, with approximately 1 in 7 children surviving 22-27 weeks GA having cerebral palsy, 1 in 16 at 28-31 weeks GA, and 1 in 140 at 32-36 weeks.

Insel and colleagues [16] found that 50 % of infants (n=160) with cerebral palsy who were 22-32 weeks gestation walked independently at age 2, and 31% were unable to walk but could sit independently. This later group has an excellent prognosis for walking.. Himmelmann and colleagues [15] examined 366 children with cerebral palsy and found that 61% were Gross Motor Function Classification System (GMFCS) [77] level 1 and 2, 8% level 3, and 31% level 4 and 5. There was no relationship between the severity of cerebral palsy and GA. Oskoui and colleagues [17] recently completed an update on the prevalence of cerebral palsy. Forty-nine studies were reviewed, encompassing cohorts of children born since 1985. The pooled prevalence of cerebral palsy per 1000 live birth was 82.25 for <28 weeks GA, 43.15 for 28-31 weeks, 6.75 for 32-36 weeks. These cohorts overall numbered 1354 children with cerebral palsy born between 1989 and 2000, predominantly followed during the first 2 years of life with a few studies reporting outcomes between 4 and 6 years. Thus, key neuroprotection strategies are required across all gestational age groups, but in particular in those who are very preterm as well as late preterm.

Antenatal Risk Factors and Neuroprotectants

In univariate analysis, O'Shea and colleagues [18] identified that antecedents of cerebral palsy in very low birth weight infants include: death of a co-twin (OR 10.5), assisted ventilation (OR5.3), hypothyroxinemia (OR 4.4), pneumothorax (OR 3.3), bronchopulmonary dysplasia (OR 3), intrauterine infections (OR 2.2), hypocarbia (OR 2.7). Protective factors that reduced risk for cerebral palsy in very low birth weight infants included: Antenatal corticosteroids (OR 0.7), magnesium sulfate (OR 0.5), preecamplesia (OR 0.4), and fetal growth restriction (OR 0.5).

Clark and colleagues [19] examined the antecedents and impact of obstetric care in the etiology of cerebral palsy. Overall, they found that prematurity, low birth-weight, infection, inflammation, and multiple gestation impacted on cerebral palsy. Neuroprotective factors included magnesium sulfate, antibiotics, tocolytics, and corticosteroids.

Multiple gestations influence both the rate of prematurity and the risk for cerebral palsy. In the Western Australia registry from 1980 to 1989, the rates of cerebral palsy in twins and triplets were examined (20). The risk of a child having cerebral palsy if he/she was a singleton was 2 per 1000, if a twin 13 per 1000, and if a triplet 76 per 1000. Death of a co-twin in a monochorionic gestation increases the risk of cerebral palsy in the surviving twin with the surviving twin having a 20% overall risk of neurological impairment after the in-utero death of the co-twin. In the surviving twin of a co-twin who died in utero, the prevalence of cerebral palsy was 96.2 per 1000 – a 15-fold increased risk and 60 times higher than compared with live-born singleton (1.6 per 1000). When both twins were born alive, the prevalence was 6.3 per 1000. Pregnancies in which the in-uterine death of co-twin or co-triplet occurred had an associated risk of cerebral palsy of 10% for twins and 29% for triplets (20,) O'Callaghan [21], examined the genetic and clinical contributions to cerebral palsy.

This was a case controlled study involving 587 children with cerebral palsy and 154 children without cerebral palsy. The evaluators wished to assess the influence of single, nucleotide polymorphic associations with cerebral palsy, as well as (SNP) maternal infant infection interactions as contributors to cerebral palsy. They found that maternal and fetal carriage of inducible nitric oxide synthase, SNP, was significantly negatively associated with cerebral palsy in infants born at less than 32 weeks gestation, after adjustment for clinical cofounders and correction for multiple testing. They concluded that maternal and child inducible nitric oxide syntheses are associated with a 50% reduced risks of cerebral palsy in infants born very preterm. There was no evidence for statistically significant SNP-SNP or SNP-maternal infections as modulators or cerebral palsy risk.

Chalak and Rouse [22] examined neuroprotective approaches before or after delivery including the use of antenatal magnesium sulfate in very preterm labor. They highlighted that in the Beneficial Effect of Antenatal Magnesium (BEAM) study that smoking doubled and, neonatal hypotension tripled the risks for CP. Severe cranial sonographic abnormalities of IVH grade 3 or 4 increased the risk of CP six-fold and PVL increased the risk 45 –fold. The potential antenatal neuroprotective factors included prevention or treatment of abruption, uterine rupture during labor and cord prolapse,decreasing maternal smoking, increased use of corticosteroids for fetal maturation, and use of magnesium sulfate. In the BEAM trial, mild cerebral palsy was decreased from 3.7% to 2.2%, moderate CP from 2.2% to 1.7% and severe CP from 1.6% to 0.5% comparing those who received magnesium sulfate to placebo. Overall in the six trials involving 2658 receiving magnesium sulfate, versus 2699 with no magnesium sulfate, the relative risk of 0.69 of all cerebral palsy. For moderate severe cerebral palsy, the relative risk was 0.64, and erythropoietin.

McIntyre and colleagues [21] examined the antecedents of cerebral palsy and perinatal death in term and late preterm singletons from a total population of singletons born at or after 35 weeks of gestation. They identified 494 with cerebral palsy and 500 neonates who were matched controls, 100 neonatal deaths, and 73 intrapartum stillbirths. They classified outcomes of neonatal death and cerebral palsy as occurring without encephalopathy, after encephalopathy, or after neonatal encephalopathy considered hypoxemic-ischemic. They then examined the contribution of potentially asphyxiated birth events, inflammation, fetal growth restriction, and malformations to neonatal outcomes and to intrapartum stillbirths. The odds of cerebral palsy after potentially asphyxiated events or inflammation were moderately increased, (OR 1.9) Birth defects were recognized in 5.5% of the control group with 16% of neonatal deaths and more than half of the cases with cerebral palsy without hypoxemic-ischemic encephalopathy. Importantly among children with cerebral palsy, potentially asphyxiated birth event, inflammation, or both were experienced by 1 in 8, while growth restriction, birth defects, or both were experienced by 1 in 2. Thus fetal growth restriction and birth defects were more substantial contributors to cerebral palsy and neonatal death than potentially asphyxial birth events and inflammation [21].

Mechanisms Underlying Cerebral Palsy and Their Detection

Two mechanisms currently underlie our understanding of abnormalities in preterm infants that contribute to cerebral palsy.[24]. The first involves cerebral perfusion and are the cardiopulmonary adaptations and regulated brain flow that are part of the immaturity of the newborn brain. Some of this brain vulnerability can be detected noninvasively by the use of sequential cranial sonography. The second mechanism is inflammatory and is mediated by cytokines. The potential trigger for these events include maternal infection including intrauterine infection, neonatal infection, postnatal sepsis, necrotizing enterocolitis, and ventilator-induced lung injury.

One of the important advances for the detection of cerebral palsy is systematic use of cranial ultrasound. Periventricular echolucency and ventricular enlargement reflect periventricular white matter injury and increase the risk of cerebral palsy by 50-fold increase in cerebral palsy.(25) Beaino [26] examined the predictors of cerebral palsy in very preterm infants in the EPIPAGE cohort. The prevalence of cerebral palsy was 61% among infants with cystic periventricular leucomalacia (PVL), 50% in infants with intraparenchymal haemorrhage (IPH), 8% in infants with grade 1 intraventricular haemorrhage (IVH), and 4% in infants without a detectable cerebral lesion. After controlling for cerebral lesions and obstetric and neonatal factors, male gender (OR 1.5) and preterm premature rupture of membranes (OR 1.7) were the predictors of cerebral palsy in very preterm infants.

McElrath [27] examined amongst 1455 infants less than 28 weeks gestation from 14 US centers the antecedents of white matter injury in the ELGAN network. White matter injury was described as abnormal cranial ultrasounds with ventriculomegaly or an echolucent legion. Overall, they found that antenatal steroids tended to lower the risk of ventriculomegaly, from 23 % to 10%. Ventriculomegaly was increased when there was preterm labor and premature rupture of fetal membranes (OR 2.3 and 3.6), compared to when infants were delivered because of preeclampsia. Between 23 and 27 weeks gestation, the presence of ventriculomegaly decreased from 21% to 6% and echolucent lesions from 11% to 5%. Concurrently, the rates of quadriplegic cerebral palsy decreased from 15% to 3%, diplegic cerebral palsy from 8% to 3% and hemiplegic cerebral palsy 4% to 1%. Overall, preterm labor doubled the risk of diplegia, cervical insufficiency tripled the risk of diplegia, and preterm labor tripled the risk for hemiplegia.

Devries and colleagues demonstrated the value of sequential ultrasounds for all infants up to 32 weeks postmenstrual age and showed a sensitivity of 95%, a specificity of 99%, and a positive predictive value of 48% for cerebral palsy at age 2. (28) They discovered that ultrasound missed 9% of those who had cerebral palsy, and 25% of children with cognitive disability. Mirimiran and colleagues compared cranial MRI at new term, 36-40 weeks, (with cranial ultrasound in infants who weighed less than 1250G and were less than 30 weeks gestation. MRI was 86% sensitive and 89% specific for predicting cerebral palsy at age 2.5 years. (29) In comparison, ultrasound was 43% sensitive and 82% specific for detecting cerebral palsy at 2.5 years.

Neonatal Risk Factors

O'Shea and colleagues (25) noted that the following neonatal morbidities increased the risk for cerebral palsy: cystic PVL (OR 33.4), IPH grade 3 (OR 3.75), IPH grade 2 (OR 2.8), IPH grade 1 (OR 1.98), gestation age GA 31-32 weeks (OR 1), GA 29-30 weeks (OR 1.6), GA 24-28 weeks (OR 2.6), male gender (OR 1.5), preterm labor or preterm premature rupture of membrane (OR 2.17), maternal hypertension (OR 0.53), respiratory distress syndrome (OR 1.98), necrotizing entercolitis (OR 2.1), bronchopulmonary dysplasia (OR 1.6), acute anaemia (OR 1.95), and postnatal corticosteroid use (OR 2.76) [20,21].

Kuban and colleagues [30] examined systemic inflammation and cerebral palsy risk in extremely preterm infants. Blood protein concentrations were sampled in the first two weeks of life.Overall, 939 infants born before 28 weeks, were evaluated. Elevations of tumor necrosis factor-alpha and its alpha receptor-1, interleukin-8, and intercellular adhesion molecule-1 for at least 2 days was associated with diplegic cerebral palsy. Persistent elevations of interleukin-6, E-selectin, or insulin-like growth factor binding protein were associated with hemiplegic cerebral palsy. Both diplegic and hemiplegic cerebral palsy were more likely among infants with a subset of inflammatory biomarkers that had previously been associated with microcephaly and cognitive disability.

Davis [31] in the NICHD Neonatal Network examined the relationship between seizures in extremely low birth-weight infants and neurodevelopmental outcomes. Infants with brain or cardiac malformations, and chromosomal abnormalities were excluded. The maternal and perinatal characteristics for the 414 children with seizures compared to the 685 without seizures included higher rates of antepartum antibiotics, vaginal delivery GA <26 weeks,AGA status and African American minority status, cardiopulmonary resuscitation and intubation in delivery room occurred more frequently in those with seizures.

Amongst those with seizures there were higher rates of bronchopulmonary dysplasia (BPD) postnatal steroids,late-onset sepsis or meningitis and,retinopathy of prematurity (ROP) Cranial sonographic brain injury was more frequent in those with seizures and included, grade 3 or 4 IVH (39% versus 10%), cystic PVL (16% versus 4%), ventriculomegaly (43% versus 14%), shunt for posthemorrhagic hydrocephalus (14% versus 2%). At 18-22 months there were more neurodevelopmental disabilities in those survivors who had experienced seizures cognitive disability (64% versus 29%), moderate to severe cerebral palsy (32% versus 5%),visual disability (43% versus14%) and impaired hearing (i11% versus 4%.) This study demonstrated that infants with clinical seizures had a greater proportion of neonatal morbidities associated with suboptimal outcomes including severe IVH, sepsis, meningitis, and cystic PVL.

Schmidt and colleagues(32) examined three neonatal complications: BPD, parenchymal brain injury on serial cranial sonogram and severe ROP. This involved 910 children who were less than 1000g birth weight and were involved in the international study of prophylactic indomethacin to prevent IVH. Among survivors at 18 months of age, 13% had cerebral palsy and 26% had developmental disability. However, rates of cerebral palsy increased to 36% for those who had parenchymal brain injury which was defined as IVH grade 3-4 ventriculomegaly or cystic periventricular leukomalacia. Also, 24% of those who had severe ROP (stage 4 or 5) and 17% of those who had BPD had cerebral palsy. Among the neonates who were free of these three morbidities, the rate of death or neurodevelopmental disability at 18 months was 18%. This occurred in a setting of mortality between 1%and 3%. In contrast, the rate of death or neurodevelopmental disability was 88% if all three impairments were present. This occurred in a setting of mortality between 9% and 10%. More than half of the children who had parenchymal brain injury or severe ROP had neurodevelopmental disability. Although the numbers were small, 78% of those who had severe brain injury and ROP had neurodevelopmental disability.

Risk Factors Associated with Surgery

Morriss examined (33), in the NICHD Neonatal Research Network, the impact of surgery on neurodevelopmental outcome of very low birth weight infants, born between 1998 and 2009. Cerebral palsy occurred in 15% of those with major surgery, 7% of those with minor surgery, and 3.% with no surgery. Neurodevelopmental disability occurred in 51% major surgery, 37% minor surgery, 24% no surgery. Overall major surgery in very low birth weight babies was independently associated with greater than a 50% increase of death or neurodevelopmental disabilities.

Term Infants

The purpose of the following section is to summarize current knowledge of the aetiology and risk factors of term cerebral palsy and includes epidemiology and current status of neuroprotection strategies.

Scientific investigation of a condition tends to focus on aetiology during serious epidemics, when prognosis is poor and the limitations of treatments are obvious to all. This is also when epidemiology is at its most productive. In the 1980's when there was a rapid increase in proportions of very and extremely preterm infants with cerebral palsy there was an explosion of research aimed at understanding the aetiology of cerebral palsy and identifying preventive interventions for these new survivors; resulting in a sustained decrease over the ensuing decades. Conversely, cerebral palsy in term born infants has been remarkable for its relatively low and stable birth prevalence between 1-1.5/1000 live births [17]. This may be one reason why so little research has focussed on cerebral palsy in term and near term infants. What has been overlooked though, are the sheer numbers associated with this stable, low birth prevalence, the poor prognosis and limited treatments. Term born infants comprise 65% of all cerebral palsy. We know that prognosis for infants born at term with cerebral palsy is one of more severe neurodevelopmental challenges and medical comorbitities compared to preterm infants with cerebral palsy. It is lifelong condition, and those who work in the area also know the limitations of current treatments that are neither curative or fully restorative.

Despite this history of a lack of urgency for research for term born infants, in the last five years there has been a renewed interest in their aetiology and treatment. Two systematic reviews about risk factors in term born infants have been published [34,35]. Since these publications a further five population studies have been published that would have been included in both systematic reviews if they were to be updated today [23,34-38]. In addition new results from the Western Australian Case Control Study (Term-CCCP) are also included in the following section. Figure 1 outlines the most important risk factors for term cerebral palsy as identified by these studies.

Preconceptional	Antenatal	Intrapartum	Neonatal
GENETICS	BIRTH DEFECTS	BIRTH ASPHYXIA	SEIZURES
Social (eg not living with baby's father; postcode)	IUGR/SGA/LOW BIRTH WEIGHT	MECONIUM ASPIRATION	NEONATAL INFECTIONS
Prior maternal concerns (eg thyroid, seizures, intellectual)	PLACENTAL ABNORMALITIES	INSTRUMENTAL DELIVERY	HYPOGLYCAEMIA
3+ previous miscarriages	INFECTIONS/ INFLAMMATION	SENTINEL EVENTS	RDS
Smoking, recreational drugs	Pregnancy complications	Abnormal fetal presentation	JAUNDICE
	Maternal disease		PERINATAL STROKE
	Multiple gestation		
	Male		

Key: BOLD CAPITALS signifies risk factors that were identified in McIntyre systematic review as always statistically significant with additional confirmation data from recent population studies; CAPITALS unbolded were identified in the Himmelmann systematic review but were not always statistically significant in McIntyre review; *Italics signifies factors that are associated with increased risk not always statistically significant from both reviews and the most recent papers.*
IUGR – Intrauterine growth restriction; SGA – small for gestational age; RDS – Respiratory distress syndrome.

Figure 1. Risk factors for term cerebral palsy.

Preconceptional Risk Factors

In the systematic review led by McIntyre,[35] investigated preconceptional risk factors were consistently reported as posing a statistically significant risk. However, the Himmelmann review [34] identified that genetics are currently receiving increased attention.

The following additional and incomplete findings also support the need for further genetic research. A novel finding from the Term-CCCP was a significant increase in risk associated with a family history of intellectual disability (OR 2.4 [1.0-5.9]) and birth defects (OR 1.7 [95% CI1.1-2.5]) that was not identified in the systematic reviews. This was also the case for a family history of cerebral palsy. Small numbers prevented this finding reaching statistical significance, but six cases (1.5%) and no controls had a family history of cerebral palsy. Poor gynaecological history may have genetic components and includes previous stillbirths, neonatal deaths and multiple miscarriages. They are all more associated with premature births and cerebral palsy. However, more than 3 previous miscarriages were reported in 10 (2%) of Term-CCCP subjects compared with 5 (1%) of controls: Odds ratio 1.9 (0.7, 5.8) suggesting that recurrent miscarriage may also be a risk factor for cerebral palsy in those born at term. Asian families living in the United States also seem to have an unexplained reduced risk of cerebral palsy [41]. Finally, males have a small increased risk of cerebral palsy in all studies that investigate it.

Reports of social situations, low socio-economic status and their affects have been inconsistent in the past, but recent studies have reported that children living without their fathers are at higher risk of cerebral palsy (OR 2.6 [95% CI 1.3-5.2]) [34], and that area of residence (postal/Zip code) is also important Additionally there were increased odds ratios (1.9 [95% CI 1.2-3.2]) in the Term-CCCP associated with maternal age under 20. Those who smoke during pregnancy are also at a small increased risk for cerebral palsy [34] and the relative cheapness of recreational drugs means that their use is also a potential risk. Data for other variables related to socio-economic status (maternal education and employment status) were missing for too many Term-CCCP subjects to enable further analysis, and other recent studies have neglected to look closely at both the social situation and socio economic status.

Antenatal Risk Factors

Antenatal causes and risk factors are considered to be the most important for term born infants [35]. The presence of birth defects was the antenatal factor with the highest odds ratio for cerebral palsy and neonatal death in the Term-CCCP [23] consistent with the systematic review [35], in particular cerebral abnormalities [34, 36]. Forty-three percent of term and late preterm singletons had at least on birth defect in the Term-CCCP but the birth defects identified were variable, and more than half had multiple defects with very few obvious patterns.

Growth restriction, being small for gestational age and low birth weight were associated with a significantly increased risk of cerebral palsy in both systematic reviews and updated papers. In the Term-CCCP study, one in two of those with growth restriction also had a birth defect [23]. More research is needed to identify if growth restriction, when on paths with other risk factors, plays an aetiological role or whether it is a consequence of the risk. Dahlseng et al. [42] recently identified that reduced size measurements of growth were associated with unilateral and diplegic cerebral palsy, and increased size were associated with quadriplegic and dyskinetic cerebral palsy.

Infections and an inflammatory response throughout pregnancy are known risk factors for cerebral palsy. One such intrauterine infection, congenital cytomegalovirus (cCMV) is known to be capable of directly causing longterm neurological impairment. The neurotropic effects seem to be worse if the infection is transmitted early in pregnancy. This is one explanation, but not a complete explanation of why some infants with cCMV are neurologically normal, while others have severe cerebral palsy and others are deaf without any motor impairments [43]. It is probable that different congenital infections work on different pathways to cerebral palsy. cCMV manifests as a severe neurodevelopmental disability manifested as spastic quadriplegica with, Gross Motor Classification System (GMFCS) [71] IV and V, epilepsy, and severe communication limitation) In contrast bacterial growth in urine and the use of antibiotics during pregnancy are associated with stroke and hemiplegia [34,37,43].

Chorioamnionitis had a wide range of central estimates in the McIntyre systematic review and reflects the different definitions employed across studies. Similarly, there were no cases of clinical chorioamnionitis in a recent Swedish study [34], and in the Term-CCCP 4% of cases were identified with a statistically non significant increased risk (OR1.8 [0.7-4]). The great majority of placentas in the Term-CCCP were not sent to pathology, so the diagnosis of chorioamnionitis relied on observations by the midwife attending the delivery. Likewise, placental investigations were not discussed in the recent Swedish population study, and they both may therefore be under ascertained.

When "maternal disease" is used as a composite variable the effect of any that may be on a causal path is washed out [44]. In the Term-CCCP, maternal anaemia (in contrast to the systematic review), hypertension and pre-eclampsia were the maternal conditions with the highest risk of cerebral palsy for the infant. Disturbance of amnionitic fluid volume (polyhydramnios or oligohydramnios) was more strongly associated with cerebral palsy in the Term-CCCP than in the systematic review of term infants. Thirteen of 19 cerebral palsy cases but none of three controls with either condition also had a birth defect.

Being a multiple birth increases a child's risk four-fold if they are born at term. However, they are at highest risk following the fetal death of a co-twin [20,44]. Placental abnormalities and events such as severe abruption are also associated with a two to fifteen-fold increased risk of cerebral palsy when they are studied, and this is an area of research that holds much hope for understanding aetiology more completely in the future [35,36,40].

Intrapartum Risk Factors

As identified in both the systematic reviews 'birth asphyxia' was the strongest risk factor identified in the Term-CCCP. There was much variation in the definition of birth asphyxia, some variably defined it as hypoxic-ischemic encephalopathy, others as experiencing an intrapartum sentinel events and some by low Apgar scores. Individual sentinel events such as cord prolapse, true knot in cord, severe shoulder dystocia and haemorrhage were also strongly associated with increased risks in the Term-CCCP and the Swedish study, but occurred rarely [34]. A tight nuchal cord was the only sentinel event that occurred without encephalopathy in the Term-CCCP, yet it was the most numerous sentinel event in controls and cerebral palsy without neonatal encephalopathy (NE).

The question remains, was tight nuchal cord on the path to cerebral palsy for these infants? Or was it a coincidence, with a completely unrelated cause. Inflammation has also been known to mimic signs of birth asphyxia. Fever during labour was not reported in the primary findings of the systematic review because only three studies reported it. The Term-CCCP confirmed this was a risk factor for cerebral palsy (OR 2.3[95% CI 0.9-6.0]).

Both systematic reviews identified a number of modes of delivery as consistently statistically significant risk factors for cerebral palsy (emergency caesareans, vacuum deliveries, breech delivery).

The Term-CCCP did not find any of these to be statistically significant risk factors with the exception of forceps delivery (OR 1.5 [1-2.1]). There were inconsistent findings in the systematic reviews for forcep deliveries. Most emergency caesarean sections are undertaken because of a prolonged labour and failure to progress, so it is possible that some emergency caesareans could be avoided by active labour strategies to reduce the second stage of labour [29]. Meconium aspiration is the only other intrapartum factor that has proved to be associated with increased risk across all studies.

Neonatal Factors

The Term-CCCP confirmed findings of the systematic review that the presence of seizures was associated with a marked increase in the odds of cerebral palsy. It is agreed that seizures do not cause the brain damage that is responsible for cerebral palsy [45]. It is less certain whether seizures can exacerbate brain damage [46].

The presence of seizures is usually one element of the definition of neonatal encephalopathy. Neonatal encephalopathy (NE) is itself a very strong risk factor for cerebral palsy. Those with a diagnosis of NE have the highest risk of cerebral palsy for any subgroup, including those born extremely preterm [34, 47]. Hypoglycaemia, infections as a newborn and jaundice requiring treatment were also confirmed by the Term-CCCP as risk factors for cerebral palsy.

Apnoeas also increased the odds of cerebral palsy in the Term-CCCP, but were not reported in the primary findings of the systematic review because it was investigated by too few studies. Subdividing term and near-term infants into those at highest risk (following NE) and those at lowest risk (receiving only routine care as a newborn) gives a more accurate picture of the research being conducted in this infant population. There has been a rapid increase of research considering those at highest risk following the discovery of cooling as a neuro-protective treatment. [47]

However exciting this line of enquiry, it has limited potential, as only 1 in 8 infants [48] of those selected for this treatment respond favourably, and the majority of term and near term infants that are subsequently described as having cerebral palsy are not eligible for this treatment.

The research world is set to test several adjuvant therapies to cooling to increase this success rate, yet little is known about the antepartum experience of infants who are depressed in the newborn period and whether this affects the manner in which they respond to cooling.

Conversely, very little research throughout the world considers the majority of term born infants with cerebral palsy that do not exhibit encephalopathy as a newborn, yet numerically this is the largest group, and two in three of this group have moderate to severe motor disability.

A Framework to Reduce the Prevalence of Cerebral Palsy, It's Motor Severity and Associated Impairments

We now summarize current research strategies for collaborative trial networks and propose a new model to accelerate findings in cerebral palsy, with a particular example for one causal path for term infants. We will propose a radical change to streamline research with the aim to reduce the rate, severity and secondary impairments in cerebral palsy.

To advance the knowledge of neuroprotective factors throughout the 21st century it is critical to accelerate the rate of phase III clinical trials focused on effectiveness and subsequent translation into clinical practice. The purpose of health and medical research is to achieve better outcomes for individuals. Better health includes increased life expectancy, quality of life, and the current research field is relying on research designs and methodology that often results in representative but small samples due to limited access to populations. In an effort to solve the challenges with recruitment, to accelerate the rate of phase III clinical trials, to achieve better outcomes for individuals at risk of cerebral palsy, current research initiatives are moving towards increased research collaboration.

There is a critical need for an increased focus on multi-site research, with an increasing number of guidelines developed, particular in the field of cancer research, to encourage consistent clinical trials programs conducting multi-disciplinary, multi-institutional clinical trials. These trial networks are mainly found within and between the United States of America [49] and Australia [50]. The Children's oncology group in the United States [51] has an established national and an international network in which member criteria, personnel service requirements, performance monitoring program and conduct of clinical research are strictly outlined in guidelines which joining organizations are expected to adhere to. This successful cancer network spans today across five of our six continents.

The key elements in the successful Children's oncology group involve the following: 1) steering committee, 2) institutional review board, 3) membership eligibility criteria, 4) established benefits and responsibilities of membership, 5) a basic reporting system and record keeping to allow participating organizations to use the open trial network for their own clinical research portfolio management, 6) access to view accrual information submitted to a clinical trial network, 7) i informed consent, 8) performance monitoring requirements with a data currency of scores of $\geq 90\%$, 9) patient eligibility, 10) ethics clearance from each participating organisation's ethics committee, 11) on-site services, 12) personnel readily accessible and 13) services readily accessible.

If the key elements, mentioned above, were employed in a multi-disciplinary and multi-institutional neuroprotective clinical trial network with the aim to open recruitment to all, theoretically research can be conducted in more hospitals with less numbers. By embedding research in normal patient care, there is an opportunity to increase the uptake of evidence based neuroprotective interventions, and allow the developing world to participate in cutting edge research and health care where feasible.

In Australia a strategic review of Health and Medical Research was conducted in 2013 [50]. The review proposed a national online approval workflow system to increase the number of portals for recruitment. To create a more efficient ethics application process, it is proposed to move towards creating 8-10 national ethics committees which should replace the numerous local ethics committees and establish and implement an national clinical trial liability insurance scheme, coordinated from a national clinical trial office within the health and medical research body. The Australian strategic review of Health and Medical Research also identified the importance of informing policy with evidence and has proposed strategies to enhance the capability of the National Health and Medical Research Council and researchers to support policy makers, by embedding researchers within government policy departments and encourage research on gaps between health policy, practice and the evidence base, and to consider new approaches to funding clinical trials [50].

A neuroprotective clinical trial network collaboration that recognizes that health is a complex, non-linear process occurring in multiple dimensions and at multiple levels and phases is presented in Figure 2. In an open trial network the primary goal is the aim is to facilitate recruitment to studies from multiple sites and organizations to advance cerebral palsy research within prevention, cure and optimal lifelong health. The primary targets include physiological, behavioural, social and cultural functions and their contributions, known and unknown, to causal

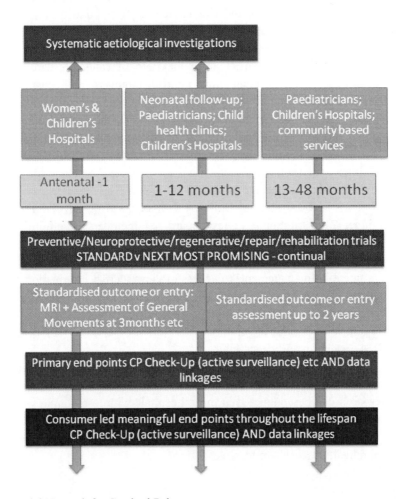

Figure 2. Neurotrial Network for Cerebral Palsy.

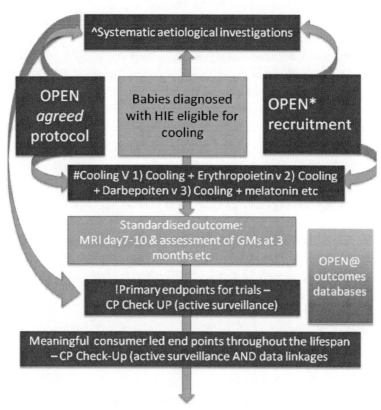

^ Aetiology researchers working with intervention trialists to help identify which infants respond best to each intervention

Cost saving opportunities – if recruitment is open to all, theoretically research can be conducted in more hospitals with less numbers per hospital. Thus research becomes a part of normal patient care, because it is doable (n=1 or 2 per hospital instead of n=50). This requires the need to overcome the barrier of ethical review for every recruiting site This can be accomplished through a memorandum of understanding with appropriate oversite and inputs. This would increase the pace of recruitment exponentially – theoretically you could recruit any number in one day and a trial that normally takes three years to recruit could have recruitment completed in a few weeks.

#This concept is one of continual testing of the "next most promising treatment" against the current "standard". Investigators would be able to add their next most promising treatment to the mix once they had data to prove their intervention safe, effective and with the potential of being more effective than the standard.

& *cost saving opportunity* - Much earlier interim endpoint

! Primary endpoint will have enough n's for a definitive answer – *major cost saving* – only one lot of analysis to complete

@ *cost saving opportunity* - Long term population databases that people could enter their data into (unique identifiers would be given at randomisation along with treatment arm)

Figure 3. Proposed HIE trials network to reduce cerebral palsy.

Research that advances in vitro and in vivo pre clinical findings from phase I to phase III are of outmost importance yet held back by the challenges in recruiting subjects. The evidence of the protective properties of hypothermia in term neonates with hypoxic ischemic encephalopathy (HIE) was established in 1998 by Gunn, Gunning, Williams and Gluckman

[52]. However, it took 13 years and 7 trials to recruit 1214 neonates and produce a meta-analysis [53]. That equates to a total of 100 infants a year across the world randomized into these trials. The results of this meta-analysis states that up to 50% still either die or have cerebral palsy. As a result, there are now seven adjuvant therapies moving toward phase III trials. How long will it to take to understand the efficacies of each treatment? In Figure 3 we propose a model that the model would increase the pace of recruitment, reduce the costs of research, and be implemented in a framework of ongoing prevention and neuroprotection trials.

Active Surveillance and Impact on Life Activities

Disability organisations and service providers, working in a family-centred framework, strive to provide co-ordinated and holistic services that best meet the needs of children and youth with cerebral palsy and their families. Families and individuals with cerebral palsy have expressed that service providers address their needs by providing information relevant to their developmental materials and family dynamics [54]. This will mean that the families require support across health, education and rehabiliation services that need to be co-ordinated over time.

In this section we describe an active surveillance program, CP Check-Up [55, 56] that extends a cerebral palsy aetiology register, with the aim to prevent secondary impairments such as pain, musculoskeletal, communication, feeding and sleep problems by addressing movement, sensation, cognition, communication and well-being in one comprehensive, co-ordinated service delivery program. This active surveillance program could also double as the long term follow up for trials as suggested in Figures 2 and 3.

The Rate of Secondary Impairments in Cerebral Palsy

The literature reports that of 3 in 4 individuals with cerebral palsy experience pain. This distress is present at all levels of physical disability [57] and starts early in life with many children with cerebral palsy needing neonatal intensive care and are exposed to painful stimuli on immature neural pain circuits [58].

Half of Australian children with cerebral palsy experience chronic pain [59] which often arises from hip dislocation which has been reported to affect 7% of walking and 60% of total body involved children [59]. Hip displacement is related to cerebral palsy sub type, age and gross motor function. Those children born with a more severe form of cerebral palsy such as spastic quadriplegia are at high risk whilst those with a mild spastic hemiplegia and ataxia are at low risk [60,61]. International evidence supporting active surveillance as a means of preventing hip dislocation and reducing contractures and other secondary impairments is well established [62-64].

Sleep problems are one of the top five parental concerns presented to paediatricians [65]. In children with cerebral palsy, sleep disturbances are related to motor impairment, pain, behavioral problems and epilepsy [66]. Despite the reported prevalence of sleep problems

(33%), screening of sleep is often inconsistently carried out, and more well-designed studies are necessary to advance evidence-based treatments in the area [67].

Dysphagia is prevalent amongst children with cerebral palsy, with observational studies reporting a prevalence of 61-99% [68,69] and parental questionnaires indicating a slightly lower prevalence between 43-89% [70,71]. However, it is recognised that parents may underestimate the presence and severity of dysphagia [68, 69]. Despite this, it is often not included in routine health encounters [70] though it significantly impacts on nutrition, recurrent pneumonias and oral health.

Very preterm and very low birth weight states are associated with reduction of white and grey matter which impacts on motor, cognitive and behavioural functioning [72]. Challenges in executive functions and social adjustment problems in cerebral palsy display, longitudinal follow-ups have been recommended to establish its impact on the individual's daily life at school and in the community. [73].

Assessment of Secondary Impairments

In the proposed active surveillance program, a variety of assessments are used to collect information across many aspects of a person's life including physical status, functional abilities, cognitive abilities and emotional health and well-being 1-2 times a year.

To assess musculoskeletal issues, ranges of motion in all major joints are measured with a goniometer. The measurements are performed in standardized positions that are described in a manual accompanying the recording form. The local physiotherapists and occupational therapists examine the child and fill in a recording form twice a year until the age of 6 years, then once a year. The cerebral palsy subtype is described according to the Cerebral Palsy Description form [74] which use modified Tardieu [75,76] to determine muscle tone. The gross and fine motor function is classified according to Gross Motor Classification System (GMFCS) [77], Manual Ability Classification System (MACS) [78] and Hand function classification (modified House) [79, 80]. Communication function is classified using Communication Functioning Classification System (CFCS) [81]. Gross Motor Function Measure (GMFM) (82)is used to record the child's mobility. Orthoses, surgery and spasticity management and muscles injected with botulinum toxin are recorded for upper and lower limb. Hand function in children with hemiplegia is assessed using Mini- Assisting Hand Assessment (mini-AHA) [83] or Assisting Hand Assessment AHA [84, 85].

To assess sleep, the Sleep Disturbance Scale [86] is used. The location of the pain, its frequency, intensity and description are reported by proxy, which often is the mother of the child [87]. Pediatric Evaluation of Disability Inventory (PEDI) [88] is used to record self-care. Swallowing and aspriation difficulties are classified using the Dysphagia Disorder Survey (DDS) [89]. Drooling is classified using the Drooling Impact Scale [90]. A child's cognition is evaluated using the standardized assessment for cognitive development, the Bayley Scale of Infant Development III (BSID) [91]. Parent well-being is assessed using Depression Anxiety and Stress Scale (DASS 21) [92] and the Relationship Quality Index [93].

Information from the assessments is collated in a secure electronic database, this enables assessment results to be compared across different time points easily and quickly. The results from the assessments are used to help understand a person's current status in order to plan and provide appropriate and timely interventions now and in the future.

Conclusion

Risks factors for cerebral palsy have been identified prior to pregnancy commencing (preconceptional), during pregnancy (antenatal), around the time of labour (intrapartum) and during the neonatal period (neonatal) and beyond. This is a complicated picture, and they do not all carry the same level of risk. The next phase of research is to identify how and when the risk factors discussed interact, and to identify appropriate and feasible opportunities for prevention. While looking for avenues for prevention, aetiology researchers need to help neuroprotective intervention researchers, as it is more than possible that aetiology will affect a baby's ability to respond favourably to treatment. We suggest that a debate occurs regarding a radical overhaul to cerebral palsy research in the form of a global clinical trial network that addresses the continuum of primary prevention through longterm management and secondary impairment prevention. Assessing outcomes that address the full range of secondary impairments over the life-course among the diversity of individuals with cerebral palsy remains challenging. Randomized clinical trials are clearly invaluable for evidence-based medicine, but are not always feasible and not affordable for every possible intervention. However, active surveillance can be a powerful method that provides an avenue for prospective follow up studies. International evidence supporting active surveillance as a means of preventing hip dislocation and reducing contractures and other secondary impairments is well established, and is currently considered best practice in the management of lower limb translational impairments. We hope that this important example will lead to other efforts to improve outcomes and supports for living a life with cerebral palsy. This strategy will be required until we have the interventions that will fully prevent and restore all individuals who experience cerebral palsy.

Acknowledgments

We would like to acknowledge Professor Eve Blair for her mentoring and allowing us to use the previously unpublished data from the Western Australian case control study of cerebral palsy and perinatal death. Dr. Msall supported in part by Illinois LEND.

References

[1]   Nelson K B & Ellenberg, J.H., *Antecedents of cerebral palsy: Multivariate analysis of risk.* New England Journal of Medicine, 1986. 315(2): p. 81-86.
[2]   Blair, E. and F. Stanley, *When can cerebral palsy be prevented? The generation of causal hypotheses by multivariate analysis of a case-control study.* Paediatr Perinat Epidemiol, 1993. 7(3): p. 272-301.

[3] .Walstab, J., et al., *Antenatal and intrapartum antecedents of cerebral palsy: a case-control study.* Aust N Z J Obstet Gynaecol, 2002. 42(2): p. 138-46.

[4] Stelmach, T., H. Pisarev, and T. Talvik, *Ante- and perinatal factors for cerebral palsy: case-control study in Estonia.* J Child Neurol, 2005. 20(8): p. 654-60.

[5] Thorngren-Jerneck, K. and A. Herbst, *Perinatal factors associated with cerebral palsy in children born in Sweden.* Obstet Gynecol, 2006. 108(6): p. 1499-505.

[6] Ahlin, K., et al., *Non-infectious risk factors for different types of cerebral palsy in term-born babies: a population-based, case-control study.* BJOG, 2013. 120(6): p. 724-31.

[7] Ahlin, K., et al., *Cerebral Palsy and Perinatal Infection in Children Born at Term.* Obstet Gynecol, 2013. 122(1): p. 41-49.

[8] Reid, S.M., et al., *Population-based studies of brain imaging patterns in cerebral palsy.* Dev Med Child Neurol, 2014. 56(3): p. 222-32.

[9] Msall ME. The panorama of cerebral palsy after very and extremely preterm birth: evidence and challenges. Clin Perinatol. 2006 Jun;33(2):269-84. Review 9. Himmelmann, K., et al., *Risk factors for cerebral palsy in children born at term.* Acta Obstet Gynecol Scand, 2011. 90(10): p. 1070-81.

[10] Rattihalli, R., L. Smith, and K. Field, Prevention of preterm births: Are we looking in the wrong place? The case for primary prevention. Archives of Disease in Childhood. *Fetal Neonatal Edition*, 2012. 97(3): p. F160-161.

[11] Chang, H.H., et al., Preventing preterm births: Analysis of trends and potential reductions with interventions in 39 countries with very hig human development index. *Lancet,* 2013. 381(9862): p. 223-234.

[12] Costeloe, K.L., et al., Short term outcomes after extreme preterm birth in England: Comparison of two birth cohorst in 1995 and 2006 (the EPICure studies). *British Medical Journal*, 2012. 4(345): p. e7976.

[13] Himpens, E., et al., Prevalence, type, distribution, and severity of cerebral palsy in relation to gestational age: a meta-analytic review. *Developmental Medicine & Child Neurology,* 2008. 50(5): p. 334-340.

[14] Surveillance of Cerebral Palsy in Europe, Surveillance of cerebral palsy in Europe: A collaboration of cerebral palsy surveys and registers. Surveillance of Cerebral Palsy in Europe (SCPE). *Developmental Medicine & Child Neurology*, 2000. 42(12): p. 816-824.

[15] Himmelmann, K., G. Hagberg, and P. Uvebrant, The changing panorama of cerebral palsy in Sweden. X. Prevalence and origin in the birth-year period 1999-2002. *Acta Paediatrica,* 2010. 99(9): p. 1337-1343.

[16] Insel, T.R., Mental disorders in childhood: Shifting focus from behavioral symtomst to neurodevelomental trajectories. *JAMA: The Journal of the American Medical Association* 2014. 311(17): p. 1727-1728.

[17] Oskoui, M., et al., An update on the prevalence of cerebral palsy: A systematic review and meta-analysis. *Developmental Medicine & Child Neurology*, 2013(55): p. 6.

[18] O'Shea, T.M. and O. Dammann, Antecedents of cerebral palsy in very low-birth weight infants. *Clinics in Perinatology*, 2000. 27(2): p. 285-302.

[19] Clark, S., M.G. Labib, and G.D.V. Hankins, Antenatal antecedents and the impact of obstetric care in the etiology of cerebral palsy. *Clinical Obstetrics & Gynecology*, 2008. 51(4): p. 775-786.

[20] Petterson B1, Nelson KB, Watson L, Stanley F. Twins, triplets, and cerebral palsy in births in Western Australia in the 1980s. *BMJ* 1993;307(6914):1239-43.

[21] O'Callaghan, M.E., et al., Genetic and clinical contributions to cerebral palsy: A multi-variable analysis. *Journal of Paediatrics and Child Health*, 2013. 49(7): p. 575-581.

[22] Chalak, L.F. and D.J. Rouse, Neuroprotective approaches: Before and after delivery. *Clinics in Perinatology*, 2011. 38(3): p. 455–470.

[23] McIntyre, S., et al., Antecedents of Cerebral Palsy and Perinatal Death in Term and Late Preterm Singletons. *Obstetrics and Gynecology* 2013. 122(4): p. 869-877.

[24] O'Shea, T.M., Cerebral palsy in very preterm infants: New epidemiological insights. *Mental Retardation and Developmental Disabilities Research Reviews* 2002. 8(3): p. 135-145.

[25] O'Shea, T.M. and O. Dammann, Antecedents of cerebral palsy in very low-birth weight infants. *Clinics in Perinatology*, 2000. 27(2): p. 285-302.

[26] Beaino, G., et al., Predictors of cerebral palsy in very preterm infants: the EPIPAGE prospective population-based cohort study. *Developmental Medicine & Child Neurology*, 2010. 52(6): p. e119-125.

[27] McElrath, T.F., et al., Maternal antenatal complications and the risk of neonatal cerebral white matter damage and later cerebral palsy in children born at an extremely low gestational age. *American Journal of Epidemiology*, 2009. 170(7): p. 819-828.

[28] De Vries, LS., et al., Ultrasound abnormalities preceding cerebral palsy in high-risk preterm infants. *J Ped*, 2004. 144(6): 815-820.

[29] Mirmiran, M., et al., Neonatal brain magnetic resonance imaging before discharge is better than serial cranial ultrasound in predicting cerebral palsy in very low birth weight preterm infants. *Pediactrics*, 2004. 114(4):992-8.

[30] Kuban, K.C.K., et al., Systematic inflammation and cerebral palsy risk in extremely preterm infants. *Journal of Child Neurology*, 2014. 18.

[31] Davis, A.S., et al., Seizures in extremely low birth weight infants are associated with adverse outcome. *The Journal of Pediatrics* 2010. 157(5): p. 720-725.

[32] Schmidt, B., et al., Impact of broncho pulmonary dysplasia, brain injury, and severe retinopathy on the outcome of extremely low-birth-weight infants at 18 months: results from the trial of indomethacin prophylaxis in preterms. *JAMA*, 2003. 289(9):1124-9.

[33] Morriss, FH. Jr., et al., Surgery and neurodevelopmental outcome of very low-birth-weight infants, *JAMA*, 2014. 168(8):746-54.

[34] Himmelmann, K., et al., Risk factors in cerebral palsy in children born at term. *Acta Obstet Gynecol Scand*, 2011. 90(10): p. 1070-1081.

[35] McIntyre, S., et al., A systematic review of risk factors for cerebral palsy in children born at term in developed countries. *Developmental Medicine & Child Neurology*, 2012. 55(6): p. 499-508.

[36] Ahlin, K., et al., Non-infectious risk factors for different types of cerebral palsy in term-born babies: A population-based, case-control study. *BJOG,* 2013. 120(6): p. 724-731.

[37] Ahlin, K., et al., Cerebral palsy and perinatal infection in children born at term. *Obstet Gynecol,* 2013. 122(1): p. 41-49.

[38] Moster, D., et al., Cerebral palsy among term and postterm births. JAMA: *The Journal of the American Medical Association*, 2010. 304(9): p. 976-982.

[39] Stoknes, M., et al., The effects of multiple pre- and perinatal risk factors on the occurrence of cerebral palsy. A Norwegian register based study. *Eur. J. Paediatr Neurol.*, 2012. 16(1).

[40] Stoknes, M., et al., Cerebral palsy and neonatal death in term singletons born small for gestational age. *Pediatrics*, 2012. 130(6): p. e1629-1635.

[41] Lang, T.C., et al., Cerebral palsy among asian ethnic subgroups. *Pediatrics*, 2012. 129: p. e992-998.

[42] Dahlseng, M.O., et al., Risk of cerebral palsy in term-born singletons according to growth status at birth. *Developmental Medicine & Child Neurology*, 2014. 56(1): p. 53-58.

[43] Smihters-Sheedy, H., et al., Congenital cytomegalovirus is associated with severe forms of cerebral palsy and female sex in a retrospective population-based study. *Developmental Medicine & Child Neurology*, 2014.

[44] Blair, E. and F. Stanley, When can cerebral palsy be prevented? The generation of causal hypotheses by multivariate analysis of a case-control study. *Paediatr Perinat Epidemiol.*, 1993. 7(3): p. 272-301.

[45] Glass, H.C. and J.E. Sullivan, Neonatal seizures. *Curr. Treat Options Neurol.*, 2009. 11(6): p. 405-413.

[46] Glass, H.C. and E. Wirrell, Controversies in neonatal seizure management. *J. Child Neurol.*, 2009. 24: p. 5.

[47] Kyriakopoulos, P., et al., Term neonatal encephalopathy antecedent cerebral palsy: A retrospective population-based study. *Eur. J. Paediatr. Neurol.*, 2013. 17(3): p. 269-273.

[48] Jacobs, S.E., et al., Cooling for newborns with hypoxic ischaemic encephalopathy. *Cochrane Database Syst Rev*, 2013. 31(1:CD003311).

[49] Children's Oncology Group. *International Associate Membership*. 2014 [cited 2014 13.07.2014].

[50] Australian Government, D.o.H.a.A., Strategic Review of Health and Medical Research - Better Health Through Research, 2013.

[51] Children's Oncology Group. *Conduct of Clinical Research for Member Institutions*. 2014 [cited 2014 13.07.2014].

[52] Gunn, A., et al., Neuroprotection with prolonged head cooling started before postischemic seizures in fetal sheep. *Pediatrics*, 1998. 102(5): p. 1098-1106.

[53] Tagin, M., et al., Hypothermia for neonatal hypoxic ischemic encephalopathy an updated systematic review and meta-analysis. *Arch. Pediatr Adolesc. Med.*, 2012. 166(6): p. 558-566.

[54] Almasri, N., et al., Profiles of family needs of children and youth with cerebral palsy. *Child Care Health Dev.*, 2011. 38(6): p. 798-906.

[55] Karlsson, P., et al. Active surveillance programs and cerebral palsy: Parent and staff experiences within a community rehabilitation setting. in Australasian Academy of Cerebral Palsy and Developmental Medicine. 2014. Hunter Valley, NSW, Australia: *Developmental Medicine and Child Neurology*.

[56] Karlsson, P. and H. Smithers-Sheedy. Family-centred care in disability services: Is active surveillance the answer?. in Australasian Academy of Cerebral Palsy and Developmental Medicine. 2014. Hunter Valley, NSW, Australia: *Developmental Medicine and Child Neurology*.

[57] Novak, I., et al., Clinical prognostic messages from a systematic review on cerebral palsy. *Pediatrics,* 2012(130): p. e1284-e1313.

[58] Fitzgerald, M., The development of nociceptive circuits. *Nat. Rev. Neurosci.,* 2005. 6: p. 507-520.

[59] Lonstein, J.E. and K. Beck, Hip dislocation and subluxation in cerebral palsy. *J. Pediatr Orthop.,* 1986. 6(5): p. 521-526.

[60] Hägglund, G., H. Lauge-Pedersen, and P. Wagner, Characteristics of children with hip displacement in cerebral palsy. *BMC Musculotskeletal Disorders,* 2007. 8: p. 101.

[61] Larnert, P., et al., Hip displacement in relation to age and gross motor function in children with cerebral palsy. *Journal of Children's Orthopaedics,* 2014. 8(2): p. 129-134.

[62] Hägglund, G., et al., Prevention of dislocation of the hip in children with cerebral palsy. *The journal of bone and joint surgery* (Br), 2005. 87(1): p. 95-101.

[63] Hägglund, G., et al., Prevention of severe contractures might replace multilevel surgery in cerebral palsy: Results of a population-based health care programme and new techniques to reduce spasticity. *Journal of Pediatric Orthopaedics,* 2005. 14(4): p. 269-273.

[64] Gordon, G.S. and D.E. Simkiss, A systematic review of the evidence for hip surveillance in children with cerebral palsy. *J. Bone Joint Surg. Br,* 2006. 88B: p. 1492-1496.

[65] Owens, J.A., The practice of pediatric sleep medicine: Results of a community survey. Pediatrics, 2001. 108: p. E51.

[66] Romeo, D.M., et al., Application of the Sleep Disturbance Scale for children (SDSC) in preschool age. *European Journal of paediatric neurology,* 2012. 17: p. 374-382.

[67] Galland, B.C., D.E. Elder, and B.J. Taylor, Interventions with a sleep outcome for children with cerebral palsy or a post-traumatic brain injury: A systematic review. *Sleep Medicine Reviews,* 2012. 16(6): p. 561-573.

[68] Otapowicz D, et al., Dysphagia in children with infantile cerebral palsy. *Advances in Medical Sciences,* 2010. 55(2): p. 222-227.

[69] Calis EA, et al., Dysphagia in children with severe generalized cerebral palsy and intellectual disability. *Developmental Medicine & Child Neurology,* 2008. 50(8): p. 625-630.

[70] Sullivan P, et al., Prevalence and severity of feeding and nutritional problems in children with neurological impairment: Oxford Feeding Study. *Developmental Medicine & Child Neurology,* 2000. 42(10): p. 674-680.

[71] Parkes J, et al., Oromotor dysfunction and communication impairments in children with cerebral palsy: a register study. *Developmental Medicine & Child Neurology,* 2010. 52(12): p. 1113-1119.

[72] de Kieviet, J.F., et al., Brain development of very preterm and very low-birthweight children in childhood and adolescence: a meta-analysis. *Developmental Medicine & Child Neurology,* 2012. 54(4): p. 313-323.

[73] Roy, A., A more comprehensive overview of executive dysfunction in children with cerebral palsy: Theoretical perspectives and clinical implications. *Developmental Medicine & Child Neurology,* 2013. 55: p. 877-884.

[74] Love, S., Better description of spastic cerebral palsy for reliable classification. *Developmental Medicine & Child Neurology* 2007. 47: p. 24-25.

Cerebral Palsy in an Era of Neuroprotection and Evidence Based Interventions 23

[75] Boyd, R.N., et al., Validity of a clinical measure of spasticity in children with cerebral palsy in a double-blinded randomized controlled trial. *Developmental Medicine & Child Neurology*, 1998. 40(Suppl 78)(7).

[76] Mackey, A.H., et al., Intraobserver reliability of the Modified Tardieu Scale in the upper limb of children with hemiplegia. *Developmental Medicine & Child Neurology*, 2004. 46: p. 267-272.

[77] Palisano, R., et al., Development and reliability of a system to classify gross motor function in children with cerebral palsy. *Developmental Medicine & Child Neurology*, 1997. 39(4): p. 214-223.

[78] Eliasson, A.C., et al., The Manual Ability Classification System (MACS) for children with cerebral palsy: Scale development and evidence of validity and reliability. *Developmental Medicine & Child Neurology*, 2006. 48: p. 549-554.

[79] Koman, L.A., et al., Quantification of upper extremity function and range of motions in children with cerebral palsy. *Developmental Medicine & Child Neurology*, 2008. 50: p. 910-917.

[80] House, J.H., F.W. Gwathmey, and M. Fidler, A dynamic approach to the thumb-in-palm deformity in cerebral palsy. *Journal of Bone and Joint Surgery*, 1981. 63A(2): p. 216-225.

[81] Cooley Hidecker, M.J., et al., Developing and validating the Communication Function Classification System for individuals with cerebral palsy. *Developmental Medicine & Child Neurology*, 2011. DOI: 10.1111/j.1469-8749.2011.03996.x.

[82] Russel, D., et al., The Gross Motor Function Measure (GMFM-66 & GMFM-88) User's Manual. 2002, London: Mac Keith Press.

[83] Greaves, S., et al., Development of the Mini-Assisting Hand Assessment: Evidence for content and internal scale validity. *Developmental Medicine & Child Neurology*, 2013. 55(1): p. 1030-1037.

[84] Krumlinde-Sundholm, L. and A.-C. Eliasson, Development of the Assisting Hand Assessment: A Rasch-built measure intended for children with unilateral upper limb impairments. *Scandinavian Journal of Occupational Therapy*, 2003. 10: p. 16-26.

[85] Krumlinde-Sundholm, L., et al., The Assisting Hand Assessment: Current evidence of validity, reliability, and responsiveness to change. Developmental Medicine & Child *Neurology*, 2007. 49(4): p. 259-264.

[86] Bruni, O., et al., The Sleep Disturbance Scale for Children (SDSC). Construction and validation of an instrument to evaluate sleep distrubances in childhood and adolescence. *J. Sleep Research*, 1996. 5(4): p. 251-261.

[87] Parkinson, K.N., et al., Pain in children with cerebral palsy: A cross-sectional multicentre European study. *Acta Paediatrica*, 2010. 99: p. 446-451.

[88] Hayley, S.M., et al., Pediatric Evaluation of Disability Inventory (PEDI). 1992: Pearsons Education Inc.

[89] Sheppard, J.J., Dysphagia disorders survey and dysphagia managment scale, users manual and test forms revised. 2002, Lake Hopatcong: NC: Nutritional managment associates.

[90] Reid, S.M., J.H. M, and D. Reddihough, The Drooling Impact Scale: A measure of the impact of drooling in children with developmental disabilities. *Developmental Medicine & Child Neurology*, 2010. 52(2): p. e23-28.

[91] Bayley, N., Bayley Scales of Infant and Toddler Development, Third Edition (Bayley-III). 2005: Pearson Education Inc.

[92] Henry, J.D. and J.R. Crawford, The short-form of the Depression Anxiety Stress Scales (DASS-21): Construct validity and normative data in a large non-clinical sample. *British journal of Clinical Psychology*, 2005. 44(2): p. 227-239.

[93] Norton, R., Measuring Marital Quality: A critical look at the dependent variable. *Journal of Marriage and the Family*, 1993. 45(1): p. 141-151.

In: Handbook on Cerebral Palsy
Editor: Harold Yates

ISBN: 978-1-63321-852-9
© 2014 Nova Science Publishers, Inc.

Chapter 2

Integration of Exergames and Virtual Reality in the Treatment of Cerebral Palsy Children

Bruno Bonnechère[1,2], Bart Jansen[3,4],
Lubos Omelina[3,5] and Serge Van Sint Jan[1,2]

[1]Laboratory of Anatomy, Biomechanics and Organogenesis (LABO),
Faculty of Medicine - Université Libre de Bruxelles, Brussels, Belgium
[2]Center for Functional Evaluation, Faculty of Medicine – Université Libre
de Bruxelles, Brussels, Belgium
[3]Department of Electronics and Informatics (ETRO),
Vrije Universiteit Brussel, Brussels, Belgium
[4]Department of Future Health, iMinds, Ghent, Belgium
[5]Institute of Computer Science and Mathematics, Slovak University
of Technology, Bratislava, Slovakia

Abstract

How to motivate children (patients) to perform their exercises during rehabilitation or at home? This is the challenge met by physical therapists in their daily professional practice with disabled patients. Indeed, a lack of motivation is one of the most frequent reasons for patients to drop out.

Commercial video games have significantly evolved over the last decade. Today computer performance and play experience allow new perspectives for rehabilitation. Thanks to new gaming controllers (Nintendo Wii Fit™, Microsoft Xbox Kinect™, etc.) video game playing has changed from a passive (i.e., the player is seated on a sofa) to an active experience: players have to move in order to interact with games.

Clinicians are now prospecting the new potential use of these games in rehabilitation mainly through testing available commercial games with patients suffering from various pathologies (e.g., cerebral palsy, brain stroke, Parkinson disease, elderly...). Physical rehabilitation must be based on active exercises, and new gaming strategy allows it.

Furthermore, the game environment is obviously a major advantage to increase patient motivation to perform their rehabilitation schemes. Today challenge is to use games as rehabilitation.

However, results of these first clinical tests using commercial video games are not as good as first expected. Several limitations appeared when using commercial video games in rehabilitation. Such games are designed for entertainment purpose and obviously do not include any therapeutically know-how and strategies. Further, the architecture of the games (i.e., tasks to achieve, visual background, etc) is not adapted for patients showing various kinds of disabilities like motor or visual disorders. For example, most games are based on scenario fast movements to succeed while such quick execution is often contraindicated during many physical rehabilitation schemes related to neurological disorders. Also, player motion accuracy requested by the player during the games is low while most therapists will aim to improve patient joint control and coordination. In short, commercial video games are not adapted for rehabilitation; contrariwise the different gaming controllers used offer interesting new perspectives for rehabilitation. The current challenge for therapists is to help the game industry to develop specific games well-adapted for specific pathologies. Since a few years specific solutions have been developed and tested with cerebral palsy children. This chapter presents an overview of the different works that have been done in the field both using commercial games as well as games specifically developed for the target group. Advantages and limits of each approach will be then discussed. Finally, the last part of this chapter will focus on global trends for future work and perspectives will be provided on how to integrate rehabilitation aspects (physiotherapy, occupational therapy) in game scenarios.

1. Introduction

1.1. Current Treatment and Management of Cerebral Palsy

The aim of this chapter is not to describe current state-of-the art treatment available for Cerebral Palsy (CP) children (an extensive review of the available treatment has been recently been published [Novak et al. 2013]). It is however important to have a brief overview of the different options and approaches available for clinicians in order to have a full overview of the problem before speaking of new technologies.

Treatment can be roughly divided into two main categories: interventional interventions and rehabilitation.

1.1.1. Interventional Interventions

Several options are possible in order to attempt reducing muscle spasticity and muscle co-contractions. We will shortly present these options.

- Oral medication (baclofen, benzodiazepine, gabapentin, sodium dantrolene, tiagabine, tizanidine…) can be used to control spasticity but adverse effects are common and long term efficacy is subject to debate (Chung et al. 2011).
- Medication can be injected directly into the muscles. In most of the case the pharmacological agent used is botilinum toxin. Botox will block the junction between the nerve and the muscles and therefore induced a decrease of muscle activity. The duration of action is limited (between 8 and 12 weeks) therefore

intensive rehabilitation program should be programmed during this period in order to maximize the benefits of this injection (Ward 2008).
- A third option is to release the medication (Baclofen) directly into the spinal cord thanks to small pump: intrathecal Baclofen. Although some benefits have been described this technique is quite dangerous and therefore patients should be selected carefully (Kolaski & Logan 2008).
- A last option is the surgical intervention. In order to avoid long term complications induced by spasticity (bones deformations, vicious attitudes…) some surgeries can be planned (e.g., bones derotation, tendon lengthening, etc). A recent review concluded that there is no level of evidence supporting multilevel surgery in the literature (McGinley et al. 2012).

1.2. The Importance of Physical Therapy

Physical therapy (PT) and occupational therapy (OT) are the two key stones of the treatment of CP children. PT is focusing on maintaining and preserving range of motion and some flexibility of the muscles while OT is focusing on increasing function. Due to the nature of the lesions (irreversible brain lesion) progresses are very slow and for some patients there is even no evolution. For patient with the most severe disability the general trends is even to a decrease of motor function (see Figure 1) (Hanna et al. 2009). In order to struggle against this long term degradation patients need to regularly performed rehabilitation exercises with physiotherapists and occupational therapists but also at home in order to maintain benefice from the previous sessions. Various approaches are possible for PT and OT depending on the trend.

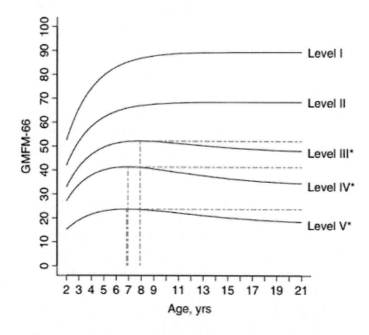

Figure 1. Evolution of motor control (evaluated by Gross Motor Function Measure) trough ages. Level I are the less disabled children and level V the most severely disabled (from Hanna et al. 2009).

One of the most popular approaches is a so-called *neurodevelopment treatment* developed by Bobath during the sixties. The main objective is to allow patient to have a greater independence by increasing global function instead of focusing on one particular joint or one particular motion (Bobath, 1967). Other approaches are massage, stretching, aerobic exercises, and strength training.

The common point of all these techniques is that they have to be performed daily, especially with severely impaired children, in order to be efficient. Except in specialized center where CP children are followed almost every time, patients have thus to perform a number of exercises at home without the supervision of a therapist.

1.3. (De) Motivation Problems

Unfortunately, at some points of the therapy – mainly during puberty, patients gets demotivated by therapy because progresses are to slow or they do not experiment any progress or feel that their state is getting worst despite they are performing rehabilitation for a long period of time. In summary, patients' own perception about their therapy might lead them to quit the rehabilitation schemes put in place in order to improve their physical status. Furthermore patients can sometimes be lost in the different treatment and approach that clinicians are trying. Figure 2shows various interventions that can be proposed to patients. We compared the rehabilitation process as a labyrinth where patients (and his family) can easily get lost it is therefore very important to inform these patients on the goals and the reason why such kind of treatment is proposed to the patients. If the patients experiment the feeling of being lost and doing things that he did not understand he will get demotivated and stopped the treatment.

However it is well known by clinicians that keeping patients motivated is one of the most important point of the treatment. In order to keep patient motivation high therapists often propose some ludic activities to their patients including challenges and awards instead of strict rehabilitation exercises only.

Although such alternatives may appear attractive, low adherence to treatment induced by lack of motivation remains an issue and is reported as being the main reason for patient dropout, failure to comply, relapse or other negative treatment outcomes (Ryan & Plant, 1995). It is estimated that only 30% of the patients, including all kind of pathologies (e.g., orthopedics, neurological, uro-genital…) regularly performed exercises at home (Sluis et al. 1993).

A systematic review on the treatment adherence identified four groups of barriers; the following points are strongly associated with a lower adherence to treatment (Jack et al. 2010): physical (low level of physical activity at aerobic capacity at baseline, low in-treatment adherence with exercise, low level of exercise adherence in previous weeks), psychological (low self-efficacy [for exercises, task and coping], high level of depression at the beginning of the treatment [baseline], no change or worse depression compared with baseline, high degree of helplessness), socio-demographic (poor social or family support for activity, greater number of barriers to exercise), clinical (worsening of pain during exercise).

In summary, patient motivation is a key element for a successful physical therapy, and it is therefore not surprising clinicians are aiming to integrate gamification, and more particularly video games, into conventional exercises therapy.

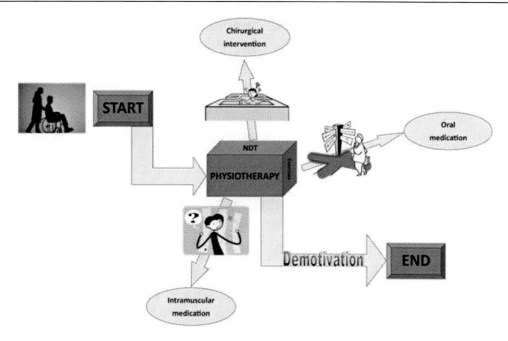

Figure 2. The labyrinth of rehabilitation leading to demotivation.

1.4. Exergames, Virtual Reality, Interactive Computer Play and Serious Games

Before explaining goals and principles of this new approach it is important to define the different terms that are used in research and literature. To our eyes the term exergames, contraction of the word exercises and games, is the best term to describe the use of video games in therapy. The term Virtual Reality (VR) is also used but this term is much wider that only doing physical exercises during rehabilitation. The aim of VR is to immerse patient in a virtual environment in order to (re)create some sensory inputs and/or putting patients in various situations that will help him to perform those kinds of activities later on in the real life. The interactive computer play is one subset of VR-based therapy wherein users can interact with virtual object in a simulated game environment (usually on a two-dimensional screen, not being immersed in 3D virtual environment) and receive real time feedback on their actions (Ni et al. 2014). The term serious gaming is used to describe the use of commercial games (e.g., Nintendo Wii™, Microsoft Xbox Kinect™) in rehabilitation.

Finally the term Serious Games (SG), defined as games designed with a primary purpose other than pure entertainment, is very often used but for some people there is one inadequacy between those two terms, according to them if a game is to serious this is not a game anymore.

Some might be surprised by the fact that, despite many different treatments are already available for CP patients (see Points 1.1 and 1.2) and thus potentially a lack of clarity in the general plan of long-term treatment, people try to add another approach to this list. Actually this is not another approach but a complement to PT, OT and home-based exercises in order to improve some weak points of those techniques.

Regardless of the term used the overall idea of introducing video games into therapy was to struggle against patient demotivation (see Point 1.3)since those therapeutically exercises are embedded and sometimes even hidden into the games. Several studies have already shown that SG can be used to increase patient's motivation during the rehabilitation process (e.g., Reid 2004, Harris & Reid 2005, Bonnechère et al. 2013).

Another advantage is that when patient is focusing on the games he is less focusing on pain or restricted motion and could therefore performed more repetitions of motions without getting bored. This point is particularly important since it is well know that the more the patient is repeating the motion the more progress he will do (Langhorne et al. 2011).

We will now summarize previous works that have been done in the field using those two main different approaches: using commercial games or specially developed one.

In order to determine in these approaches (commercial and specially developed games) are efficient a literature review was performed. The research paper ended the first December 2013.

Only Randomized Clinical Trial (RCT) and cohort studies were included. Based on the results of these studies and of our own personal experience of the development and use of SG for CP children we will then discuss the current advantages and limits of this approach.

2. The Use of Commercial Games

2.1. Available Technology

The industry of commercial video games has increased significantly over the last decade. Dramatic changes in performance of the computer, but also, and more important for rehabilitation, the way of playing the video games has changed over the last few years. Thanks to new unconventional gaming controllers (etc.) the way of playing video games has changed from a passive (the player is seated on a sofa) to an active way: players have to move in order to interact with games.

Clinicians have quickly found out the new potential use of these games in rehabilitation and have tested available commercial games with patients suffering from various pathologies (e.g., cerebral palsy, stroke, Parkinson disease, elderly…).

2.2. Clinical Studies

Currently there are three commercial games devices that allow patients, or gamers, to interact with the games: the Microsoft Xbox Kinect™ (Kinect), the Nintendo Wii Balance Board™ (Wii) (with or without Balance Board) and the PlayStation 2 and 3 with Eye Toy™. The Kinect was released on November 2010 and the Wii on July 2007 and the Eye Toy in 2003 and 2007 (for PlayStation 2 and 3 respectively). The way of controlling the games and the different potential option in rehabilitation of those two devices are different: the Kinect required proper joint control and coordination while the Wii is more used to train balance and posture. Therefore we presented separately the results of the study.

2.2.1. Microsoft Xbox Kinect™

Currently, despite high clinical potential only one paper was found on the use of the Kinect for CP rehabilitation. One of the possible reasons is that the Kinect was only released at the end of 2010. Some time is required in order to know how to use the product in clinics, then organize a clinical trial and finally published the results. Obviously, it is expected that clinical papers will be soon published in this field.

In 2013 Luna-Oliva et al. tested to integrate 8 weeks of commercial video games into the conventional physiotherapy programs. They focused on the motor skills (balance and gait parameters) and fine dexterity motions and observed significant statistical improvement after the 8 weeks of training. Due to the study design it is however impossible to determine if these results are due to the integration of games or due to the increase of rehabilitation's time.

2.2.2. Nintendo Wii™

Most of the studies using commercial games have been done with the Wii and are focusing on balance training with the Balance Board.

One RCT was found using Wii Sport and Wii Fit™ (Sharan et al. 2012). Sixteen CP children were allocated into one group receiving SG along the conventional therapy and one group receiving only conventional therapy. Patients in the SG groups shows significant improvement for balance and the level of participation, satisfaction and cooperation were significantly higher is this interventional group.

Six cohorts studies were find, all of them were published in 2012 and 2013.

Before testing the clinical relevancy of commercial games in rehabilitation researchers have investigated the level of energy expenditure achieved during this kind of exercises in order to see if it could be an alternative to aerobic and fitness training. Howcroft et al. (2012) tested Wii Sports games with 17 children (GMFCS I) and found a light to moderate physical activity level achieved during these games. Another study (Robert et al. [2013]) has studied the exercises intensity reached during four different games (jogging, cycling, snowboarding and skiing). A group of 10 CP children and a control group of 10 healthy children were included in the study. The authors didn't find differences between the 4 sports and no difference were found between CP and control group.

Concerning (potential) clinical benefits of the Wii four studies have been included:

Ramstrad & Lygnegard (2012) tested the use of Wii Fit in a group of 18 CP children (GMFCS I-II) during 5 weeks of training (30 minutes a day, 5 days a week). The authors tried to bring out a change in balance and posture after this training. No statistical significant difference was found before and after the training.

Jelsma et al. (2013) tried the Wii Fit with a population of 14 CP children (GMFCS I-II) during three weeks but contrariwise the previous study they applied this program instead of conventional therapy, not as a complement. Authors found significant improvement in balance performance after this relatively short training. Authors also pinpointed the fact that young patients preferred to play games compared to conventional physical rehabilitation exercises.

Tarakci et al. (2013) also tested the use of Wii fit with 14 CP children (GMFCS I-III). Patients were included in a 12 weeks training program (two sessions per weeks. Various tests (one leg standing test, functional reach test, timed-up and go test, 6-mon walking test) were used to compare balance before and after interventions. Authors found statistically significant improvement for each tests after the intervention.

Only one study (Winkels et al. [2013]) tested the Wii games controlled with hand(not with the balance board) for 12 weeks (two sessions per weeks) with 15 CP children (GMFCS I-III) to test whether or not these games could be used to increase upper limb dexterity of function. The author didn't show any improvement of the quality of upper extremity motion but they found a significant increase of convenience in using upper limbs during functional activity of daily living.

2.2.3. The PlayStation™

Two cohort studies were found about the use of PlayStation 2 for CP children.

Like for the Wii the first study on the use of PlayStation was more focused on energy expenditure and crude analysis of the type of motion that has been performed during the games. Sandlund et al. (2011) tested the use of PlayStation with 15 CP children (GMFCS I-III) during 4 weeks (5 sessions per week). After this period authors concluded that the games promote physical activity (light to moderate intensity) and enhance motor performance. The same team (Sandlund et al. [2013]) repeated this protocol. They analysis kinematics of the subjects (using motion analysis system) during the games and found a significant increase in precision and movement control during the games after the 4 weeks period of training. Unfortunately we didn't know if these progresses are only during the games or if there is a transfer during activity of daily living.

2.2.4. Other

We also found two RCT using commercially available games solutions. Note that there solutions are available for public but are, more or less, adapted for patients.

Ritterband-Rosenbaum et al. (2012) tested the MiTii solution (MiTii development) in a RCT. 40 CP children were randomly allocated to the intervention group (30 minutes of daily training) or a control group (normal physical activity). The MiTii system is composed by a pen-tablet and patients have to move object on the tablet to reach some points. After the training the authors observed a significant decrease of compensatory motions of the upper limbs. Chen et al. (2012) tested the use of a virtual cycling system with 28 CP children (GMFCS I-II) allocated in the intervention group (40 minutes of training on virtual cycling, 3 sessions per week during 12 weeks) or a control group (general physical activity 3 sessions a weeks for 12 weeks). Authors observed a significant improvement of knee muscle strength in the intervention group but no difference in the test of motor proficiency. In 2013 the same team presented more results of this study. They investigated bone mineral density of the lumbar spine and femur in both group and observed a greater femoral bone density in the intervention group compared to control group after specific training.

2.3. Conclusion on the Use of Commercial Games

The main objective of commercial games is mostly entertainment and enjoyment, except for some few games that aimed to promote physical activity and fitness (Wii Fit, Kinect Move...). Therefore, many patients are attracted by these ludic platforms, but their physical disorders are often a limitation. Indeed there are several problems with the use of commercial games in rehabilitation:

- *Visual complexity*: Background and graphics tend to be more and more realistic, the players are literally immersed into the games. Lots of patients have visual impairment and/or low cognitive levels and it is difficult for them to focus on the task they need to perform because they are distracted by the environment.
- *Speed based*: Most of the commercial games are based on speed reaction time or the speed of motion. However, high motion speed is clinically contraindicated form many disorders
- *Non configurable*: Generally the level of difficulty is automatically increasing during the games but it is not possible to configure the way of controlling the games (e.g., amplitudes needed to reach the goal, select only one joint to control one particular motion...).
- *Not therapeutically relevant*: Physiotherapy is a therapy induced by motion, so in theory it is good to move. Except that there are some schemes and relevant therapeutically exercises that need to be performed. Most of the time motions that need to be performed during the games are not the same as those one performed during rehabilitation session.

Despite these negatives points we have seen in the previous section that they have some evidence in the literature supporting the use of commercial video games in the treatment of CP children. Nevertheless we think that specific solutions, taking into account the needs of CP children rehabilitation, could be much more efficient. We will now discuss this aspect in the next section.

3. The Use of Specifically Developed Games

3.1. Why Is It Important? ...and Needed!

The first obvious reason is to solve, some of, the limitations about the use of commercial games that have been described in section 2.3. The most important think is the lack of configuration in the games, not only for the difficulty levels but also for the way of controlling the games.

Each pathology requires specific approach in rehabilitation; clinicians will not adopt the same strategy with patients suffering from CP or from multiple sclerosis for example. Therefore clinicians must be able to modify the games in order to reproduce the same relevant therapeutic schemes with the SG.

And of course inside one particular pathology each patient is very unique and presented various clinical signs with more or severity, this is particularly true with CP children where patients present very heterogeneous clinical signs. Some patients are only suffering for local spastic problem inducing limited range of motion one upper limb while other patients are almost not able to move. An ideal situation would be that those two patients could be able to play the same games with adapted configuration. Ranges of motions required to accomplish the games must be configured separately for each patients and each selected joint but also the starting position must be defined (in case of malicious posture or bones/joints deformations) in order to allow patients to succeed in the games. If patients cannot succeed in the games they will of course get frustrated and demotivated.

3.2. Clinical Studies

Two RCT we found in the literature testing some developed solutions in the conventional treatment of CP children.

Akhutina et al. (2003) is, to our best knowledge, the first study on the use of SG in the rehabilitation of CP children. This is a computer-based system focusing on motor and cognitive aspects. 45 CP children were included in this study and played games 6 to 8 times for 30-60 minutes during one month or some non-specific rehabilitation training. After the intervention authors didn't find difference on computer based test but they find significant improvement in the Benton Judgement of Line orientation tests in the intervention group.

Reid & Campbell (2006) tested specially developed games with 31 CP children (GMFCS I-V) during 8 weeks (one session of 90 minutes per week) and a control group receiving standard of care (physiotherapy and occupational therapy). In term of performance (Quality of Upper Extermity Skills Test, Canadian Occupational Performance Measure) no statistical difference was found between both groups. Authors found significant difference in the social acceptance score in the intervention group.

Most of the studies were cohort studies, seven of then we found.

Reid (2004) tested the playfulness of games on CP. Results showed that virtual environment stimulated motivation and internal control of these patients. These works were followed by another one (Harris & Reid [2005]) also showing that exergames seems to be a promising medium to increase patients' motivation during rehabilitation.

Chen et al. (2007) tested a system focusing on hand rehabilitation with 4 CP children. The intervention lasted for 4 weeks (2-3 sessions per week). Results indicated that 3 of the 4 children showed improvement in the quality of reaching performance and that these results were partially maintained four weeks after the intervention.

Golomb et al. (2010) also tested a system for upper limb and finger rehabilitation with 3 hemiplegic CP children. Intervention lasted for 3 weeks (5 sessions per week). There was a significant improvement in the function of the plegic limb and in bone density. Authors also did functional imaging of the brain (MRI) that showed that there was a spatial extent of the activation in the motor cortex after the training.

Kirshner et al. (2011) tested the feasibility of integrating games in the rehabilitation of CP children (one session on 60 minutes per week during 2 weeks) and evaluated enjoyment and score of CP children compared to healthy control group. Results point that both group enjoyed playing games and that, unsurprisingly, CP children have lower score in the game.

Wu et al. (2011) tested a haptic device combined with VR, 12 CP children (GMFCS I-III) were included for 18 sessions of 60 minutes of training. Authors observed a significant increase in both active and passive motion, in motor control performance, in functional capability, in balance and in mobility.

Green & Wilson (2012) tested their VR system with 8 CP children 30 minutes a day during 4 weeks. Authors used results and scores provided during the games (precision, reaction time...), specific tests for the upper limbs (functional grasp and release, ABILHAND-Kids...) and questionnaire to evaluate participation and engagement. They observed a significant improvement of upper limb function and activity participation after rehabilitation.

3.3. Conclusion on the Use of Specifically Developed Games

Specifically developed games for the treatment of CP children has been created and tested over the last decade. Despite ten years of development the level of evidence supporting these techniques, commercial or developed games, is weak and there is no clear evidence to support this kind of approach in rehabilitation. Paradoxically this situation is not an exception in CP rehabilitation, actually there is a lack of high level evidence supporting most of the more popular intervention (see Section 1.1.1).

Several explanations are possible: CP is due to non-evolutive lesion in the brain therefore progresses, if any, are very slow (for some techniques it required years before seeing any impact) and most of the clinical trials last for maximum one year in general, one other point is that there is no one CP but there is a large variety of clinical presentation and severity of this disease therefore the treatment needs to be adapted for each and every patients unfortunately this "practical clinical approach" is against the scientific approach where a strict protocol must be followed for each patients.

A last point that can be raised it that due to the highly heterogeneous forms of CP and the size of the expected progresses the sample size required in obtained to show any benefice must be important and required thus multicentric studies, such kind of studies are more difficult to planned (for both ethical, practical and financial reason).

Concerning SG all the above reasons are, of course, also applicable but there are also two major points that could definitely play a role: people's mind and financial issues. These points are going to be discussed in the next section.

4. What Are the Next Steps?

Predicting the future is difficult. Several directions can be however expected based on previous studies and on the general societal trends. Before going any further there is one major barrier that needs to be stride over before any potential development of SG: the people mind! It is difficult to change people's habits and thinking, in particular in the health domain. It is natural, and scientific, to have questions and doubts about the use of new techniques in medicine and rehabilitation but people must be aware and opened to change. However we are currently stuck in a vicious circle: clinicians do not want to use exergames because they said that this is not validated but in order to validate those tools patients and clinical centers must be deeply involved in the validation process.

In the vast majority of the cases, at least at the early phases of the project, research and development are done at university level. The transition between a university research project and the release of largely available product is not a clear valorization path.

There are plenty of reasons to explain that:

- *Time consuming*: Finding funding and shareholders but also develop a stable and user friendly solution instead of a beta version used for testing.
- *Financial issues*: Developed and launch start-up required money (product development, marketing, sales…). You need to find investors that believed in the project and are ready to take some risks.
- *Other interests*: People working at university are mainly interested in academic research and teaching, and are less proned to be involved in entrepreneurship, business development and marketing strategies required to launch a company.

Once the products are available another important issue is to know who is going to pay for the developed products and services: the clinicians, the patients or both of them? Furthemore, national health services and health insurance are not (yet) organized reimbursement for treatment based on SG.

Another major issue to solve remains the motivation problem. It is well known that when you are trying something new in rehabilitation (new techniques, new devices…) patients are willing to use them and are enthusiastic. Furthermore clinicians that tested these systems are also enthusiastic and take time to test the system with patients. Most of the studies found in the literature are relatively short and therefore there is no information about the use on long term of the exergames. However we have seen that rehabilitation of CP children is a very long and difficult process, therefore one challenge is to develop games that must remain simple and clinically oriented but also remained fun, challenging and modifiable.

Another point, directly link to the last one, is the "competition" against commercial video games. For the patients with severe disability is a not a problem because they are not able to play with commercial games and are thus very happy to play with adapted video games. But for CP children with less disability (GMFCS I-II) they are able to play most of the commercial games (even if there are not adapted for them and sometimes even contraindicated for their specific problem) and find thus adapted games quite boring.

To illustrate this point we conducted a small study with 10 CP children (GMFCS I) who were invited to play 5 specially developed mini-games (from the ICT4rehab project, http://www.ict4rehab.org) for 20 minutes a day during 5 consecutive days and then 10 minutes of commercial games (Microsoft Kinect Adventures). We asked them which games they preferred, results are presented in Figure 3 and did not require any further comments!

Patients were asked to assess on Visual Analog Scales the level of enjoyment (0 = no enjoyment, 10 = highest enjoyment), the level of pain (0 = worst pain, 10 = complete absence of pain) and the level of boredom (0 = no boredom, 10 = maximal boredom) during conventional PT sessions and during specially-developed exergames.

Compared to conventional PT, games showed a higher level for enjoyment, a significantly lower level of pain feeling and a not-significative decrease of the level of boredom (Figure 4). These results confirm thus the fact that exergames can motivate patients and that there are less concentrated on the pain and less bored by the repetition of movements when they are immersed in the games.

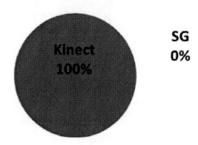

Figure 3. CP children preference between specially developed games and commercial games.

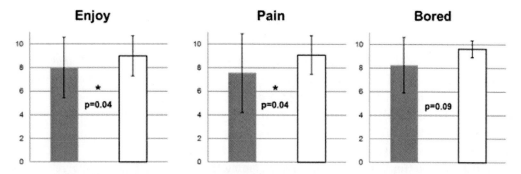

Figure 4. Results of psychological tests during conventional PT exercises (grey color) and exergames (white color) P-values are results of Wilcoxon's tests (adapted from Bonnechère et al. 2013).

Conclusion

Despite more than a decade of research, supplementary research is request to objectively assess the efficiency of SG use in rehabilitation compared to conventional therapeutical schemes used with CP patients. This chapter explained the reasons behind the current lack of scientific evidence supporting the efficacy of exergames in rehabilitation: complexity of the management and treatment of CP children, multidisciplinary approach, heterogeneous clinical presentation... However, because of the non-evolutive nature of Cerebral Palsy it is difficult to quantify changes in patients' conditions. Therefore clinical efficacy is not the only question that needs to be answered during a large-scale clinical use, here is a (non-exhaustive) list:

- Which patients (age group, pathology...) are most likely to receive such kind of treatments and have a favorable outcome?
- How many sessions per weeks are needed? What is the best duration of these sessions?
- Concerning the motivation, would the patients still want to play the games after several months or would they be tired of them?

- Do the exergames be played under the supervision of a therapist or can the patients play alone?
- Can these exergames be counter-productive for the patients (wrong execution, compensatory motions, etc)
- Are there any adverse effects (e.g., seizure) that could occur during these exergames?

In conclusion, many prospective work remains to be achieved before having all the objective elements in hand to be able to decide whether or not exergames can be integrated into the conventional treatment of CP children. This decision should be made taking into account available and future scientific research. It must be stressed that the use of SG for the rehabilitation of other patient categories (who are presenting evolutive disorders such as cerebro-vascular accidents, orthopedic traumas, etc.) should show more easily quantifiable progresses although here too more scientific and clinical evidence should be collected.

References

Akhutina T, Foreman N, Krichevets A, Matikka L, Narhi V, Pylaeva N, Vahakuopus J. Improving spatial functioning in children with cerebral palsy using computerized and traditional game tasks. *Disabil. and Rehabil*. 2003; 25(24):1361-71.

Bobath B, The very early treatment of cerebral palsy. *Dev. Med. Child. Neurol*. 1967; 9(4): 373-90.

Bonnechère B, Jansen B, Omelina L, Da Silva L, Mougeat J, Heymans V, Vandeuren A, Rooze M, Van Sint Jan S. Use of serious gaming to increase motivation of cerebral pasly during rehabilitation. *Eur. J. Paediatr. Neurol*. 2013; 17(1): S32.

Chen CL, Chen CY, Liaw MY, Chung CY, Wang CJ, Hong WH. Efficacy of home-based virtual cycling training on bone mineral density in ambulatory children with cerebral palsy. *Osteoporos. Int*. 2013; 24(4):1399-406.

Chen CL, Hong WH, Cheng HY, Liaw MY, Chung CY, Chen CY. Muscle strength enhancement following home-based virtual cycling training in ambulatory children with cerebral palsy. *Res. Dev. Disabil*. 2012 ;33(4):1087-94.

Chen YP, Kang LJ, Chuang TY, Doong JL, Lee SJ, Tsai MW, Jeng SF, Sung WH. Use of virtual reality to improve upper-extremity control in children with cerebral palsy: a single-subject design. *Phys. Ther*. 2007; 87(11):1441-57.

Chung CY, Chen CL, Wong AM. Pharmacotherapy of spasticity in children withcerebral palsy. *J. Formos. Med. Assoc*. 2011;110(4):215-22.

Finley M, Combs S. User perceptions of gaming interventions for improving upper extremity motor function in persons with chronic stroke. *Physiother. Theory Pract*. 2013; 29(3): 195-201.

Golomb MR, Warden SJ, Fess E, Rabin B, Yonkman J, Shirley B, Burdea GC. Maintained hand function and forearm bone health 14 months after an in-home virtual-reality videogame hand telerehabilitation intervention in an adolescent with hemiplegic cerebral palsy. *J. Child. Neurol*. 2011;26(3):389-93.

Green D, Wilson PH. Use of virtual reality in rehabilitation of movement in children with hemiplegia--a multiple case study evaluation. *Disabil. Rehabil*. 2012;34(7):593-604.

Hanna SE, Rosenbaum PL, Bartlett DJ, Palisano RJ, Walter SD, Avery L, Russell DJ.Stability and decline in gross motor function among children and youth with cerebral palsy aged 2 to 21 years. *Dev. Med. Child. Neurol.* 2009; 51(4): 295-302.

Harris K, Reid D. The influence of virtual reality on children's motivation. *Can. J. Occup. Ther.* 2005; 72(1): 21-29.

Harris K, Reid D. The influence ofvirtual reality play on children's motivation. *Can. J. Occup. Ther.* 2005;72(1):21-9.

Howcroft J, Klejman S, Fehlings D, Wright V, Zabjek K, Andrysek J, Biddiss E. Active video game play in children with cerebral palsy: potential for physical activity promotion and rehabilitation therapies. *Arch. Phys. Med. Rehabil.* 2012; 93(8):1448-56.

Jack K, McLean SM, Moffett JK, Gardiner E. Barriers to treatment adherence in physiotherapy outpatient clinics: a systematic review. *Man Ther.* 2010;15(3):220-8.

Jelsma J, Pronk M, Ferguson G, Jelsma-Smit D. The effect of the Nintendo Wii Fit on balance control and gross motor function of children with spastic hemiplegic cerebral palsy. *Dev. Neurorehabil.* 2013; 16(1): 27-37.

Kirshner S, Weiss PL, Tirosh E. Meal-Maker: a virtual meal preparation environment for children with cerebral palsy. *Eur. J. Spec. Needs Educ.* 2011; 26 (3): 323-336.

Kolaski K, Logan LR. Intrathecal baclofen in cerebral palsy: A decade of treatment outcomes. *J. Pediatr. Rehabil. Med.* 2008; 1(1): 3-32.

Langhorne P, Bernhardt J, Kwakkel G. Stroke rehabilitation. *Lancet.* 2011;377(9778):1693-702.

Luna-OlivaL, Ortiz-Gutiérrez RM, Cano-de la Cuerda R, Piédrola RM, Alguacil-Diego IM, Sánchez-Camarero C, MartínezCulebras Mdel C. Kinect Xbox 360 as a therapeutic modality for children with cerebral palsy in a school environment: a preliminary study. *Neuro Rehabilitation.* 2013; 33(4): 513-21.

McGinley JL, Dobson F, Ganeshalingam R, Shore BJ, Rutz E, Graham HK. Single-event multilevel surgery for children with cerebral palsy: a systematic review. *Dev. Med. Child. Neurol.* 2012;54(2):117-28.

Ni L, Fehlings D, Biddiss E. Design and evaluation of virtual-reality based therapy games with dual focus on therapeutic relevance and user experience for children with cerebral palsy. *Games Health J.* 2014; 3(3): 162-171.

Novak I, McIntyre S, Morgan C, Campbell L, Dark L, Morton N, Stumbles E, Wilson SA, Goldsmith S. A systematic review of interventions for children with cerebral palsy: state of the evidence. *Dev. Med. Child. Neurol.* 2013; 55(10): 885-910.

Ramstrand N, Lygnegård F. Can balance in children with cerebral palsy improve through use of an activity promoting computer game? *Technological Health Care.* 2012; 20(6): 501-10.

Reid D, Campbell K. The use of virtual reality with children with cerebral palsy: a pilot randomized trial. *Ther. Recreation J.* 2006; 40(4): 255-268.

Reid D. The influence of virtual reality on playfulness in children with cerebral palsy: a pilot study. *Occup. Ther. Int.* 2004; 11(3): 131-44.

Reid D. The influence of virtual reality on playfulness in children with cerebral palsy: a pilot study. *Occup. Ther. Int.* 2004; 11(3):131-44.

Ritterband-Rosenbaum A, Christensen MS, Nielsen JB. Twenty weeks of computer-training improves sense of agency in children with spastic cerebral palsy. *Res. Dev. Disabil.* 2012; 33(4):1227-34.

Robert M, Ballaz L, Hart R, Lemay M. Exercise intensity levels in children with cerebral palsy while playing with an active video game console. *Phys. Ther.* 2013; 93(8):1084-91.

Ryan RM, Plant RW. Initial motivations for alcohol treatment: relations with patient characteristics, treatment involvement, and dropout. *Science.* 1995; 20(3): 279-297.

Sandlund M, Domellöf E, Grip H, Rönnqvist L, Häger CK. Training of goal directed arm movements with motion interactive video games in children with cerebral palsy - A kinematic evaluation. *Dev. Neurorehab.* 2013. [Epub ahead of print].

Sandlund M, Waterworth EL, Häger C. Using motion interactivegamesto promote physical activity and enhance motor performance in children with cerebral palsy. *Dev. Neurorehab.* 2011; 14(1):15-21.

Sharan D, Ajeesh PS, Rameshkumar R, Mathankumar M, Paulina RJ, Manjula M. Virtual reality based therapy for post operative rehabilitation of children with cerebral palsy. *Work.* 2012; 41 (S1):3612-5.

Sluis EM, Kok GJ, van der Zee J. Correlates of exercise compliance in physical therapy. *Phys. Ther.* 1993; 73(11): 771-82.

Tarakci D, Ozdincler AR, Tarakci E, Tutuncuoglu F, Ozmen M. Wii-based Balance Therapy to Improve Balance Function of Children with Cerebral Palsy: A Pilot Study. *J. Phys. Ther. Sci.* 2013;25(9):1123-1127.

Ward, A.B. Spasticity treatment with botulinum toxins. *J. Neural Tra*nsm. 2008; 115(4): 607–616.

Winkels DG, Kottink AI, Temmink RA, Nijlant JM, Buurke JH. Wii™-habilitation of upper extremity function in children with Cerebral Palsy. An explorative study. *Dev. Neurorehabil.* 2013; 16(1): 44-51.

Wu YN, Hwang M, Ren Y, Gaebler-Spira D, Zhang LQ. Combined passive stretching and active movement rehabilitation of lower-limb impairments in children with cerebral palsy using a portable robot. *Neurorehabil. Neural. Repair.* 2011; 25(4):378-85.

In: Handbook on Cerebral Palsy
Editor: Harold Yates

ISBN: 978-1-63321-852-9
© 2014 Nova Science Publishers, Inc.

Chapter 3

Unilateral Cerebral Palsy: Epidemiology, Etiology, Imaging and Treatment of Hand Function Problems

Lucianne Speth M.D.[1,2,], and Hans Vles M.D. Ph.D.[3,4]*

[1]Adelante, Pediatric Rehabilitation, Valkenburg, the Netherlands
[2]Adelante, Centre of Expertise in Rehabilitation and Audiology,
Hoensbroek, the Netherlands
[3]Maastricht University Medical Centre, Department of Neurology,
Maastricht, the Netherlands
[4]Maastricht University, Research School GROW, Department of Neurology,
Maastricht, the Netherlands

Abstract

Cerebral Palsy (CP) describes a group of permanent disorders of development of movement and posture, causing activity limitation, that are attributed to non-progressive disturbances that occurred in the developing fetal or infant brain. The prevalence of CP remains constant over the last years at 2.11 per 1000 live births. Unilateral spastic CP (uCP), also called hemiplegic CP, has a prevalence of 0.6 per 1,000 live births, and amounts to about 30% of the CP subtype proportion. In children with a birth weight of 2,500g or more, there is an increase of the uCP subtype.

The definition of CP gives no etiological explanation. However, with the introduction of modern neuro-imaging, we are more informed in detail about the different etiological and risk factors. Different etiology will have different consequences with concern to cortical and sub-cortical re-organization.

---

[*]l.speth@adelante-zorggroep.nl.

In this review chapter we will focus on a vascular event (hypoxic ischemic, HI or stroke) as a cause for uCP, using definitions related to gestational age.

Ultrasound (US) and Magnetic Resonance Imaging (MRI) are not only of importance in studying etiology but also can be of help to determine the time the insult took place.

The clinical presentation of uCP is variable due to the severity and localization of the lesion, associated pathology and the aspect of the incident: chronic HI versus acute asphyxia. With the introduction of new neuro-imaging techniques, such as functional MRI (fMRI) and Diffusion Tensor Imaging (DTI), we are more informed about the relation of structure and function and the possibilities of neuronal adaptation. This is of utmost clinical importance, because the way the re-organization of neuronal networks (ipsi or contra lateral) takes place and the severity and localization of the lesion correlates with hand function and bimanual performance and even influences therapy outcome.

Developmental disuse is a problem typically occurring in uCP and also influencing therapy outcome. Evidence of several treatment modalities of unilateral hand function problems in children with unilateral CP, i.e., bimanual intensive goal directed treatment, constraint induced movement therapy and botulinum toxin A treatment, will be discussed.

Definition

Cerebral Palsy (CP) describes a group of permanent disorders of development of movement and posture, causing activity limitation, that are attributed to non-progressive disturbances that occurred in the developing fetal or infant brain. The motor disorders of cerebral palsy are often accompanied by disturbances of sensation, perception, cognition, communication, and behavior; by epilepsy, and by secondary musculoskeletal problems [1].

Epidemiology

According to a systematic review and meta-analysis the prevalence of CP remains constant over the last years at 2.11 per 1000 live births despite the increased survival of at risk preterm infants [2].

Unilateral spastic CP (uCP), also called hemiplegic CP, has a prevalence of 0.6 per 1,000 live births, and amounts to about 30% of the CP subtype proportion [3]. MRI findings most often observed in uCP are periventricular white matter lesions (PWML), focal periventricular gliosis or post-hemorrhagic porencephalic lesions in 36%, cortical or deep gray matter lesions, mainly infarcts of the middle cerebral artery (MCA) in 31% and brain maldevelopments, mainly focal cortical dysplasia or unilateral schizencephaly in 16% of the cases. PWML occur significantly more often in preterm uCP than in term (86% vs. 20%) and cortical or deep gray matter lesions significantly less often (0% vs 41%). Brain maldevelopments occur in preterm uCP nearly as often as in term uCP (14% vs. 16%) [3]. In a Canadian study of 213 children with CP 31.8% had the hemiplegic neurological subtype. Of the children with uCP 18.3% had PWML, 12.7% brain malformation, 26.8% cerebro vascular accidents, 19.7% gray matter injury, 2.8% intracranial hemorrhage, 15.5% non-specific and 4.2% had normal neuro imaging findings. Due to an underrepresentation of premature born children in the cohort in this study, there was less PWML [4]. Trends in the prevalence of CP in children born with a birth weight of 2,500 g or above in Europe show a decrease in the bilateral spastic-CP subtype and an increase in uCP, with a stable prevalence of CP of 0.99 per 1,000 live birth in 1998 and a significant decrease in neonatal mortality. The prevalence of uCP increased significantly from 0.37 to 0.46. The type of CP was spastic in 84.9% of cases (bilateral in 45.7%, unilateral in 39.2%) [5].

Incidence, Etiology and Clinical Presentation of Perinatal Stroke

Focal brain injury occurs most frequently as a consequence of infarction of the left MCA, or more rarely as a consequence of cerebral sinus venosus thrombosis (CSVT). Neurodevelopmental morbidity occurs in over 50% of the children [6]. With an incidence of 1/2800 to 1/5000 new births, perinatal arterial ischemic stroke (PAIS) is the most frequent form of cerebral infarction in children [7]. Perinatal ischemic stroke is defined as a group of heterogeneous conditions in which there is focal disruption of cerebral blood flow secondary to arterial or cerebral venous thrombosis or embolization, between 20 weeks of fetal life through the 28th postnatal day, confirmed by neuroimaging or neuropathologic studies. Three subcategories can be distinguished: fetal ischemic stroke, diagnosed before birth from fetal imaging or in stillbirths on the basis of neuropathological examination; neonatal ischemic stroke, diagnosed after birth and on or before the 28th postnatal day (including in preterm infants); presumed perinatal ischemic stroke, diagnosed in infants over 28 days of age in whom it is presumed (but not certain) that the ischemic event occurred sometime between the 20th week of fetal life through the 28th postnatal day. The hypothesis is that an infarction that occurred later in infancy or childhood would have been symptomatic at the time of the first occurrence.

Risk factors for PAIS are: thrombotic history, infertility, previous pregnancy related disorders in the mother; first pregnancy, primiparity, twin pregnancy, pre-eclampsia, gestational diabetes, chorioamnionitis, premature rupture of membranes; signs of fetal distress, intervention during delivery (notably emergency caesarean section); male sex, extreme birth weight, polycytemia, hypoglycemia, meningitis, congenital heart disease, extra-corporeal membrane oxygenation in the newborn; lipoprotein (a) > 30 ng/ml, factor V Leiden and factor II G20210A mutation, antiphospholipid antibodies in either mother or child.

60% of the infants present early symptoms. In more than 90% the presenting symptoms are tonic/clonic seizures, focal in 74%, leading to a status epilepticus in one third of the infants. 46 of 100 infants had a persistently altered tone, 36 a decreased level of consciousness, and 16 had focal deficit. Confirmation of a suspected infarct from an ultrasound (US) scan should be done directly with magnetic resonance imaging (MRI), which provides further insight into the timing of the infarct and in the outcome. The development of the MRI findings during the first 3 days show there is a short time frame in which the neonatal stroke occurs, and makes the hypothesis of a placento-cerebral embolism during pregnancy prior to labor less probable. 67% of the infants with corticospinal tract involvement on MRI developed hemiplegia (uCP) versus 6% of those without. 26% of these infants with neonatal stroke, who were followed until 24 months of age, had motor impairments, mostly uCP.

In 40% of the infants with PAIS the clinical presentation is delayed. All these children present at the age of 5 months with motor problems as early handedness, decreased hand use, rigidity of the upper limb or fisting, which has been well observed by the parents while playing or dressing. 14 to 25% of these children present with seizures. The timing of the clinically silent vascular event leading to stroke is uncertain in these patients in the pre- or perinatal period. Also there is uncertainty regarding the mechanisms of the event. In some cases the images show a clear arterial ischemic pattern of injury (presumed perinatal ischemic stroke), but in other cases the findings are more equivocal and some cases suggest periventricular venous infarction, primary parenchymal hemorrhage, or even a non-vascular mechanism [7]. Golomb et al. found that 76 of 111 children with PAIS (68%) had cerebral palsy, most commonly hemiplegic (66/76; 87%) [8]. Both delayed presentation (presumed perinatal infarction) and male sex were associated with CP. Most of the children with perinatal co morbidities were children with neonatal presentation.

Imaging in Relation to Reorganization and Hand Function

De Vries et al. mentioned the additional value of diffusion weighted MRI (DW-MRI) to establish cortical tract injury in newborn infants with PAIS. The presence of increased signal intensity at the posterior limb of the internal capsule and the cerebral peduncles is followed by Wallerian degeneration and development of uCP [9]. This is in agreement with Staudt et al. finding a correlation of the total lesion volume and degree of Wallerian degeneration of the pyramidal tract at the anterior portion of the posterior limb of the internal capsule at the MRI scan, with motor impairment of the hand in adults with congenital hemi paresis due to periventricular lesions [10].

Central motor reorganization in hemiplegic CP was first investigated by Carr et al. using focal transcranial magnetic stimulation (TMS) of the cortex. Two types of reorganization patterns were found. In both forms TMS demonstrated novel ipsilateral pathways form the undamaged motor cortex to the hemiplegic hand. Ipsilateral projections were not found from the damaged motor cortex. In subjects who had intense mirror movements, the corticospinal axons descending from the ipsilateral cortex had branched abnormally projecting to each side of the spinal cord. This was not the case in subjects without mirror movements. Good EMG responses in the hand after TMS of the contralateral cortex corresponded to good hand function whereas absent EMG responses meant poor hand function unless mirror movements were present [11].

Holmström et al. studied the relationship between brain lesions, cortico-motor projections and hand function in children with uCP [12]. There was no relation between mirror movements and hand function and performance, although the children with clear sensory problems performed poorly on hand function assessments. Children with mild PWML performed better than children with severe (>50%) white matter loss or children with gray matter lesions. In the majority of these severely affected children, there was also involvement of the basal ganglia or the thalamus. Children with contralateral motor projections to their hemiplegic hand showed better hand function than children with ipsilateral projections. Also children with mixed projections performed better than children with ipsilateral projections.

Strong mirror movements were only present in children with ipsilateral projections. In the group with white matter lesions, all children with contralateral motor-projection patterns had mild or moderate white-matter loss, whereas all children with ipsilateral projections had severe white-matter loss. All children with basal ganglia abnormalities, irrespective of whether the primary lesion was in the periventricular white matter or in the cortical gray matter, were in the group with ipsilateral motor projections to the hemiplegic hand. Although the most impaired hand function was seen in the ipsilateral motor projection group, some children in this group had fairly good ability [12]. With diffusion tensor imaging (DTI) of corticofugal fibers clear correlations between hand function and performance in uCP and the size of the contralateral corticospinal tract in the cerebral peduncle and the anterior part of the posterior limb of the capsula interna were found [13, 14].

Better hand function, measured with the Melbourne Assessment of Upper Limb Function (MUUL) [15], was found in children with PWML than in those with gray matter lesions [16]. This was also a conclusion of Holmefur et al., who measured hand function development from 1.5 to 8 years of age with the Assisting Hand Assessment (AHA) [17, 18]. Their most important finding was that the absence of a concurrent lesion to the basal ganglia and thalamus had the highest predictive power of better development of hand function, independent of the basic type of lesion. The extent of white-matter damage also predicted hand function development. Rose et al. found a significant negative correlation from a reduction of volume of the precentral gyrus of children with congenital hemiplegia due to periventricular damage and preserved corticospinal tract projections from the damaged hemisphere with bimanual performance, measured with the AHA [19]. They also concluded that the sensorimotor thalamic pathways correlated more significantly with paretic hand functions than did the corticospinal tracts.

Developmental Disregard and Treatment Options of Unilateral Impairments in Hand Function

An often-occurring problem in children with uCP is developmental disregard. Learned-non-use was for the first time described by Taub in stroke patients, based on his experimental research with deafferentation of one limb by dorsal rhizotomy in monkeys [20]. He introduced Constraint-Induced Movement Therapy (CIMT) in stroke patients to improve training and use of the affected arm by restraining the non-affected arm. Charles et al. also used the term learned-non-use in their publication about the effect of CIMT in children with uCP [21]. Unlike adults with hemiplegia, who have had functional use of the upper extremities before the time of the insult; children with uCP have not used the involved upper limb typically from birth. DeLuca et al. introduced the term developmental disregard in their case study of the effect of CIMT in a young developing child [22]. Rather than learned-non-use, a child may not develop neural pathways involved in movement because of the lack of ability to experience age-appropriate sensorimotor stimuli that lead to the development of upper extremity skills.

CIMT has proven to be an effective treatment option in children with uCP to improve bimanual performance [23, 24]. Also bimanual intensive movement therapy, BIMT, or HABIT, as Charles and Gordon called it, has proven to have a positive effect on bimanual performance, measured with the AHA [25]. Comparing CIMT and BIMT, both treatment options lead to improvement in unilateral capacity and bimanual performance with no clear difference between these treatment options, yet CIMT seems to have more effect on unilateral capacity and BIMT on bimanual performance [26, 27, 28]. In their review of intensive upper limb therapy Andersen et al. concluded that although CIMT and BIMT have similar improvements in unilateral capacity and bimanual performance outcomes, considering participant and caregiver goal achievement, evidence favors a bimanual approach [29]. They discussed type and duration of restraint of the unaffected limb in CIMT, and age of treatment. BIMT is an option in children with severe hand function impairments, or children who have clear bimanual goals in which the assistance of the affected hand is needed. In both treatment options, intensity of treatment influences outcome. After botulinum toxin A (BoNT-A) injections CIMT offered no added value compared to less intensive bimanual occupational therapy (OT) in improving bimanual performance [30].

According to the Cochrane review BoNT-A injections in the upper limb in uCP clearly reduce spasticity and improve range of motion [31]. Comparing BoNT-A and OT aimed at improving bimanual skills with OT alone, the effect on unilateral capacity is questionable. Review of the pooled data showed small positive effects at the MUUL and the Quality of Upper Extremities Skills Test (QUEST) [32] at three months after BoNT-A, which disappeared at 6 months. No bimanual performance outcome measures were used. There were clear positive effects at Goal Attainment Scaling (GAS) and limited positive effects at the Canadian Occupational Performance Measure (COPM). Olesch et al. studied very young children (mean age 3 years 8 months) with uCP. They found no significant differences between BoNT-A + OT and OT alone at the QUEST, but also positive effects at GAS of BoNT-A + OT [33].

Effects of Several Treatment Modalities on Brain Structure and Imaging

Comparing the therapeutic response of BoNT-A injections with physiotherapy with physiotherapy alone using DTI and clinical scores in diplegic CP children a significant change in motor and sensory fiber bundle sizes and improvement in clinical scores were found due to physiotherapy, but no additional effect of BoNT-A was found [34]. In a study investigating whether the type of cortical reorganization (identified by TMS) influenced the efficacy of CIMT in adolescents with uCP, both patients controlling their affected hand via ipsilateral corticospinal projections from the contralesional hemisphere and patients with preserved crossed corticospinal projections from the affected hemisphere to the affected hand significantly improved in quality of upper extremity movements. This was accompanied by a significant gain of speed in patients with preserved crossed projections, whereas patients with ipsilateral projections tended to show speed reduction [35]. The patients with preserved contralateral projections had a unilateral corticosubcortical infarction in the MCA territory and those with ipsilateral projections from the contralesional hemisphere had PWML. In a later publication of this research group about the same study population, two types of exercise-induced neuroplasticity were revealed [36]. Individuals with ipsilateral corticospinal projections had a decrease in transsynaptic premotor cortex excitability (measured by TMS) and a decrease in synaptic activity of the primary motor cortex during active movements of the paretic hand (measured by functional MRI) after CIMT, whereas patients with contralateral projections after CIMT showed an increase in primary motor cortex excitability and also in activation in the sensorimotor cortex. Both individuals with ipsilateral and those with contralateral projections showed evidence for significant increase in synaptic activity of the sensory cortex during stimulation of the paretic hand (measured with magneto encephalography) after CIMT. Also after CIMT, Islam et al. found improvement in movement speed of the affected hand and in bimanual performance, measured with the AHA, but not in MUUL scores, irrespective of corticomotor projection patterns [37]. In their study with kittens, in which the primary motor cortex activity was blocked unilaterally during a critical postnatal period, Friel et al. found that early training of the affected limb in combination with restraint of the unaffected limb restored the corticospinal tract (CST) connections, improved primary motor cortex (M1) activity and increased spinal interneuron number on the contralateral, relative to the ipsilateral side, and abrogated limb control impairments [38]. Delayed training in adolescence restored CTS connections and M1 activity, but not contralateral spinal interneuron numbers or motor performance. Restraint alone only restored CST connectivity.

Conclusion

UCP has a prevalence of 0.6 per 1,000 live births and amounts to about 30% of the CP subtype proportion. In children born with a birth weight of 2,500 g or above there is an increase in prevalence.

MRI findings most often observed in uCP are PWML, gray matter lesions, mainly infarcts of the MCA, and brain maldevelopments.

PAIS is the most frequent form of cerebral infarction in children. Risk factors for PAIS are mentioned. 60% of the infants with PAIS have early symptoms, mostly tonic/clonic seizures; in 40% there is a delayed clinical presentation at the age of 5 months with motor problems as early handedness.

There is a correlation of the total lesion volume and degree of Wallerian degeneration of the pyramidal tract at the anterior portion of the posterior limb of the internal capsule at the MRI scan, with motor impairment of the hand. There are two types of central motor reorganization in uCP. Children with contralateral motor projections to their hemiplegic hand have better hand function than children with ipsilateral projections. Strong mirror movements are only present in children with ipsilateral projections. All children with basal ganglia abnormalities, irrespective of whether the primary lesion is in the periventricular white matter or in the cortical gray matter, are in the group with ipsilateral motor projections to the hemiplegic hand. Better hand function was found in children with PWML than in those with gray matter lesions. The absence of a concurrent lesion to the basal ganglia and thalamus has the highest predictive power of better development of hand function, independent of the basic type of lesion. The sensorimotor thalamic pathways correlate more significantly with paretic hand functions than the corticospinal tracts.

An often-occurring problem in children with uCP is developmental disregard. Comparing CIMT and BIMT, both treatment options lead to improvement in unilateral capacity and bimanual performance with no clear difference between these treatment options, yet CIMT seems to have more effect on unilateral capacity and BIMT on bimanual performance. Comparing BoNT-A and OT aimed at improving bimanual skills with OT alone, the effect of BoNT-A on unilateral capacity is questionable.

Individuals with ipsilateral corticospinal projections had a decrease in transsynaptic premotor cortex excitability and a decrease in synaptic activity of the primary motor cortex during active movements of the paretic hand after CIMT, whereas patients with contralateral projections after CIMT showed an increase in primary motor cortex excitability and also in activation in the sensorimotor cortex. Both individuals with ipsilateral and those with contralateral projections showed evidence for a significant increase in synaptic activity of the sensory cortex during stimulation of the paretic hand after CIMT. In an animal study early training of the affected limb in combination with restraint of the non-affected limb is more effective in restoring central nervous system structure, than training in adolescence or restraint alone.

Therefore, knowing the type of cortical reorganization pattern can be useful in the choice of the treatment modality, although improvement of bimanual performance after CIMT was obtained irrespective of the corticomotor projection pattern. Neural plasticity mechanisms in the developing brain are enhanced, which have positive and negative implications. Exercise leads to improvement of trained skills by reorganization of neuronal networks with more effect if training takes place at younger age, in which there is a post-natal burst in synaptogenesis followed by activity-dependent pruning of excessive synapses later in the post-natal period. Due to the vulnerability associated with plasticity of the developing brain, environmental enrichment has a positive effect on learning and memory ability, but sensory deprivation has negative effects, because developing neurons are dependent on a stable level of neuronal depolarization and are vulnerable to loss of stimulation by excitatory neurotransmitters [39]. Increasing skilled activity of the affected limb in bimanual performance from an early age on seems to be important to improve optimal regeneration of the CST and promote possible contralesional hemisphere cortical projections. Restricting movement of the less affected upper limb for long periods of time without training of the affected limb may disrupt the normal development of the CST and its cortical projection patterns. Therefore, restriction of the less affected upper limb should be done moderately at early age. Training of the affected limb from early age on, as an assisting hand in bimanual play and meaningful skills to achieve bimanual goals, seems to be supported by this evidence.

References

[1] Rosenbaum P, Paneth N, Leviton A, Goldstein M, Bax M, Damiano D, Jacobsson B: A report: the definition and classification of cerebral palsy April 2006. *Dev. Med. Child Neurol.*, 2007;49(109): 8–14.

[2] Oskoui M, Coutinho F, Dykeman J, Jette N. An update on the prevalence of cerebral palsy: a systematicreview and meta-analysis. *Developmental Medicine & Child Neurology,* 2013; 55: 509–519.

[3] Krägeloh-Mann I, Cans C. Review Article. Cerebral palsy update. *Brain & Development,* 2009, 31: 537–544.

[4] Towsley K, Shevell MI, Dagenais L on behalf of the REPAQ consortium. Population-based study of neuroimaging findings in children with cerebral palsy. *European Journal of Paediatric Neurology,* 2011; 15: 29-35.

[5] Selier E, Surman G, Himmelmann K, et al. Trends in prevalence of cerebral palsy in children born with a birthweight of 2,500 g or over in Europe from 1980 to 1998. *Eur. J. Epidemiol,* 2010; 25:635-642.

[6] Rutherford MA, Ramenghi LA, Cowan FM. Neonatal Stroke. Review. *Arch Dis Child Fetal. Neonatal. Ed.,* 2012; 97: F377-F384.

[7] Chabrier S, Husson B, Dinomais M et al. New insights (and new interrogations) in perinatal arterial ischemic stroke. Mini review. *Thrombosis research* 2011; 127: 13-22.

[8] Golomb MR, Garg BP, Saha C, Azzouz F, Williams LS. Cerebral palsy after perinatal arterial ischemic stroke. *J. Child Neurol.,* 2008; 23: 279–86.

[9] De Vries LS, Van der Grond J, Van Haastert IC, Groenendaal F. Prediction of Outcome in New-born Infants with Arterial Ischemic Stroke Using Diffusion-Weighted Magnetic Resonance Imaging. *Neuropediatric s,* 2005; 36: 12–20.

[10] Staudt M, Niemann G, Grodd W, Krägeloh-Mann I. The Pyramidal Tract in Congenital Hemiparesis: Relationship between Morphology and Function in Periventricular Lesions. *Neuropediatrics,* 2000; 31: 257-264.

[11] Carr LJ, Harrisson LM, Evans AL, Stephens JA. Patterns of central motor organization in hemiplegic cerebral palsy. *Brain,*1993; Oct. 116: (Pt 5) 1223-47.

[12] Holmström L, Vollmer B, Tedroff K, Islam M et al. Hand function in relation to brain lesions and corticomotor-projection pattern in children with unilateral cerebral palsy. *Developmental Medicine & Child Neurology,* 2010, 52: 145–152.

[13] Bleyenheuft Y, Grandin CB, Cosnard G, Olivier E, Thonnard JL. Corticospinal Dysgenesis and Upper-Limb Deficits in Congenital Hemiplegia: A Diffusion Tensor Imaging Study. *Pediatrics,* 2007;120;e1502-e1511.

[14] Holmström L, Lennartsson F, Eliasson AC, Flodmark O et al. Diffusion MRI in corticofugal fibers correlates with hand function in unilateral cerebral palsy. *Neurology,* 2011; 77 August 23: 775-783.

[15] Randall M, Carlin JB, Chondros P, Reddihough D. Reliability of the Melbourne assessment of unilateral upper limb function. Dev Med Child Neurol 2001; 43: 761–67.

[16] Feys H, Eyssen M, Jaspers E, et al. Relation between neuroradiological findings and upper limb function in hemiplegic cerebral palsy. *Eur. J.Paediatr. Neurol.,* 2010; 14: 167-177.

[17] Holmefur M, Kits A, Bergström, Krumlinde-Sundholm L et al. Neuroradiology Can Predict the Development of Hand Function in Children With Unilateral Cerebral Palsy. *Neurorehabilitation and Neural. Repair,* 2013; 27(1): 72-78.

[18] Krumlinde-Sundholm L, Eliasson A. Development of the Assisting Hand Assessment: A Rasch-built measure intended for children with unilateral upper limb impairments. *Scand. J.OccupTher.,* 2003; 10:16–26.

[19] Rose S, Guzetta A, Pannek K, Boyd R. MRI Structural Connectivity, Disruption of Primary Sensorimotor Pathways, and Hand Function in Cerebral Palsy. *Brain Connectivity,* 2011; 1(4): 309-316.

[20] Taub E, Uswatte G, Pidikiti R. Constraint-induced movement therapy: A new family of techniques with broad Application to Physical Rehabilitation-A Clinical Review. *J.Rehabil. Res. Dev.,* 1999 Jul;36(3):237-51. Review.

[21] Charles J, Lavinder G, Gordon AM. Effects of Constraint-Induced Therapy on Hand Function in Children with Hemiplegic Cerebral Palsy. *PediatrPhysTher.*, 2001 Summer; 13(2): 68-76.

[22] DeLuca S, Echols K, Landesman Ramey S, Taub E. Pediatric Constraint-Induced Movement Therapy for a Young Child With Cerebral Palsy: Two Episodes of Care. *PhysTher.,*2003; 83:1003-1013.

[23] Hoare BJ, Wasiak J, Imms C, Carey L. Constraint-induced movement therapy in the treatment of the upper limb in children with hemiplegic cerebral palsy. *Cochrane Database of Systematic Reviews,* 2007, Issue 2. Art. No.: CD004149.

[24] Aarts PB, Jongerius PH, Geerdink YA, van Limbeek J, Geurts AC. Effectiveness of Modified Constraint-Induced Movement Therapy in Children With Unilateral Spastic Cerebral Palsy: A Randomized Controlled Trial. *Neurorehabil Neural. Repair.,* 2010; 24: 509-18.

[25] Gordon AM, Schneider JA, Chinnan A, et al: Efficacy of a hand-arm bimanual intensive therapy (HABIT) in children with hemiplegic cerebral palsy: a randomized control trial. *Dev. Med. Child Neurol.*, 2007; 49:830-838.

[26] Gordon AM, Hung YC, Brandao M, Ferre CL, Kuo HC, Friel K, Petra E. Bimanual Training and Constraint-Induced Movement Therapy in Children With Hemiplegic Cerebral Palsy: A Randomized Trial. *Neurorehabil. Neural. Repair.,* 2011; 25: 692-702.

[27] Sakzewski L, Ziviani J, Abbott JF, Macdonell RA, Jackson GD, Boyd RN. Randomized trial of constraint-induced movement therapy and bimanual training on activity outcomes for children with congenital hemiplegia. *Developmental Medicine & Child Neurology,* 2011; 53: 313–320.

[28] Deppe W, Thuemmler K, Fleischer J, Berger C, Meyer S, Wiedemann B. Modified constraint-induced movement therapy versus intensive bimanual training for children with hemiplegia – a randomized controlled trial. *Clinical. Rehabilitation,* 2013; 27(10), 909-920.

[29] Andersen JC, Majnemer A, O'Grady K, Gordon AM. Intensive Upper Extremity Training for Children with Hemiplegia: From Science to Practice. *SeminPediatrNeurol,* 2013; 20: 100-105.

[30] Hoare B, Imms C, Villanueva E, Rawicki HB, Mattyas T, Carey L. Intensive therapy following upper limb botulinum toxin A injection in young children with unilateral cerebral palsy: a randomized trial. *Developmental Medicine & Child Neurology,* 2013; 55: 238–247.

[31] Hoare BJ, Wallen MA, Imms C, Villanueva E, Rawicki HB, Carey L. Botulinum toxin A as an adjunct to treatment in the management of the upper limb in children with spastic cerebral palsy (UPDATE). *Cochrane Database Syst. Rev.,* 2010 Jan 20;(1): CD003469. Review.

[32] 32.DeMatteo C, Law M, Russell D, Pollock N, Rosenbaum P, Walter S. The Reliability and Validity of the Quality of Upper Extremity Skills Test. *Phys&OccTher in Pediatrics,* 1993; 13(2): 1-18.

[33] Olesch CA, Greaves S, Imms C, Reid SM, Graham HK. Repeat botulinum toxin-A injections in the upper limb of children with hemiplegia: a randomized controlled trial. *Developmental Medicine &Child Neurology,* 2010, 52: 79-86.

[34] Chaturvedi SK, Rai Y, Chourasia A, Goel P, et al. Comparative assessment of therapeutic response to physiotherapy with or without botulinum toxin injection using diffusion tensor tractography and clinical scores in term diplegic cerebral palsy children. *Brain & Development,* 2013, 35: 647-653.

[35] Kuhnke N, Juenger H, Walther M, Mall V, Staudt M. Do patients with congenital hemiparesis and ipsilateral corticospinal projections respond differently to constraint-induced movement therapy? *Developmental Medicine & Child Neurology,* 2008, 50: 898-903.

[36] Juenger H, Kuhnke N, Braun C, UmmenhoferF, et al. Two types of exercise-induced neuroplasticity in congenital hemiparesis: a transcranial magnetic stimulation, functional MRI, and magnetoencephalographic study. *Developmental Medicine & Child Neurology,* 2013, 55: 941-952.

[37] Islam M, Nordstrand L, Holmström L, Kits A, Forssberg H, Eliasson AC. Is outcome of constraint-induced movement therapy in unilateral cerebral palsy dependent on corticomotor projection pattern and brain lesion characteristics? *Developmental Medicine & Child Neurology,* 2014, 56: 252–258.

[38] Friel K, Chakrabarty S Kuo HC, Martin J. Using Motor Behavior during an Early Critical Period to Restore Skilled Limb Movement after Damage to the Corticospinal System during Development. *The Journal of Neuroscience,* 2012, 32 (27): 9265-9276.

[39] Johnston MV. Plasticity in the Developing Brain: Implications for Rehabilitation. *Dev.Disabil. Res. Rev.,* 2009, 15: 94-101.

In: Handbook on Cerebral Palsy
Editor: Harold Yates

ISBN: 978-1-63321-852-9
© 2014 Nova Science Publishers, Inc.

Chapter 4

The Problem Patella of Crouch Gait in Adolescents with Cerebral Palsy

Prof. Tim O'Brien, Damien Kiernan and Rory O'Sullivan
The Gait Laboratory, Central Remedial Clinic, Clontarf, Dublin, Ireland

Abstract

The purpose of this review is to demonstrate the etiology and effects of patellar fractures in adolescents with crouch gait. We describe the correlation between these fractures and Gait Laboratory kinematic and kinetic data. These fractures are not incidental findings as they are always associated with a significant deterioration in gait. The kinematic and kinetic data that accompanies displaced fractures are typical of knee extensor disruption.

The more common oblique fracture through the distal pole of the patella is caused by an increased bending force on the patella while the increased traction of crouch can also result in a sleeve fracture. We outline the surgical options for treatment of knee extensor disruption.

Introduction

The patella is the largest sesamoid bone in the human body. Developing in the quadriceps muscle tendon it has a quadrilateral appearance and articulates with the femoral condyles. The distal part gives attachment to the patellar tendon. Thus the patella transmits great forces from the strongest muscle, the quadriceps, to the patellar tendon.

Its function is to assist the quadriceps in knee extension by providing a fulcrum for the quadriceps. People who have the patella surgically removed have subjective and objective quadriceps weakness due to the loss of this fulcrum [1, 2]. However, this same fulcrum causes problems for those who walk with crouch knees.

The Etiology and Diagnosis of Patellar Fractures in Crouch Gait

The problem of fracture of the patella in Cerebral Palsy and the deterioration in gait that accompanies them has been known since 1985 [3]. At that time objectively describing this associated gait deterioration was not possible.

As a result confusion remains regarding the significance and treatment of these fractures which some have even described as "fragmentation" rather than fracture [4, 5]. A Gait Laboratory captures and displays kinematic, kinetic and other temporal data that accurately defines gait. Some have dismissed patellar fractures as of no consequence in Cerebral Palsy (CP) patients but we strongly dispute this. In our experience patellar fracture with knee extensor disruption is the commonest cause of acute gait deterioration in adolescents with CP. It is more likely that these fractures are dismissed as insignificant when there is no associated objective gait data [4, 5].

Over the last 25 years we in the National Gait Laboratory have collected data on clients with CP and other conditions that affect gait and documented changes in gait as these children develop. The Gait Laboratory accurately defines crouch gait where the knees are flexed during stance. Because of the fulcrum effect of the patella crouch gait results in increased bending and traction forces through the patella. As a result the fulcrum effect of the patella becomes a disadvantage in crouch gait.

In crouch gait the Gait Laboratory data demonstrates how the Ground Reaction Force is displaced behind the knee instead of through the knee in normal walking at mid stance (Figure 1).

As a result of this the quadriceps muscle needs to contract to prevent the knee from buckling at a time in the gait cycle when it is normally silent. The increased power generated by the quadriceps is identified in the kinetic graph from the force plate and knee kinematic data. It is this burst of abnormal power generation that alerts us to the potential for damage to the patella in children with crouch.

In normal gait the knee flexes to 10-15 degrees in early stance so that weight transfer to the supporting lower limb is smooth(Figure 2). The knee then extends with a short concentric contraction of the quadriceps until such quadriceps power is no longer needed in the second half of stance. However, in those who walk in crouch, i.e., with flexed knees, the quadriceps needs to continue contracting to prevent the knee from buckling. We identify this enormous strain on the quadriceps in the Gait Laboratory as an internal extension force (Figure 2). In turn this force becomes a bending force as well as a traction force on the patella.

When the bending force on the patella exceeds the strength of the patellar bone it fractures. The fracture is usually located in the distal third of the patella which is not supported by the articulation with the femoral condyles (Figure 3 A & B). Indeed this last point of patellar contact with the femoral condyles acts as a fulcrum making it a pivotal point for bending forces. The fracture propagates from the anterior cortex of the patella and travels distally and obliquely across the patella (Figure 3C).

The fracture should not be confused with an ossification centre which forms a bipartite patella as this is always located proximally. When the fracture is complete the knee extensor mechanism stops functioning effectively. This is associated clinically with the development of a knee flexion contracture, patella alta, increased knee crouch and a typical knee kinematic and kinetic profile [6] (Figure 4).

The proximal patella retains its attachment to the quadriceps and displaces proximally resulting in patella alta. The non-specific gait features include reduced gait speed and reduced stance time of the involved lower limb.

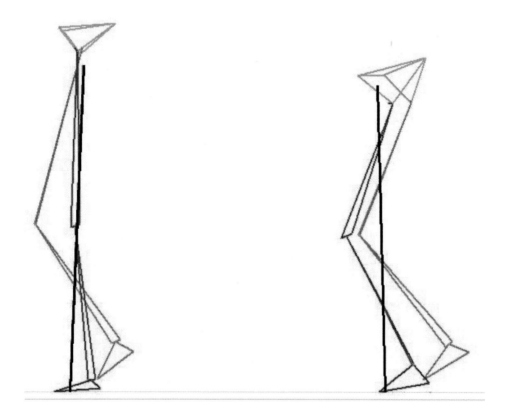

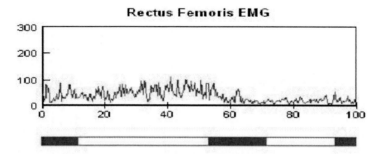

Figure 1. Stick figures of normal midstance of the the right lower limb (Red) and of crouch. The GFR is the black line going through the right knee in the normal stance and behind the right knee in crouch stance. The EMG shows continuous rectus femoris (quadriceps) activity during crouch stance compared to the normal activity designated by the red blocks. Rectus EMG activity of one gait cycle is shown. The first 60 percent is stance followed by 40 percent swing.

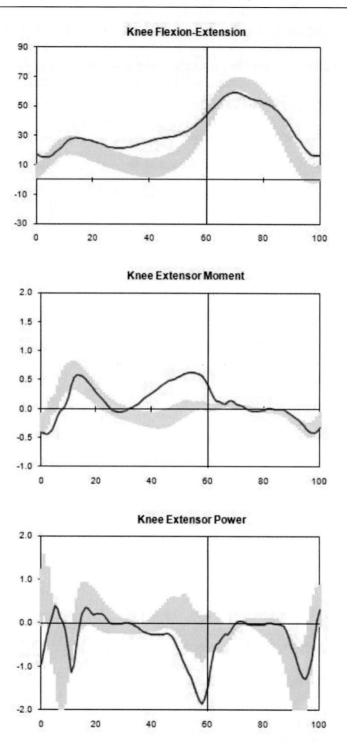

Figure 2. Each panel represents a single gait cycle. The vertical line at 60 percent divides stance (0 to 60) from swing (60 to 100). Top. Sagittal kinematic graph of knee crouch. Normal values are in shaded areas. The knee remains abnormally flexed in mid to late stance. Middle: Demonstrating the increased moment in late stance and Bottom: Kinetic graph showing the a burst of power in late stance. Normal values are in shaded areas.

The Problem Patella of Crouch Gait in Adolescents with Cerebral Palsy 57

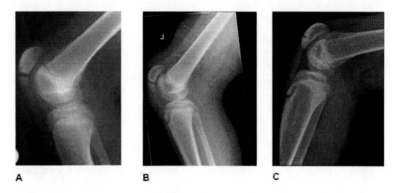

Figure 3. A & B. Radiographs of two teenage boys who developed similar patellar fractures causing Knee Extensor Disruption (KED). C. Radiograph demonstrating propagation of fracture from the anterior cortex of the patella.

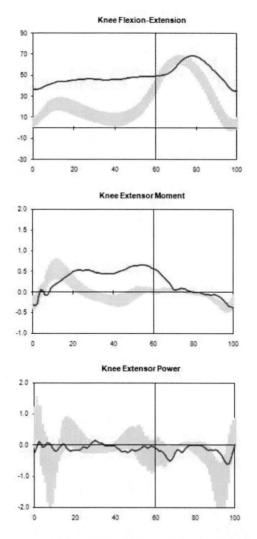

Figure 4. Top. Kinematic profile typical of KED with loss of shock absorption in early stance and increased crouch. Compare with Figure 2. Bottom. Power graph demonstrating loss of quadriceps function.

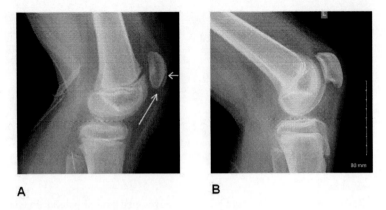

Figure 5. A. Typical radiographic appearance of an acute sleeve fracture. B. Radiographic appearance of a healed sleeve fracture with double anterior cortex and distal spur.

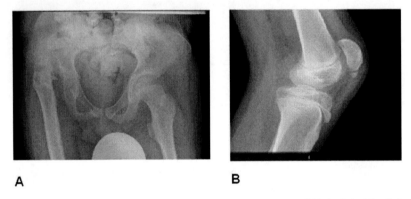

Figure 6. A Pelvic radiograph of a 14 year old boy showing an untreated high right hip dislocation. B Radiograph of his left knee demonstrating distal patellar fracture and some periosteal reaction.

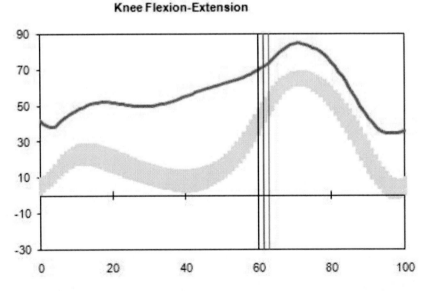

Figure 7. Sagittal left knee kinematics of same boy as in Figure 6 showing knee crouch throughout stance.

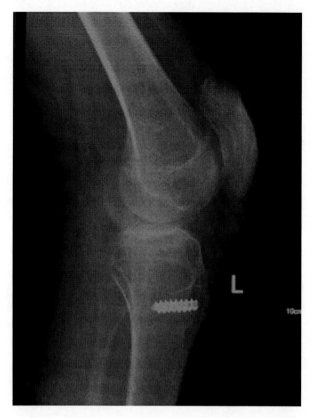

Figure 8. Lateral radiograph of a late presentation of a patellar fracture. The fracture healed with deformity and elongation of the patella. It was decided to transfer the tibial tubercle distally to improve quadriceps function.

The increased traction force generated by crouch can result in pulling the patellar tendon from its attachment to the tibial tubercle [7], or stripping the periosteum from the patella and displacing the patella superiorly. This latter situation is referred to as a sleeve fracture and is much less common in crouch gait than the bending fracture described above (Figure 5 A & B). This fracture heals by forming a typical double anterior patellar cortex and a distal spur from the patella if not displaced too much (Figure 5 B). When displaced significantly it also results in patella alta.

Crouch gait is the common factor in these two types of patellar fractures. Most commonly we see these fractures in C P where independent walking and involvement in sport is encouraged even in the presence of crouch knees [8].

While spasticity may play a role in promoting the development of these fractures due to co-contraction of opposing muscles (the quadriceps and the hamstrings) we believe that knee crouch plays the major role. This is demonstrated by a case report of a boy who walked in left knee crouch to compensate for a 4 centimeter leg length discrepancy due to an untreated high right hip dislocation. The crouch knee fractured the patella in an otherwise normal leg (Fig 6 A & B). The left knee kinematic data demonstrates severe crouch with the features of knee extensor disruption (Figure 7).

These fractures are not always accompanied by a complaint of knee pain. In our retrospective report of knee extensor disruption in CP we found that only half of the patients had complained of knee pain. Even when they complained of knee pain they were more likely to have had pelvic XRays rather than knee XRays because of the strong association between CP and hip dysplasia.

This tendency to XRay the hip initially might also be due to the fact that knee pain is often the presenting symptom of hip disease owing to the phenomenon of referred pain. The fracture of the patella is always accompanied by a noticeable deterioration in gait. This explains why we diagnose this problem so regularly in the Gait Laboratory to which the patients are referred to assess the gait deterioration and where the condition has a diagnostic kinematic and kinetic profile.

Indeed, it is the practice in our Gait Laboratory to advise all our clients with crouch gait to seek an urgent review with us if a sudden deterioration of gait is noticed by carers or if the client complains of knee pain.

Treatment

Fractures of the patella as a result of crouch gait require the same urgent treatment as those fractures that are the result of a traumatic event. Unfortunately, when these fractures are not accompanied by pain and the deterioration in gait goes unnoticed, there is a tendency, in our opinion, to treat these fractures sub- optimally.

Allied to this is the suggestion by some that these fractures are of no clinical significance as mentioned above. The following is our recommended approach to treatment of the various presentations.

1. When the patient presents acutely and is known to have CP the fracture should be surgically reduced and fixed with tension band wiring. We recommend that the ipsilateral hamstrings are injected with botulinum toxin under the same anesthetic. Apply a soft knee extension brace to allow an early post operative rehabilitation exercise program begin.
2. When the diagnosis is delayed and there is a non-union of the fracture there is likely to be a fixed flexion contracture of the knee which complicates the treatment approach. While the fracture is approached surgically by excision of the non-union, freshening the bone surfaces and internally fixing the reduced fracture with tension band wiring, we recommend that a distal femoral extension osteotomy be considered and performed simultaneously to correct significant knee fixed flexion deformities that are greater than 20 degrees and considered unlikely to respond to conservative treatment. For flexion deformities that are less than 20 degrees and likely to respond to physiotherapy botulinum toxin should be administered to the hamstrings.
3. Finally, a complex situation may exist in a very late presentation where the patellar fracture has united though elongated (Figure 8). There is a choice of approach to be considered in this circumstance, either to reconstruct the patella or to transfer the tibial tubercle distally. Any co-existing fixed flexion deformity will need to be approached as in 2 above.

Conclusion

Fractures of the distal pole of the patella are common in adolescents with crouch gait. Cerebral Palsy is the most common cause of crouch gait but these fractures occur in other conditions that result in knee crouch and they do not need to have associated spasticity. Fracture of the patella is the commonest cause of acute gait deterioration in CP adolescents. The deterioration in gait that accompanies the displaced fractures shows quadriceps insufficiency which is termed Knee Extensor Disruption. In the absence of a complaint of knee pain a high index of suspicion is required to diagnose this condition. The Gait Laboratory plays a major role in the assessment and monitoring of CP adolescents with crouch gait.

References

[1] Sutton FS Jr, Thompson CH, Lipke J, Kettelkamp DB. The effect of patellectomy on knee function. *J. Bone Joint Surg. Am.* 1976 Jun;58(4):537-40.

[2] S. Einola, A. J. Aho, and P. Kallio. Patellectomy After Fracture: Long-Term Follow-Up Results With Special Reference to Functional Disability 1976, Vol. 47, No. 4, Pages 441-447

[3] Lloyd-Roberts GC, Jackson AM, Albert JS. Avulsion of the distal pole of the patella in cerebral palsy. A cause of deteriorating gait. *J. Bone Joint Surg. Br.* 1985;:252–4.

[4] Rosenthal RK, Levine DB. Fragmentation of the distal pole of the patella in spastic cerebral palsy. *J. Bone Joint Surg. Am.* 1977 Oct;59(7):934-9.

[5] Topoleski TA, Kurtz CA, Grogan DP. Radiographic abnormalities and clinical symptoms associated with patella alta in ambulatory children with cerebral palsy. *J. Pediatr. Orthop.* 2000 Sep-Oct;20(5):636-9.

[6] O'Sullivan R, Walsh M, Kiernan D, et al. The knee kinematic pattern associated with disruption of the knee extensor mechanism in ambulant patients with diplegic cerebral palsy. *Clin. Anat.* 2010;:586–92.

[7] Yahya Elhassan, Damien Kiernan, Tim Lynch, Tim O Brien Bilateral knee extensor disruption in severe crouch gait. *BMJ Case Rep.* 2013 Jun27; DOI:10.1136/bcr-2013-010337.

[8] Elhassan Y, O'Sullivan R, Walsh M, O Brien T. Knee extensor disruption in mild diplegic cerebral palsy: a risk for adolescent athletes. *BMJ Case Rep.* 2013 Feb 20;2013. pii: bcr2012008120. doi: 10.1136/bcr-2012-008120.

In: Handbook on Cerebral Palsy
Editor: Harold Yates

ISBN: 978-1-63321-852-9
© 2014 Nova Science Publishers, Inc.

Chapter 5

Infant Cerebral Palsy in Hemiplegic Children: Treatment Options and Outcome

Melissa Rosa-Rizzotto, M.D., Ph.D., Cristina Ranzato, Ph.D. and Paola Facchin, M.D., Ph.D.

Epidemiology and Community Medicine Unit, Paediatrics Department
University of Padua, Padova, Italy

Abstract

Cerebral palsy (CP) describes a group of disorders of the development of movement and posture, causing activity limitation, that are attributed to non progressive disturbances that occurred in the developing fetal or infant brain. CP is the leading cause of childhood disability affecting function and development. This disorder affects the development of movement and is believed to arise from nonprogressive disturbances in the developing fetal or infant brain. In addition to the motor disorders that characterize cerebral palsy, which may limit a patient's activities, individuals with cerebral palsy often display epilepsy, secondary musculoskeletal problems, and disturbances of sensation, perception, cognition, communication, and behavior.

CP is characterized by sensorimotor dysfunction as manifested by atypical muscle tone, posture and movement. Severity of impairment varies widely, depending on the site and severity of brain damage.

Hemiplegia is a unilateral physical impairment, is a common type of CP accounting for 36-40% of all CP. Typically, the upper limb is more involved than the lower, with impairments of spasticity, sensation and reduced strength.

One of the most disabling symptoms of hemiplegia is unilaterally impaired hand and arm function, which affects self-care activities such as feeding, dressing, and grooming. The impairment of the hand is often the result of damage to the motor cortex and corticospinal pathways responsible for the fine motor control of the fingers and hand. Thus, skilled independent finger movements do not develop typically in children with hemiplegia. During tasks that require fine manipulation, such children often use several fingers, and often show abnormal hand posturing as well as reduction in distal strength and dexterity.

Sensory disturbances can occur as well, further complicating any motor impairment. Furthermore, children with hemiplegia due to cerebral palsy (CP, the most motorically studied subtype of hemiplegia) have difficulty with the timing and coordination of reaching movements, grasping, movement planning, and a deficient capacity to modulate postural adjustments during reaching.

The resulting sensory and motor impairments in children with hemiplegia compromise movement efficiency. Such children often tend not to use the affected extremity, resulting in a developmentally learned non-use of the involved upper extremity that can be termed 'developmental disuse.

Typically, rehabilitation techniques have focused on teaching and reinforcing compensatory strategies that encourage use of the non-involved upper extremity to decrease functional limitations. Strong evidence for the successful application of any therapeutic approach is lacking. Recent evidence suggests that children with hemiplegic CP can improve motor performance if provided sufficient practice. This finding indicates that intensive practice may improve function in the involved upper extremity that could lead to increased use in daily life.

In the last decades, several treatment approaches have been employed to improve upper limb function in hemiplegic CP.

The chapter provides a review of current efficacy of the most recent treatment approaches, including a focus on Constraint Induced Movement Therapy and bimanual intensive rehabilitation approach.

Cerebral Palsy in Children

Cerebral palsy (CP) describes a group of disorders of the development of movement and posture, causing activity limitation, that are attributed to non progressive disturbances that occurred in the developing foetal or infant brain. [1, 2, 3] It is characterized by sensorimotor dysfunction as manifested by atypical muscle tone, posture and movement. [4] Severity of impairment varies widely, depending on the site and severity of brain damage. [5,6] A recent systematic review [7] held by McIntyre & colleagues identified ten risk factors in term-born infants as statistically significant predictors of CP: placental abnormalities, major and minor birth defects, low birthweight, meconium aspiration, instrumental/emergency caesarean section, birth asphyxia, neonatal seizures, respiratory distress syndrome, hypoglycaemia, and neonatal infections. The literature reviewed in term of prevention and occurrence reduction, identified birth asphyxia (1/6-9 CP births) as the unique risk factor for term-born infants for which a post-event treatment is currently available. In this case, CP can be prevented if the infant receives hypothermia within 6 hours of the causal event.

Hemiplegia is a unilateral physical impairment, [8], is the most common type of CP accounting for 36-40% of all CP. Typically, the upper limb is more involved than the lower, with impairments of spasticity, sensation and reduced strength. [9, 10]

One of the most disabling symptoms of hemiplegia is unilaterally impaired hand and arm function, which affects self-care activities such as feeding, dressing, and grooming. [11] The impairment of the hand is often the result of damage to the motor cortex and corticospinal pathways responsible for the fine motor control of the fingers and hand. [12, 13] Thus, skilled independent finger movements do not develop typically in children with hemiplegia. During tasks that require fine manipulation, such children often use several fingers, and often show abnormal hand posturing as well as reduction in distal strength and dexterity. [9, 12, 14, 15]

Sensory disturbances can occur as well, further complicating any motor impairment. [16, 17] Furthermore, children with hemiplegia due to cerebral palsy (CP, the most motorically studied subtype of hemiplegia) have difficulty with the timing and coordination of reaching movements, grasping, movement planning, and a deficient capacity to modulate postural adjustments during reaching. [18]

The resulting sensory and motor impairments in children with hemiplegia compromise movement efficiency. Such children often tend not to use the affected extremity, resulting in a developmentally learned non-use of the involved upper extremity that can be termed 'developmental disuse'. [9, 18, 19, 20]

Typically, rehabilitation techniques have focused on teaching and reinforcing compensatory strategies that encourage use of the non-involved upper extremity to decrease functional limitations. [9] Strong evidence for the successful application of any therapeutic approach is lacking. [19] Recent evidence suggests that children with hemiplegic CP can improve motor performance if provided sufficient practice. This finding indicates that intensive practice may improve function in the involved upper extremity that could lead to increased use in daily life. [19, 21]

Epidemiology

Cerebral palsy is the most common physical disability of childhood with a prevalence of approximately 2-3.5 per 1000 newborns, [22, 23, 24, 25] in most developed countries. [26]. Prevalence in developing countries seems to be similar, but data sources are not well defined. Methods of identifying CP children and causal factors and the effects of disability need to be better established. [27, 28]

In 1998, fourteen centres in eight European countries started a network called Surveillance of Cerebral Palsy in Europe (SCPE). [29] After reaching consensus about the criteria to classify CP, they presented the prevalence rates in six countries, and more detailed prevalence estimates of 13 areas. [30] In Table 1 a summary of the prevalence estimates of CP of the SCPE, as well as from some other north-western Europe countries, is given. [29] As can be concluded from this table the prevalence and the trends in time of CP are comparable in these countries. [31, 32]

The prevalence of CP rises in time from well below 2.0 per 1000 life births in the 70s to well above 2.0 in the 90s. Boys form a small majority (58%). It seems fair to assume that these European data are not very different from findings in other parts of the world. [22] For example, the prevalence of CP in China is reported to be 1.6 per 1000 children under age 7. [33, 34, 35] In Mississippi (USA) 2.12 per 1000 inhabitants were diagnosed with CP with a higher prevalence for males, and a, non-significant, higher prevalence in black people. [36] The prevalence of CP in Australia is 2.0 to 2.5 per 1000 live births. [37] The prevalence of CP among low-birthweight children is higher than among normal birthweight children. [5, 26]

Table 1. Prevalence of cerebral palsy in Northwest Europe

Country	Birth year	Prevalence per 1000 lifebirths
Northeast England	1964-1968	1.68
	1969-1973	1.39
	1974-1978	1.71
	1979-1983	2.00
	1984-1988	2.27
	1989-1993	2.45
Scotland	1984-1989	2.10
Norway	1977-1981	1.91
	1982-1986	1.98
	1987-1991	2.05
Denmark	1979-1986	2.80
	1987-1990	2.40
Sweden	1979-1982	2.17
	1990-1993	2.20
	1991-1994	2.12
The Netherlands	1977-1979	0.77
	1980-1982	1.00
	1983-1985	1.84
	1986-1988	2.44

Modified form Odding E et al. Disabil Rehabil. 2006.[25]

Clinical Main Characteristics and Classification

Motor impairment is obligatory for the diagnosis CP. In people with hemiplegic CP the prevalence of additional impairments is 42%. Common additional impairments are cognitive impairments, epilepsy, sensory, endocrine and urogenital impairments. [5,38] Table 2 gives a summary of the data about the most common impairments associated with CP, crude prevalence rates are given.

Table 2. Prevalence of impairments among children with cerebral palsy

Impairment	%
Motor	100
Cognitive [IQ<70]	23-44
Sensibility	44-51
Speech	42-81
Visual [moderate = 6/18-6/60D; severe ≤ 6/60D]	62-71
Hearing [moderate = 45-70 dB loss; severe = 70 dB loss]	25
Epilepsy	22-40
Growth	23
Weight	52
Urinary incontinence	23.5

Modified form Odding E et al. Disabil Rehabil. 2006 [25]

As can be seen in Table 2, a large proportion of people with CP have some kind of cognitive impairment. [39] The prevalence varies with the type of CP and especially increases when epilepsy is present. In severely disabled CP children, 97.7% are profoundly mentally impaired. But, since 1976 the prevalence of severe mental retardation has decreased significantly. About 40% of children with hemiplegic CP have normal cognitive abilities, while children and adolescents with tetraplegic CP are generally severely intellectually impaired. [5, 38]

There is no association between IQ level and memory scores and location of brain damage (left or right). Nonverbal learning impairments, characterized by good language abilities and week visual-spatial abilities with fear of new situations and stepwise development, are common. [5, 38, 40]

Behavior problems are five times more likely in children with CP (25.5%) compared with children with no known health problem. [41] The odds ratio for behavior problems of children with CP without mental retardation is 4.9. The attention deficit hyperactivity disorder (ADHD) is more common among children with CP. Other specific behavior problems in children with CP are dependency, being headstrong, and hyperactivity in general. [42]

A large minority of people with CP has epilepsy, and the prevalence varies with the type of motor impairment. It is most common among the hemi- and tetraplegics. [12]

Sensibility and senses may be affected as well. [12] Stereognosis and two-point discrimination of the hands is impaired in 44–51% of all children with CP (astereognosia in 20%). Term children tend to be more severely affected. Sensory impairments are most common among hemiplegic CP people. Nine out of 10 hemiplegic children have significant bilateral sensory deficits. Stereognosis and proprioception are the chief modalities affected bilaterally. The extent of sensory loss does not mirror the severity of the motor deficit. Chronic pain is reported by 28% of the adults with CP, versus 15% of the adults in the general population. [43] Impairment of speech is common and strongly associated with the type and severity of the motor impairment. The most common impairment is dysarthria but aphasia occurs also. [44]

Ophthalmic abnormalities are present in 62% of CP children. [45] Low visual acuity is reported in 71% of children with CP. Because ophthalmological examination cannot explain the low visual acuity of the vast majority, there is a high probability of cerebral visual disturbance. [46]

Impairments in hearing do occur but less often than the other impairments; however, data are very scarce. [47]

Peculiar radiological features may be observed in children affected by cerebral palsy. [14,48] MRI brain abnormalities can be classified into four groups: i.e., group 1: brain malformations; group 2: cortical-subcortical lesions; group 3: abnormalities of the periventricular white matter; and group 4: postnatal brain-injuries. In groups 1 and 2 the severity of hemiplegia is mainly moderate, while it is mild in groups 3 and 4. [49, 50]

Mental retardation occurs in one-third of children in groups 1 and 4, less often in the other two. Seizures occur in half of the children in groups 1 or 2, while the incidence was lower in the other two. In very low-birthweight children (500 – 1499 g) periventricular leukomalacia, and secondly, intraventricular hemorrhage are predictive of cerebral palsy and of functional outcome. [49] Among all CP categories, abnormal cranial ultrasound is most strongly associated with hemiplegia, normal cranial ultrasounds with diplegia. [49] In children with bilateral spastic CP hypoperfusion in the thalamus or cerebellar hemispheres is found. Mildly decreased perfusion is associated with mild delays in gross motor development, while almost all children with severe hypoperfusion show severe developmental delay. [49]

CP Treatment Main Targets

Clinicians dedicate considerable time and resources towards upper limb rehabilitation. [51, 52, 53] In the last years, high-quality dedicated research and CP evidence base have dramatically increased providing professionals, patients and their families with newer, safer and more effective interventions. High levels of evidence existed in the literature summarizing intervention options for children with CP leading to an exponential increase in the number of systematic reviews published [54] revealing the emergence of highly effective prevention interventions. [55, 56]

Motor Disorders

Description. Children affected by CP usually present developmental delay and motor deficits: the distinction between a progressive clinical course and a static one is crucial. The main result of this disorder is the limitation of activity, and may be accompanied by disturbances of sensation, cognition, communication, perception and /or behaviour, and/or by a seizure disorder. Cerebral palsy can be classified according to motor types: spastic, ataxic, dyskinetic or mixed; by site: hemiplegia, diplegia, triplegia or quadriplegia; or by severity of effect on motor function. Motor deficits of children with CP often include: delayed motor milestones; persistent primitive reflexes; spasticity or hypotonia; abnormal walking pattern and movement; and early hand dominance. [5]

Children with *spastic CP* have increased tone in the muscles: spasticity is a velocity dependant increased muscle tone with hyperreflexia resulting from hyperexcitability of the stretch reflex, resulting in unusual postures and/or abnormal movements, and it can lead to muscle stiffness, functional impairment and finally atrophy. [57] Spasticity will be described in the following paragraph. Children with *hemiplegic CP* may show hand dominance before the usual age of 18 months. [58] The gait of children with *diplegic CP* is characterized by flexed posture at the hips and knees. [59] Complications may include joint contractures, hip dislocation and scoliosis. Children with *ataxic CP* are unsteady, wobbly and uncoordinated. [60] Children with *dyskinetic CP* have involuntary, uncontrolled, recurring and occasionally stereotyped movements. [61]

In addition, children with CP are more likely to have other developmental disabilities including hearing and visual problems, mental retardation, speech and language delay, epilepsy, and chronic ill health, such as poor growth and frequent chest infection resulting from oromotor problems, described in the next paragraphs.

About 65% to 90% of children with CP survive to adulthood. In these adults, chronic pain due to musculoskeletal deformities, overuse syndromes, arthritis and degenerative changes (commonly over the hip, knee, ankle, lumbar and cervical spine) are common. [62] Mild physical involvement, presence of vocational training and good family support are the several positive indicators for future employment. [63]

Intervention. Appropriate interventions for CP are dictated by patient's functional ability, severity, pattern of motor disorder, associated pain and discomfort, and age. The general approach and management include parent education, facilitation of normal motor development and function, prevention of complications such as deformities and disabilities and associated medical conditions, as well as to provide necessary environment modifications at home and school with community integration and family adjustment. [64, 65]

Physical and occupational therapy for these children are usually employed and can be based on the principles of neuroplasticity, motor learning, patterning, postural balance, muscle strengthening or stretching. [66]

Physical therapy focuses on gross motor skills (sitting, standing, walking, wheelchair mobility, transfers and community mobility), while occupational therapy address the visual and fine motor skills that enable coordinated functions of ADL and play (eating, self-care, clothing, writing, play). [67]

Forced use and constraint induced movement therapy as well as bimanual intensive training can increase the use of the affected arm in tasks solving in hemiplegic CP. These techniques will be described below.

In CP management a crucial role is played by education and training for the child, family as well as immediate caretakers on the management of cerebral palsy, for optimal care of the child. [68, 69]

Spasticity

Description. Motor interventions aim to change the overactive elements of the upper motor neuron syndrome by reducing the effect of increased muscle tone or improving the fluidity of motor control. Their effects might be temporary, as with oral medication, or permanent as in most surgical interventions. The most relevant options of management are. [70] Physical therapy, Orthoses, Pharmacological therapy (Oral drugs, Botulinum toxin type A, Continuous pump-administered intrathecal baclofen), Surgery. [26] The paucity of randomized controlled trials lead to weak evidence for most of these interventions, also because of the effect of comorbidities. Management of spasticity can be challenging with a wide variety of possible therapeutic interventions. The treatment must be goal oriented, such as to assist with mobility, reduce or prevent contractures, improve positioning and hygiene, and provide comfort. Each member of the child's multidisciplinary team, including the child and both parents, should participate in the serial evaluations and treatment planning.

Intervention. Offering and formulating a tailored physical therapy program means to choose among: task-focused active-use therapy (i.e., constraint-induced movement therapy followed by bimanual therapy to enhance manual skills); muscle-strengthening therapy (i.e., repetitive exercises performed against resistance towards a defined goal); Postural management strategies. Moreover, physical therapy intervention need to be reassessed at regular intervals to ensure that the programme remains appropriate to patient's needs. [71]

Orthoses may improve posture, upper limb function, walking efficiency; may prevent development of contractures, hip migration; may relieve discomfort or pain. They could be considered for: upper limb spasticity (i.e., elbow, rigid wrist, hand function); ankle–foot (CP patients with serious functional limitations to improve foot position for sitting, transfers between sitting and standing, and assisted standing); body trunk (i.e., scoliosis or kyphosis). [72]

CP patients may benefit from treatment with oral drugs: in children with dystonia, which contributes significantly to problems with posture, function and pain, the drug treatment considered are trihexyphenidyl, levodopa or baclofen; oral diazepam or oral baclofen could be considered in the management of discomfort or pain and/or muscle spasms. [73]

Botulinum toxin type A could be used to treat focal spasticity of the upper limb. [74]

Continuous pump-administered intrathecal baclofen is recommended in case of problems related to pain or muscle spasms, posture or function and self-care, in patients typically affected by moderate or severe motor function problems and bilateral spasticity affecting upper and lower limbs. [75]

Selective dorsal rhizotomy represents the most relevant and frequent surgical intervention in order to improve walking ability in ambulant individuals with bilateral involvement: some dorsal spinal nerve rootlets are resected, thereby downregulating the overactive spinal reflex. [76] There is lack of evidence concerning the long-term outcomes after this irreversible treatment. [77]

Children affected by CP, suffer also of the presence of associated impairments and functional limitations that affects child's outcome. When seeking to prognosticate the severity of CP and plan intervention and treatment, it results fundamental to assess associated impairments. Many patients, in fact, will have a number of impairments, and the presence of these impairments complicates therapy, decreases health status and quality of life for the individual and their family, and increases costs for the family and to society. [78] The most relevant impairment are summarized below. [79]

Epilepsy

Description. The prevalence of epilepsy is 5 times more common in patients with CP compared to normal children. [80] Epilepsy can potentially severely limit the quality of life for CP patient and their family. [81] Epilepsy occurs in up to 36% of individuals with CP, [82] showing an onset in the first year of life in 70% of the cases. [83] In 2% of CP patients, their epilepsy will be resolved by the time they turn 5 years of age. For those whose seizures are not resolved, epilepsy is a lifelong condition. Rates of epilepsy are higher in those with: spasticity born at term compared with preterm (48% vs 28%); bilateral compared with unilateral (34–87% vs 23%); and those with intellectual impairment compared with no intellectual impairment (61% vs 19%). [47, 84]

Intervention. No specifically addressed trials on evidence in CP. Since high quality evidence exists in non-CP populations and there are high risks of adverse events from uncontrolled seizure. Several new Anti-Epileptic Drugs (AEDs) are useful to control seizures. Patients with CP and epilepsy tend to require multiple AEDs to control the seizures and tend to have prolonged seizures. [85]

On the other side, any deterioration in motor function may be related to toxic effects of AEDs: sodium channel blockers particularly carbamazepine, lamotrigine, oxcarbazepine, and phenyoin may negatively affect coordination. [86]. For children with CP, multiple factors (low sunlight exposure, low level of weight bearing, and inadequate calcium and vitamin D intake) contribute to the development of vitamin D deficiency state and AEDs can further increase the risk of rickets, interfering with vitamin D metabolism. Calcium, phosphate, and vitamin D levels as well as bone density should be regularly monitored in children on chronic AED therapy. Calcium and vitamin D supplementation may be appropriate in this high risk population.

Intellectual Impairment

Description. 50% of individuals with CP have an intellectual impairment and between 20 and 30% have a severe intellectual impairment. There is a relationship between the severity of CP and mental retardation: children with spastic quadriplegic CP have greater degree of intellectual impairment than those with spastic hemiplegia. [87] Formal assessment of intellect is essential for a child affected by CP. [88]

Intervention. They are referred to occupational therapy, including: animal-assisted therapy service animals to provide companionship and assist with independence, e.g., seizure first aid, door opening, crossing roads; to improve socialization and leisure; reduced stress, anxiety and loneliness. [89, 90]

Communication

Description. Communication disability can have a major impact on the individual with CP and their family. Impairment in this domain can impact on both understanding of language and expression. For individuals who have severe communication impairment, social isolation and poor self-esteem can result. Between 20 and 30% of people with CP are nonverbal which means that systems to support other forms of communication are required. [91, 92, 93] [They are more likely to be non-verbal if they are non-ambulatory (57%) compared to those who are able to walk (4%). [94]

Intervention. CP patients are often referred to speech and language therapy services, to maximize their communication skills and help them to take an independent interaction. [95] This can include introducing augmentative and alternative communication systems, such as symbol charts or speech synthesizers, as well treating children's natural forms of communication. [96, 97] Augmentative and alternative communication (AAC) systems, which can range from low/light technology systems such as signing or use of alphabet charts to high technology systems such as speech generating devices, may be used to communicate. Improved participation in education, communication and play are treated via alternative computer access. [98] On the other side, no firm evidence exists of the effectiveness of speech and language therapy to improve the speech of children with early-acquired dysarthria. [99]

Vision

Description. Vision impairments can range from mild requiring glasses, to functionally blind. About 5–12% of individuals with CP have a severe impairment, or are functionally blind. Another 30% will have a mild to moderate vision impairment. The visual impairment includes retinopathy of prematurity, myopia, strabismus, glaucoma, and amblyopia. [100, 101]

Intervention. The recommended screening includes acuity, eye movement, fundoscopy, and serial ophthalmological assessments routinely. [102]

Hearing

Description. Hearing impairments can range from mild to bilateral deafness (2% of people with CP. Other hearing impairments occur in a further 10% [6]. Assessment of hearing in children with CP should be thorough and done early, as it can impact greatly on their ability to learn and achieve milestones.

Intervention. The recommended screening includes behavioral audiometry, auditory-evoked brainstem responses (it should be performed before or shortly after discharge from the neonatal intensive care unit as well as for every preterm baby), or transient evoked oto-acoustic emission. [103]

It should always be considered in CP patients to be submitted to cochlear implantation. These patients are potential limited/non-users. Closer cooperation between children, children's family, children's school and the cochlear implant team is essential. [104]

Hemiplegic CP treatment options

The therapies for hemiplegic CP are based on a variety of theoretical constructs, with different treatment elements, although some overlap may exist between therapies as well as variation in the content. [105]. For most treatment approaches for upper limb dysfunction in children with hemiplegic CP there is a paucity of evidence. Growing evidence was found for the use of casting combined with occupational therapy, as well as for *botulinum toxin type A* (BTX-A) combined with occupational therapy, [106] although there were only a small number of trials investigating these interventions, and some had very small samples. Many of the effect sizes for individual treatments had wide confidence intervals indicating a variable response to therapy. [105] A large effect size was noted for *botulinum toxin type A* combined with *occupational therapy* at 1 month, and this was partially maintained at 6 months. [106]

The management options are summarized in Table 3 and include different types of physiotherapy and occupational therapy such as Motor Learning approach; conductive education; peripheral splinting and casting; focal and generalized pharmacotherapy (such as botulinum toxin type A injections or intrathecal baclofen); and surgery aimed at improving upper limb function or reducing deformity. [105]

Behavioural and Environmental Treatments

Behavioural therapies [107, 108, 109] such and standard occupational therapy [120, 121] may have small effects that appear to be enhanced by augmentation with additional intervention (e.g., bivalved casts). [106] Newer therapies such as BTX-A have a greater magnitude of effect at 1 month, although the results are not sustained to the same level at 6 months follow-up. Further research is required to evaluate the effects of combinations of treatments over longer time intervals, utilizing a broader range of outcome measures. [106] To date, no large randomized studies of functional outcome have been completed with comparison to placebo therapy or 'no' occupational therapy. One difficulty is that ethical considerations may not permit such studies in young children with CP. Another difficulty is interpreting the content of therapy as well as the intensity delivered across trials. [144, 145]

Table 3. Treatment options for upper limb dysfunction in children with cerebral palsy

Type of treatment approach	Type of rehab options
Behavioural and environmental treatments [107,108,109]	**Bimanual training** **Conductive education [110,111,112]** **Constrain Induced Movement Therapy [113,114,115,116,117]** **Context-focus therapy** **Fitness training** **Functional training** **Motor learning [118,119]** **Occupational therapy [120,121]** Physiotherapy [122,123] **Strength training [124,125,126]**
Peripheral splinting & casting [127]	**Casting for ankle range motion** **Hip surveillance**
Special seating [128,129,130,131,132]	
Electrophysical agents	Neuromuscular Electrical Stimulation [133,134,135] EMG biofeedback [136,137]
Pharmacological [105,138]	Phenol [139] **Botulinum Toxine A [140,106]** **Diazepam** Baclofen oral **Anticonvulsivants** **Bisphosphonates**
Pharmacological – generalized spasticity management [105 138]	Intrathecal Baclofen [141]
Surgery [142]	**Selective dorsal Rhizotomy [52,143]**

(in **bold** mostly efficacious treatments).

Two very detailed studies with a range of validated objective outcome measures evaluating the efficacy of conductive education (CE) programmes [110, 111, 112] against traditional NDT programmes of rehabilitation [120, 121] have been completed which examine many aspects of function, including upper extremity measures. [144]

In two large studies, the effects of standard occupational therapy on the acquisition of fine motor skills and functional outcomes were studied over 1 year. [120,146] Attainment of visual motor skills were influenced by the intensity of sessions with play goals, fine motor skills were influenced by peer interaction, while play goals and functional outcomes were influenced by emphasis on self-care activities. CIMT and other intensive training will be described below.

Pharmacological – Generalized Spasticity Management

The main generalized approaches (pharmacotherapy and surgery) to spasticity management in children with CP are *continuous intrathecal baclofen (ITB)* [147] and selective dorsal rhizotomy (SDR). [105] The predominant effect is in the lower limbs, however, anecdotal reports of higher placement of the ITB catheter tip have suggested improvements in the upper limbs. Several reports have documented a reduction in spasticity with intrathecal baclofen treatment, but none has shown improvements in range of motion in the upper limbs or signs of improved functional skills in comparative trials. [105]

Surgery

Prospective studies without control groups investigating the effects of *selective dorsal rhizotomy* surgery for the upper limbs have yielded equivocal results. [52] Although there have been some subjective reports of improvements in arm function and activities of daily living (ADL) in small numbers of children with CP, larger investigations have demonstrated only small changes in functional performance. In more severely impaired children there has been one subjective report of improved posture in the affected upper limb as well as reduced arm pain. The only study to compare continuous intrathecal baclofen with selective dorsal rhizotomy in matched pairs showed that upper limb spasticity improved with both of these interventions, [148] although this was not translated to improvements in the performance of functional tasks such as reaching, grasping and dressing. [105]

Electrophysical Agents

A relatively new area of treatment for the upper limb in children with CP is *neuromuscular electrical stimulation (NMES)* of antagonist muscles. In two case studies, positive improvements in bimanual hand function were reported. In a larger study, improved functional outcomes were demonstrated with combined use of NMES and dynamic bracing. More recently, improvements in speed of completion of functional tasks such as turning over cards, stacking draughts and placing objects in a container was demonstrated with NMES alone. [105]

Pharmacological - Focal

Wall and colleagues were the first to report use of BTX-A in the upper limbs of five children with CP. Injection to the adductor pollicus was coupled with rigid splinting and led to improvements in hand function (key grip, precision grip), precision pinch, palmar grip and the performance of bimanual tasks. These functional improvements were carried over to effective use of the hemiplegic hand at school, home and play. BTX-A have been shown to be effective in reducing muscle stiffness using resonant frequency. [105,149]

Botulinum toxin A (BTX-A) injections work by blocking the release of acetylcholine at the neuromuscular junction, reducing focal spasticity.

Children with cerebral palsy receiving intramuscular injection, in the lower limbs, of BTX-A have not been shown to have clinically relevant improvement beyond 1 year. [150]

Despite 20 years of clinical use few are the studies investigating long-term BTX-A effects. [151, 152, 153, 154, 155]

Treatment with botulinum toxin A may improve local spasticity control (care, comfort, positioning, hygiene, tolerance of orthotic devices) in the short term. [156]

The positive features of upper motor neuron (UMN) syndrome with BTX-A, may lead to a lack of consideration of those negative features of UMN syndrome. Moreover, it seems to be that contractures are not decreased with BTX-A even though adequate reduction of clinical spasticity. [157] Stiffness of muscles continue despite BTX-A treatment. [158]

It remains uncertain whether repeat cycles of treatment with BTX-A leads to atrophy and irreversible weakness of muscles in already compromised neuromuscular system. [159]

Although considered safe by the US Food and Drug Administration, BTX-A can produce adverse effects in target and non-target muscles.

Recent investigation has shown that repeated injection of BTX-A in experimental rabbit leads to: percentage reduction of contractile material; primarily fat replacement; weakness and loss of muscle strength in the quadriceps of an in the injected muscle groups, and in the uninjected contralateral side. Those investigation suggest that repeat BTX-A injections cause muscle atrophy and loss of contractile tissue in target muscles and also in non-target muscles that are far removed from the injection site. [160]

Recent Advances

Promising developments in cell therapy for infantile cerebral palsy by transplantation of autologous umbilical cord blood are documented in recently published manuscripts, [161,162,163], the early developmental stage of this new therapeutic concept seems to lead to further options of treatment. [164]

Jensen and Hamelmann, [163], describe the case and the follow up of a 2.5 yrs child with a global ischemic brain damage resulting in a persistent vegetative state, treated with autologous cord blood and active rehabilitation. After 40 months of follow up, it appears that autologous transplantation of cord blood cells may in part have contributed to the remarkable functional neuroregeneration observed leading to the idea that cord blood transplantation may be an additional and causative treatment of pediatric cerebral palsy after brain damage. Intravenous autologous cord blood therapy for infantile cerebral palsy is safe from a clinical point of view. However, based on the preliminary uncontrolled clinical data available, it appears only to be effective in certain cases. It is important to notice that in the majority of uncontrolled cases it was not effective. In the future, there is the need to identify as the group of brain disorder responding as the therapeutic window, in which this therapy may be effective.

Not Recommended for Standard Care

The following treatments, according to a recent review, [55] are not recommended for standard care of children with CP: craniosacral therapy, hip bracing, hyperbaric oxygen, NDT, and sensory integration.

Conclusions

Recent training studies in animals and in adults who have had a stroke suggest that 'forced use training' or 'constraint induced movement therapy' may be more effective than conventional upper limb treatment. This group of cognitive neurorehabilitation therapies has evolved to encompass the issues of 'learned nonuse'. The elements of constraint induced (CI) movement therapy are constraint of the unaffected limb to encourage use of the affected limb, massed practice of the affected limb, and use of intensive shaping techniques to train use of the affected limb. The details of this new treatment approach are discussed in the following paragraph. [105, 165]

In conclusion, management of the upper limb in children with CP is both resource-intensive and costly. [105] As well as the healthcare costs, a heavy time commitment is required from both the people with CP and their carers to ensure that therapy goals are achieved and maintained. Despite the investment of time, resources, personnel and funding, there remains a paucity of randomized clinical trials evaluating management options. [105] The interventions currently with the best evidence are occupational therapy and serial casting, although outcomes of these remain similar, with only small treatment effects. There is also growing evidence to support the use of BTX-A for reducing upper limb spasticity and improving function in children with CP. The effects of BTX-A are most evident during the period of maximum chemodenervation, in the first 3–4 weeks after injection. Intramuscular injection of BTX-A alone is not guaranteed to enable a child to use the hemiplegic limb and it is recommended that it be used in conjunction with physiotherapy and occupational therapy training. Upper limb surgery aims to correct deformity, improve cosmesis and improve functional outcomes. These outcomes with upper limb surgery may be of an order of magnitude greater than occupational therapy or BTX-A; however, no randomized or controlled trials have been undertaken. [105]

Effective use of the upper limb impacts on educational outcomes, independence in activities of daily living and vocational options for many children with CP. Development of effective therapy regimes and evaluation of their efficacy with randomized controlled trials therefore require immediate attention. [105, 166]

Constraint Induced Movement Therapy

Children with unilateral cerebral palsy experience difficulties with unimanual and bimanual upper limb function, impacting independence in daily life. Targeted upper limb therapies such as constraint-induced movement therapy, bimanual training, and combined approaches have emerged in the last decade, [167], in particular interest in constraint-induced movement therapy (CIMT) for children with hemiplegic CP has increased dramatically. The number of publications has grown in this period from a few single case studies to over 70 studies, with many RCTs.

Classical CIMT involves application of a full arm cast to the unimpaired upper limb which is worn for a certain amount of time during the day and for a stated number of days/weeks, with no shared consensus on dosing. This intervention is combined with an intensive practice program for the affected upper extremity. According to some Authors, this is the most effective intensive practice to improve the use and quality of fine manipulation of the impaired limb or to reduce the developmental disregard phenomenon.

The Biological Basis

Constraint Induced Movement Therapy (CIMT) is based on earlier primate unilateral deafferentation studies. Monkeys were observed not to use the deafferented limb unless the intact limb was restrained, and they practiced tasks using the involved limb for to 2 weeks. The animals were also observed using the deafferented limb if movement of the limb was encouraged via shaping, a behavioural training technique in which a desired motor behaviour is approached in small steps by successive approximations. As these monkeys regained functional use of the deafferented limb following restraint or shaping techniques, lack of use of the involved limb was considered a result of initial unsuccessful attempts to use it. [168] Taub defined this behaviour as *"learned non-use"* and proposed that restraint of the intact limb or use of shaping techniques would overcome the learned non-use and lead to increased "real-life" function in the involved limb. [169] Further studies with deafferented monkeys were conducted to delineate the learned non-use and forced use paradigms. Constraint of the less affected upper extremity of monkeys deafferented in uterus and at birth also shows increased use of the deafferented extremity, suggesting that learned non-use can be prevented if the constraint is applied early during development. [169]

Influences on Neural Plasticity

Since CIMT has been shown to modify brain activity, especially in the affected motor and premotor cortexes, and interconnections from undamaged hemispheric structures can be engaged, there is a need to explore mechanisms through which CIMT can induce neuroplasticity. [169] Further questions involve the possible presence of neural substrates that impede movement initiation and whether these substrates might be susceptible to modification with CIMT.

The perspective of Taub and co-workers [169] is that specific behavioral retraining will reduce basic impairments as more normal function is restored. Under the learned nonuse paradigm, cortical or subcortical pathology affecting motor output (as well as reduced limb cortical representation) would result in poor function, even if the potential for use existed. Frustration, fatigue, and teaching of compensatory strategies (defined as learning to use the better upper extremity in the interest of time, convenience, and demonstration of ability) inevitably would produce learned nonuse behavior and, consequently, little initiative to use the impaired hand.

The additional factors supplied by Sunderland and Tuke [170] are referred to as "compensatory learning". This form of compensation is different from the compensatory use of the better limb. Specifically, compensatory learning includes behavioural factors, such as attention, motivation, and perceived sense of effort, that contribute to a patient's reacquisition of unique motor skills through attention, motivation, effort, and control over motor outflow from preserved or accessible pathways. This new skill capability thus may facilitate restoration of the cortical representation of movement through task practice. Therefore, this model would suggest that overcoming learned non-use and improved compensatory learning both contribute to limb use after CIMT. One could deduce that factors such as attention and sense of effort are emergent behaviours that are manifested during CIMT training. Although this behavioural linking of concepts is indeed intriguing, the model does call into question a fundamental concern about whether all non-use is indeed learned. Several factors are still unclear, for example the variations in neuronal synaptic behaviour (neuromodulation), alterations in neurotransmitter regulation, and the impact of previous behaviours (movement experience) on skill reacquisition.

Recently, neuroimaging techniques, in particular the functional Magnetic Resonance Imaging (fMRI), have been used to study the cortical reorganization following rehabilitation treatment and it opened new opportunities to verify the changes induced by different approaches. You and colleagues [171] reported in an hemiplegic child a shift in the functional MRI laterality index to the controlateral hemisphere after virtual reality treatment with bimanual activities.

In a study carried out by Sutcliffe and colleagues, [172], an hemiplegic child treated with CIMT showed at fMRI bilateral sensorimotor activation before and after treatment and a shift in the laterality index from ipsilateral to controlateral hemisphere after therapy.

In CP children, cortical modifications usually occur in the very early phases both in the affected and unaffected hemispheres. In some patients, the ipsilateral corticospinal projections – normally transient – are not withdrawn, but persist and they allow the patient to control the paretic hand ipsilaterally, while in other patients the crossed projections are preserved so that they can control their hand with the affected hemisphere. In this second case, the sensorimotor loop is preserved and seems to be crucial for effective motor learning during CIMT.

Some Authors have hypothesized that patients with different types of corticospinal organization - whether the patient has an ipsilateral or a controlateral control of the affected limb - could respond differently to CIMT. The results suggest that CIMT can influence the time required to execute the task (e.g., Contra group patients are faster that Ipsi group patients). [173, 174]

A study was recently published and the aim was to explore individual variations in outcome of hand function after constraint-induced movement therapy (CIMT) in relation to the organization of corticomotor projection and brain lesion characteristics in participants with unilateral cerebral palsy (CP). Sixteen participants were enrolled with a age range 10-16 years with unilateral CP; they participated in a 2-week CIMT day camp (63 h). Transcranial magnetic stimulation was used to explore the corticomotor organization, and brain lesion characteristics were described by visual assessment of conventional structural magnetic resonance images. Improvements were found in all types of corticomotor projection patterns, i.e., contralateral, mixed, and ipsilateral. There was no relationship between functional improvement and brain lesion characteristics. Authors concluded that individuals with CP experience improved motor outcomes after CIMT, independent of corticomotor projection pattern and lesion characteristics. [175]

In another study a standardized pediatric CIMT protocol (4 weeks, 120 h of constraint) was used on 10 children with unilateral CP who were younger than 5 years. Diffusion Tensor Tractography (DTT) was performed in five participants before and after the intervention. In two patients, the affected corticospinal tract (CST) visible on pretreatment DTT became more prominent on posttreatment DTT. In one patient, the affected CST was not visible on pretreatment DTT, but was visible on posttreatment DTT. All the clinical outcomes significantly improved in the CIMT group compared with the control group. Changes in the properties of the affected CST on DTT were accompanied with improved arm function after CIMT in the children with CP. [176]

Clinical Evidence of Efficacy in Adults

Constraint-Induced Movement Therapy (CIMT) are relatively recent therapeutic interventions for individuals with hemiplegia that involve restraint of the non-involved upper extremity and intensive practice with the involved upper extremity. Increasing evidence indicates that these interventions are effective in reducing motor deficits in the involved upper extremity and increasing functional independence in adults with hemiplegia resulting from stroke.

Two early studies in adults with hemiplegia examined the effects of forced use on the involved upper extremity. Subsequent studies involving adults following stroke utilized restraint in addition to the shaping technique as a clinical intervention to examine changes in involved upper-extremity function. Gradually the intervention was refined and eventually termed "constraint-induced movement therapy". Forced use and CI therapy involve restraint and practice using the involved upper extremity.

Although restraint is common to both techniques, the types of practice provided during the restraint period are different. By definition, placing a restraint on the non-involved upper extremity would result in practice of the involved hand and arm for any movement performed. The practice is unstructured, and the intensity of the practice is dependent on the individual wearing the restraint. Constraint-induced therapy, however, involves a structured practice period (typically 6 hours in duration) that includes shaping and repetitive task practice.

A review by Cochrane examining 19 RCTs on 619 adults concluded that CIMT has moderately positive effects on disability at the end of treatment. [177] These benefits were demonstrated on other outcomes such as improvement of limb motor function and motor impairment. Patients who seem to benefit most are those with active wrist and finger extension, with limited pain or spasticity. Nonetheless, it is still to be cleared up if CIMT maintains efficacy in the longer term follow-up and if the effect observed can be entirely attributed to CIMT itself rather than on the amount and quality of repetitive exercise.Repetitive task practice involves functional tasks that are performed continuously over a specific period, and overall feedback is provided at the end of the task. Subsequent studies of CI therapy examined the efficacy of this intervention for improving involved upper extremity use with different types of restraint, different types of intervention, different outcome measures, and in people with chronic, acute, and sub-acute stroke.

Neuroimaging and transcranial magnetic stimulation studies of the brain prior to and after CI therapy have demonstrated differences in cortical organization around the infarct site after the intervention. These differences led to hypotheses regarding central nervous system (CNS) plasticity in adulthood and the role of CI therapy in cortical reorganization. Overall, the results of these adult studies suggest that following stroke, CI therapy and forced use may be able to improve upper extremity function.

Clinical Evidence of Efficacy in Children

Recently, constraint-induced therapy have been applied to children with hemiplegia, with moderate success. At the beginning most studies were case studies or were small-scale studies, but due to the initial promising results, research on this issue has increased rapidly.

The aim of CIMT consists of an attempt of reversing the behavioral suppression of movement in the affected upper limb. According to a Cochrane review, [178] evidence on this treatment is very poor and limited, since all currently available trials reveal methodological limitations and a need for additional research to support the application of this treatment.

The term CIMT and the child-friendly version mCIMT (modified CIMT) describe an intervention that can be applied with numerous variants with regard to: method of restraint, length of restraint (per day, number of weeks), type and duration of therapy, intervention environment (home, school, or clinic), and intervention provider (therapist, parent, or teacher).

As extensively underlined in the Cochrane review, [178] all currently available trials in children differ significantly in terms of methodological quality, sample sizes, treatment and assessment tools. The first significant variant regards the method used to restrain the non-affected limb: a broad range of techniques has been used from a glove or mitt, [179] to slings, [180, 181] short arm casts [182] and long arm casts. [183] Secondly, treatment programs vary in intensity and typology, ranging from 2 months of intervention 7 days per week, [183] 2 hours per day [179] to twice weekly in 30 minute-sessions for 6 weeks. [182] Moreover, there is inconsistency in the length of time the child's non-affected limb is restrained, varying from 6 hours per day, all day, [182, 183] for a period of 10 days, [181] to two months. [179] Furthermore, treatment programs range from no increase in routine occupational therapy or physiotherapy [182] to 8 hours of therapy per day, [184] although there is currently no evidence that improvement is correlated to the time spent wearing the restraint during the treatment session. [179] The treatment setting can either be the home, [180, 185] pre-school, [179] a day camp, [186] the hospital or university clinic [181] or a combination of these environments. In general, all the settings described modulate differently the role and type of intervention required from parents or caregivers. Nonetheless, there is still insufficient support for the use of a specific device, technique or program. [178]. Moreover, Taub & Wolf [187] suggested that the impact on CIMT outcomes is probably related more to intensity of treatment, than to the treatment principle itself. Although limited information was available on this issue, children's response to treatment may also be influenced by age, diagnosis, severity of motor and sensory impairment, co-morbidities, presence and impact of mirror movements, cognitive abilities and behavior. [178, 179] The clinical significance of study results so far was unclear also due to the lack of valid and reliable tools to measure the outcome, particularly the functional use of the hemiplegic hand in bimanual tasks. [178, 179]

In most cases for the comparison group no treatment or very basic treatment is provided, leading to a possible overestimation of the surplus value of CIMT (usually combined with an intensive rehabilitation program) compared to other treatment options. In our opinion, this comparison does not allow to distinguish the Constraint's effects from those of intensive rehabilitation and therefore assess the real effectiveness of Constraint Therapy.

Some published randomized controlled trials [188] raised the question of whether similar intensive practices can be elicited without the restraint and whether this might result in even better functional results. This hypothesis was supported by Gordon and colleagues, [189] who published a randomized trial demonstrating that bimanual intensive treatment results in a better outcome if compared to no treatment.

Since its first applications in children case reports more than 70 studies have been published, but a wide diversity in study design, CIMT characteristics (CIMT protocol, dosing, combined rehab programs, control group, type of casting) make it extremely different to draw conclusions and to choose a model of CIMT to implement in current clinical practice.

Increasing evidence however supports the benefits of CIMT on motor capacity, including quality, speed and dexterity of upper limb movements, functional motor performance, i.e., the spontaneous use of impaired limb in unimanual and bimanual tasks, and functional independence in performing ADL. [141, 188, 179, 182, 183, 190, 191, 192, 193, 194, 195, 196, 197, 198, 199, 200, 201, 202, 203, 204, 205, 206, 207] A recent trial on 45 children designed to investigate the long-term effects of home-based constraint induced therapy (CIT) on motor control underlying functional change in children with unilateral cerebral palsy (CP) demonstrated that the home-based CIT induced better spatial and temporal efficiency (smoother movement, more efficient grasping, better movement preplanning and execution) for functional improvement up to 6 months after treatment than traditional rehab [208] Both groups received a 4-week therapist-based intervention at home. The home-based CIT involved intensive functional training of the more affected upper extremity during which the less affected one was restrained, while the traditional rehab involved functional unimanual and bimanual training.

Further research for CIMT application in current clinical practice is clearly needed.

Intensive Bimanual Training

Intensive models of therapy achieved modest to strong effects to improve upper limb function compared to usual care. The promising result shown with CIMT and unimanual intensive treatment have led Authors to raise the question whether similar results could be achieved without restraining the unaffected limb.

In general, Intensive Bimanual Training is developmentally focused and it takes into account principles of motor learning tailored on child's age to progressively train the utilization of the affected limb.

The environment, through the achievement of bimanual tasks, is used to force the child to use the affected hand to solve the task. According to some Authors bimanual training is more "physiological" and less invasive than CIMT and should be helpful in directly translate the functional improvements in ADL. [167]

Charles et al. have developed a child-friendly form of intensive bimanual training, called HABIT (hand-arm bimanual intensive therapy): this approach aims at improving to ameliorate the quantity and quality of affected hand use in solving bimanual tasks. [209]

To date there are fewer studies exploring efficacy or bimanual intensive training rather than CIMT, but the results obtained by now are very promising. When compared one-another, both CIMT and bimanual intensive training have shown similar results in improving unimanual capacity and bimanual performance outcomes in CP children. [195, 196, 197, 198, 203]

In particular, while CIMT seems to be better for improving unimanual goals or coordination with the removal of possible compensation of the unaffected hand, bimanual intensive training seems to be better for improving bimanual coordination and goal performance. [210,211] Studies seem to demonstrated that bimanual intensive training is more effective for children with milder impairments and that could be employed for those children who do not tolerate the restraining.

Intensive bimanual training, although is much more challenging for therapists, it includes tasks and activities that in general are more interesting for the child and more ecologically relevant maximally capturing the child interest.

Future Research Challenges on CIMT and Intensive Training

Results of currently available clinical studies have contributed to estimate the effectiveness of CIMT in cerebral palsy, presently the optimal ingredients for successful CIMT practice are not completely known.

Furthermore, when mCIMT has been compared to a similar dose of intensive bimanual treatment, both intervention obtained similar improvements and resulted by far better that a traditional rehab approach. [210] This sustains the hypothesis that the dose of therapy may be the relevant ingredient, rather than the type of treatment, for example unimanual training with a casting device vs bimanual training.

CIMT and Intensive Bimanual training are not anymore considered mutually exclusive: they can be performed concurrently o sequentially (CIMT first, followed by Bimanual Intensive Training) in order to allow gains in unimanual capacity to be translated directly into bimanual activities.

Recently an hybrid specific protocol has been describe for an ongoing trial: COMBIT, combined mCIMT and bimanual intensive training. [212]

In 2014, Eliasson and colleagues, [213], have published an expert consensus providing suggestions for future research, in the light of an overview of what is known about constraint induced movement therapy (CIMT), mostly in comparison with bimanual intensive training in children with unilateral cerebral palsy (CP), to identify current knowledge gaps and strengths. In the paper also some methodological consideration were written suggesting advices for future study designs and the use of validated outcome measures, for researches comparison purposes.

The areas of highest priority for research implementation include the exploration of long-term outcomes and persistence of CIMT improvements and mostly if the CIMT effect transfers in improvement in bimanual performance and ADL, the effect of dosage, the effect of repeated CIMT, and the impact of predictive factors, such as age, on the response to CIMT.

Some key questions still looking for a clear answer are proposed: type of restraint matters? Amount of training matters? Type of structured training matters? Environment and context of the training matters? Provider of structured training matters? Key components of intervention seem to include collaborative goal setting with families and intensive repetitive, incrementally challenging, task practice.

Also the characteristics of children who achieve clinically meaningful outcomes remain unclear and it is still to be explored the role of age in influencing outcome, the importance of severity of impairment and the function of lesion characteristics and corticospinal projections in improvement.

The CIMT construct is complex, and much remains unknown. It is unclear whether a specific model of CIMT demonstrates superiority over others and whether dosage of training matters. Future research should build upon existing knowledge and aim to provide information that will help implement CIMT in various countries with different healthcare resources and organizational structures.

Across all studies of CIMT, there are consistent positive findings. Nonetheless, no international guidelines exist for the implementation of CIMT into clinical practice, and very little is known about what the effect of treatment means in a child's life.

References

[1]   Badawi N, Keogh JM. Causal pathways in cerebral palsy. *J. Paediatr. Child Health.* 2013;49(1):5-8.

[2]   Kavcic A, Vodusek DB. The definition of cerebral palsy, April 2006. *Dev. Med. Child Neurol.* 2008;50(3):240.

[3]   Rosenbaum P, Paneth N, Leviton A, Goldstein M, Bax M, Damiano D, Dan B, Jacobsson B. A report: the definition and classification of cerebral palsy April 2006. *Dev. Med. Child Neurol.* Suppl. 2007;109:8-14.

[4]   Basu AP. Early intervention after perinatal stroke: opportunities and challenges. *Dev. Med. Child Neurol.* 2014;56(6):516-21.

[5]   Van Hus JW, Potharst ES, Jeukens-Visser M, Kok JH, Van Wassenaer-Leemhuis AG. Motor impairment in very preterm-born children: links with other developmental deficits at 5 years of age. *Dev. Med. Child Neurol.* 2014;56(6):587-94.

[6]   Surman G, Hemming K, Platt MJ, Parkes J, Green A, Hutton J, Kurinczuk JJ. Children with cerebral palsy: severity and trends over time. *Paediatr. Perinat. Epidemiol.* 2009;23(6):513-21.

[7]   McIntyre S, Taitz D, Keogh J, Goldsmith S, Badawi N, Blair E. A systematic review of risk factors for cerebral palsy in children born at term in developed countries. *Dev. Med. Child Neurol.* 2013;55(6):499-508.

[8]   Bickerstaff ER. Aetiology of acute hemiplegia in childhood. *BMJ.* 1964;2(5401):82-7.

[9]   Kesar TM, Sawaki L, Burdette JH, Cabrera MN, Kolaski K, Smith BP, O'Shea TM, Koman LA, Wittenberg GF. Motor cortical functional geometry in cerebral palsy and its relationship to disability. *Clin. Neurophysiol.* 2012;123(7):1383-90.

[10] Jaspers E, Desloovere K, Bruyninckx H, Molenaers G, Klingels K, Feys H. Review of quantitative measurements of upper limb movements in hemiplegic cerebral palsy. *Gait. Posture.* 2009;30(4):395-404.

[11] Walusinski O, Neau JP, Bogousslavsky J. Hand up! Yawn and raise your arm. *Int. J. Stroke.* 2010;5(1):21-7.

[12] Burtner PA, Leinwand R, Sullivan KJ, Goh HT, Kantak SS. Motor learning in children with hemiplegic cerebral palsy: feedback effects on skill acquisition. *Dev. Med. Child Neurol.* 2014;56(3):259-66.

[13] Domellöf E, Rösblad B, Rönnqvist L. Impairment severity selectively affects the control of proximal and distal components of reaching movements in children with hemiplegic cerebral palsy. *Dev. Med. Child Neurol.* 2009;51(10):807-16.

[14] Wittenberg GF. Experience, cortical remapping, and recovery in brain disease. *Neurobiol. Dis.* 2010;37(2):252-8.

[15] Wittenberg GF. Motor mapping in cerebral palsy. *Dev. Med. Child Neurol.* 2009;51 Suppl 4:134-9.

[16] Kirkpatrick EV, Pearse JE, Eyre JA, Basu AP. Motor planning ability is not related to lesion side or functional manual ability in children with hemiplegic cerebral palsy. *Exp. Brain Res.* 2013;231(2):239-47.

[17] Steenbergen B, Gordon AM. Activity limitation in hemiplegic cerebral palsy: evidence for disorders in motor planning. *Dev. Med. Child Neurol.* 2006;48(9):780-3.

[18] Malhotra S, Pandyan AD, Day CR, Jones PW, Hermens H. Spasticity, an impairment that is poorly defined and poorly measured. *Clin. Rehabil.* 2009;23(7):651-8.

[19] Pandyan AD, Radford K, Ashford S, Bateman A, Burton C, Connell L, Gibson A, Harris N, Hoffman K, Nair R, Shaw L, Turton A, Tyson SF, van Wijck F. NICE on rehabilitation. New guidelines on rehabilitation likely to restrict practices and stifle innovation. *BMJ.* 2013;347:f4876.

[20] Ashford S, Slade M, Malaprade F, Turner-Stokes L. Evaluation of functional outcome measures for the hemiparetic upper limb: a systematic review. *J. Rehabil. Med.* 2008;40(10):787-95.

[21] Steenbergen B, Verrel J, Gordon AM. Motor planning in congenital hemiplegia. *Disabil. Rehabil.* 2007;29(1):13-23.

[22] Himmelmann K. Epidemiology of cerebral palsy. *Handb. Clin. Neurol.* 2013;111:163-7.

[23] Pakula AT, Van Naarden Braun K, Yeargin-Allsopp M. Cerebral palsy: classification and epidemiology. *Phys. Med. Rehabil. Clin. N. Am.* 2009;20(3):425-52.

[24] Krägeloh-Mann I, Cans C. Cerebral palsy update. *Brain Dev.* 2009;31(7):537-44.

[25] Odding E, Roebroeck ME, Stam HJ. The epidemiology of cerebral palsy: incidence, impairments and risk factors. *Disabil. Rehabil.* 2006;28(4):183-91.

[26] Colver A, Fairhurst C, Pharoah PO. Cerebral palsy. *Lancet.* 2014;383(9924):1240-9.

[27] Ibrahim SH, Bhutta ZA. Prevalence of early childhood disability in a rural district of Sind, Pakistan. *Dev. Med. Child Neurol.* 2013;55(4):357-63.

[28] Gladstone M. A review of the incidence and prevalence, types and aetiology of childhood cerebral palsy in resource-poor settings. *Ann. Trop. Paediatr.* 2010; 30(3):181-96.

Infant Cerebral Palsy in Hemiplegic Children: Treatment Options and Outcome 85

[29] Surveillance of Cerebral Palsy in Europe. Surveillance of cerebral palsy in Europe: a collaboration of cerebral palsy surveys and registers. Surveillance of Cerebral Palsy in Europe (SCPE). *Dev. Med. Child Neurol.* 2000;42(12):816-24.

[30] Platt MJ, Krageloh-Mann I, Cans C. Surveillance of cerebral palsy in Europe: reference and training manual. *Med. Educ.* 2009;43(5):495-6.

[31] Pharoah PO. Dyskinetic cerebral palsy in Europe: trends in prevalence and severity, on behalf of the SCPE Collaboration. *Arch. Dis. Child.* 2009;94(12):917-8.

[32] Gainsborough M, Surman G, Maestri G, Colver A, Cans C. Validity and reliability of the guidelines of the surveillance of cerebral palsy in Europe for the classification of cerebral palsy. *Dev. Med. Child Neurol.* 2008;50(11):828-31.

[33] Liu JM, Li S, Lin Q, Li Z. Prevalence of cerebral palsy in China. *Int. J. Epidemiol.* 1999;28(5):949-54.

[34] Wang B, Chen Y, Zhang J, Li J, Guo Y, Hailey D. A preliminary study into the economic burden of cerebral palsy in China. *Health Policy.* 2008;87(2):223-34.

[35] Zhang WF, Xu YH, Yang RL, Zhao ZY. Indicators of child health, service utilization and mortality in Zhejiang Province of China, 1998-2011. *PLoS One.* 2013;8(4):e62854.

[36] LeBlanc MH, Graves GR, Rawson TW, Moffitt J. Long-term outcome of infants at the margin of viability. *J. Miss. State Med. Assoc.* 1999;40(4):111-4.

[37] Reddihough DS, Baikie G, Walstab JE. Cerebral palsy in Victoria, Australia: mortality and causes of death. *J. Paediatr. Child Health.* 2001;37(2):183-6.

[38] Shevell MI. Current understandings and challenger in the management of cerebral palsy. *Minerva Pediatr.* 2009;61(4):399-413.

[39] Shevell MI, Dagenais L, Hall N; REPACQ Consortium. Comorbidities in cerebral palsy and their relationship to neurologic subtype and GMFCS level. *Neurology.* 2009;72(24):2090-6.

[40] van Bakel M, Einarsson I, Arnaud C, Craig S, Michelsen SI, Pildava S, Uldall P, Cans C. Monitoring the prevalence of severe intellectual disability in children across Europe: feasibility of a common database. *Dev. Med. Child Neurol.* 2014;56(4):361-9.

[41] Vargus-Adams JN, Martin LK. Measuring what matters in cerebral palsy: a breadth of important domains and outcome measures. *Arch. Phys. Med. Rehabil.* 2009;90(12):2089-95.

[42] Boulet SL, Boyle CA, Schieve LA. Health care use and health and functional impact of developmental disabilities among US children, 1997-2005. *Arch. Pediatr. Adolesc. Med.* 2009;163(1):19-26.

[43] Vogtle LK. Pain in adults with cerebral palsy: impact and solutions. *Dev. Med. Child Neurol.* 2009;51 Suppl 4:113-21.

[44] Hemsley B, Balandin S, Togher L. 'I've got something to say': interaction in a focus group of adults with cerebral palsy and complex communication needs. *Augment Altern. Commun.* 2008;24(2):110-22.

[45] Saavedra S, Joshi A, Woollacott M, van Donkelaar P. Eye hand coordination in children with cerebral palsy. *Exp. Brain Res.* 2009;192(2):155-65.

[46] Sandfeld Nielsen L, Jensen H, Skov L. Risk factors of ophthalmic disorders in children with developmental delay. *Acta Ophthalmol.* 2008;86(8):877-81.

[47] Himmelmann K, Beckung E, Hagberg G, Uvebrant P. Gross and fine motor function and accompanying impairments in cerebral palsy. *Dev. Med. Child Neurol.* 2006;48(6):417-23.

[48] Zimmerman RA, Bilaniuk LT. Neuroimaging evaluation of cerebral palsy. *Clin. Perinatol.* 2006;33(2):517-44.

[49] Rose J, Butler EE, Lamont LE, Barnes PD, Atlas SW, Stevenson DK. Neonatal brain structure on MRI and diffusion tensor imaging, sex, and neurodevelopment in very-low-birthweight preterm children. *Dev. Med. Child Neurol.* 2009;51(7):526-35.

[50] Kułak W, Sobaniec W, Kubas B, Walecki J, Smigielska-Kuzia J, Bockowski L, Artemowicz B, Sendrowski K. Spastic cerebral palsy: clinical magnetic resonance imaging correlation of 129 children. *J. Child. Neurol.* 2007;22(1):8-14.

[51] Wittenberg GF. Neural plasticity and treatment across the lifespan for motor deficits in cerebral palsy. *Dev. Med. Child Neurol.* 2009;51 Suppl 4:130-3.

[52] Tilton A. Management of spasticity in children with cerebral palsy. *Semin. Pediatr. Neurol.* 2009;16(2):82-9.

[53] Hägglund G, Wagner P. Development of spasticity with age in a total population of children with cerebral palsy. *BMC Musculoskelet Disord.* 2008;9:150.

[54] Straus S, Haynes RB. Managing evidence-based knowledge: the need for reliable, relevant and readable resources. *CMAJ.* 2009;180(9):942-5.

[55] Novak I, McIntyre S, Morgan C, Campbell L, Dark L, Morton N, Stumbles E, Wilson SA, Goldsmith S. A systematic review of interventions for children with cerebral palsy: state of the evidence. *Dev. Med. Child Neurol.* 2013;55(10):885-910.

[56] Morgan C, Novak I, Badawi N. Enriched environments and motor outcomes in cerebral palsy: systematic review and meta-analysis. *Pediatrics.* 2013;132(3):e735-46.

[57] Kothari R, Singh R, Singh S, Jain M, Bokariya P, Khatoon M. Neurophysiologic findings in children with spastic cerebral palsy. *J. Pediatr. Neurosci.* 2010;5(1):12-7.

[58] Charles J. A more definitive measure of upper limb capacity for children with unilateral cerebral palsy. *Dev. Med. Child Neurol.* 2014;56(6):513.

[59] Davies BL, Kurz MJ. Children with cerebral palsy have greater stochastic features present in the variability of their gait kinematics. *Res. Dev. Disabil.* 2013;34(11):3648-53.

[60] Musselman KE, Stoyanov CT, Marasigan R, Jenkins ME, Konczak J, Morton SM, Bastian AJ. Prevalence of ataxia in children: a systematic review. *Neurology.* 2014;82(1):80-9.

[61] Ryan SE, Sawatzky B, Campbell KA, Rigby PJ, Montpetit K, Roxborough L, McKeever PD. Functional outcomes associated with adaptive seating interventions in children and youth with wheeled mobility needs. *Arch. Phys. Med. Rehabil.* 2014;95(5):825-31.

[62] Moll LR, Cott CA. The paradox of normalization through rehabilitation: growing up and growing older with cerebral palsy. *Disabil. Rehabil.* 2013;35(15):1276-83.

[63] Reddihough DS, Jiang B, Lanigan A, Reid SM, Walstab JE, Davis E. Social outcomes of young adults with cerebral palsy. *J. Intellect. Dev. Disabil.* 2013;38(3):215-22.

[64] Cahill-Rowley K, Rose J. Etiology of impaired selective motor control: emerging evidence and its implications for research and treatment in cerebral palsy. *Dev. Med. Child Neurol.* 2014;56(6):522-8.

[65] Wallen M, Hoare B. Can goal setting be isolated from activity-focused intervention in cerebral palsy? *Dev. Med. Child Neurol.* 2014;56(5):503.

[66] Taub E, Uswatte G. Importance for CP rehabilitation of transfer of motor improvement to everyday life. *Pediatrics.* 2014;133(1):e215-7.

[67] Kumban W, Amatachaya S, Emasithi A, Siritaratiwat W. Effects of task-specific training on functional ability in children with mild to moderate cerebral palsy. *Dev. Neurorehabil.* 2013;16(6):410-7.

[68] Schenker R, Sutton A. Researching conductive education. *Dev. Med. Child Neurol.* 2014;56(4):402-3.

[69] Whittingham K, Bodimeade HL, Lloyd O, Boyd RN. Everyday psychological functioning in children with unilateral cerebral palsy: does executive functioning play a role? *Dev. Med. Child Neurol.* 2014;56(6):572-9.

[70] Kent RM. Cerebral palsy. *Handb. Clin. Neurol.* 2013;110:443-59.

[71] Meghi P, Rossetti L, Corrado C, Maran E, Arosio N, Ferrari A. Core elements of physiotherapy in cerebral palsy children: proposal for a trial checklist. *Eur. J. Phys. Rehabil. Med.* 2012;48(1):123-33.

[72] Montero SM, Gómez-Conesa A. Technical devices in children with motor disabilities: a review. *Disabil. Rehabil. Assist. Technol.* 2014;9(1):3-11.

[73] Montané E, Vallano A, Laporte JR. Oral antispastic drugs in nonprogressive neurologic diseases: a systematic review. *Neurology.* 2004;63(8):1357-63.

[74] Chaléat-Valayer E, Parratte B, Colin C, Denis A, Oudin S, Bérard C, Bernard JC, Bourg V, Deleplanque B, Dulieu I, Evrard P, Filipetti P, Flurin V, Gallien P, Héron-Long B, Hodgkinson I, Husson I, Jaisson-Hot I, Maupas E, Meurin F, Monnier G, Pérennou D, Pialoux B, Quentin V, Moreau MS, Schneider M, Yelnik A, Marque P. A French observational study of botulinum toxin use in the management of children with cerebral palsy: BOTULOSCOPE. *Eur. J. Paediatr. Neurol.* 2011;15(5):439-48.

[75] Vles GF, Soudant DL, Hoving MA, Vermeulen RJ, Bonouvrié LA, van Oostenbrugge RJ, Vles JS. Long-term follow-up on continuous intrathecal Baclofen therapy in non-ambulant children with intractable spastic Cerebral Palsy. *Eur. J. Paediatr. Neurol.* 2013;17(6):639-44.

[76] Kan P, Gooch J, Amini A, Ploeger D, Grams B, Oberg W, Simonsen S, Walker M, Kestle J. Surgical treatment of spasticity in children: comparison of selective dorsal rhizotomy and intrathecal baclofen pump implantation. *Childs Nerv. Syst.* 2008;24(2):239-43.

[77] Grunt S, Becher JG, Vermeulen RJ. Long-term outcome and adverse effects of selective dorsal rhizotomy in children with cerebral palsy: a systematic review. *Dev. Med. Child Neurol.* 2011;53(6):490-8.

[78] Novak I, Hines M, Goldsmith S, Barclay R. Clinical prognostic messages from a systematic review on cerebral palsy. *Pediatrics.* 2012;130(5):e1285-312.

[79] Pruitt DW, Tsai T. Common medical comorbidities associated with cerebral palsy. *Phys. Med. Rehabil. Clin. N. Am.* 2009;20(3):453-67.

[80] Sellier E, Uldall P, Calado E, Sigurdardottir S, Torrioli MG, Platt MJ, Cans C. Epilepsy and cerebral palsy: characteristics and trends in children born in 1976-1998. *Eur. J. Paediatr. Neurol.* 2012;16(1):48-55.

[81] Michelsen SI, Uldall P, Kejs AM, Madsen M. Education and employment prospects in cerebral palsy. *Dev. Med. Child Neurol.* 2005;47(8):511-7.

[82] Arnaud C, White-Koning M, Michelsen SI, Parkes J, Parkinson K, Thyen U, Beckung E, Dickinson HO, Fauconnier J, Marcelli M, McManus V, Colver A. Parent-reported quality of life of children with cerebral palsy in Europe. *Pediatrics.* 2008;121(1):54-64.

[83] Dragoumi P, Tzetzi O, Vargiami E, Pavlou E, Krikonis K, Kontopoulos E, Zafeiriou DI. Clinical course and seizure outcome of idiopathic childhood epilepsy: determinants of early and long-term prognosis. *BMC Neurol.* 2013;13:206.

[84] Carlsson M, Hagberg G, Olsson I. Clinical and aetiological aspects of epilepsy in children with cerebral palsy. *Dev. Med. Child Neurol.* 2003;45(6):371-6.

[85] Mert GG, Incecik F, Altunbasak S, Herguner O, Mert MK, Kiris N, Unal I. Factors affecting epilepsy development and epilepsy prognosis in cerebral palsy. *Pediatr. Neurol.* 2011;45(2):89-94.

[86] Smith MC. Optimizing therapy of seizures in children and adolescents with developmental disabilities. *Neurology.* 2006;67(12 Suppl 4):S52-5.

[87] Russman BS, Ashwal S. Evaluation of the child with cerebral palsy. *Semin. Pediatr. Neurol.* 2004;11(1):47-57

[88] McIntyre S, Morgan C, Walker K, Novak I. Cerebral palsy--don't delay. *Dev. Disabil. Res Rev.* 2011;17(2):114-29.

[89] Winkle M, Crowe TK, Hendrix I. Service dogs and people with physical disabilities partnerships: a systematic review. *Occup. Ther. Int.* 2012;19(1):54-66.

[90] Tessier DW, Hefner JL, Newmeyer A. Factors related to psychosocial quality of life for children with cerebral palsy. *Int. J. Pediatr.* 2014;2014:204386.

[91] Arnaud C, White-Koning M, Michelsen SI, Parkes J, Parkinson K, Thyen U, Beckung E, Dickinson HO, Fauconnier J, Marcelli M, McManus V, Colver A. Parent-reported quality of life of children with cerebral palsy in Europe. *Pediatrics.* 2008;121(1):54-64.

[92] Darrah J, Wiart L, Magill-Evans J, Ray L, Andersen J. Are family-centred principles, functional goal setting and transition planning evident in therapy services for children with cerebral palsy? *Child Care Health Dev.* 2012;38(1):41-7.

[93] Parkes J, McCullough N, Madden A. To what extent do children with cerebral palsy participate in everyday life situations? *Health Soc. Care Community.* 2010;18(3):304-15.

[94] Shevell MI, Dagenais L, Hall N; REPACQ CONSORTIUM. The relationship of cerebral palsy subtype and functional motor impairment: a population-based study. *Dev. Med. Child Neurol.* 2009;51(11):872-7.

[95] Parkes J, Hill N. The needs of children and young people with cerebral palsy. *Paediatr. Nurs.* 2010;22(4):14-9.

[96] Pennington L, Goldbart J, Marshall J. Speech and language therapy to improve the communication skills of children with cerebral palsy. *Cochrane Database Syst. Rev.* 2004;(2):CD003466.

[97] Branson D, Demchak M. The use of augmentative and alternative communication methods with infants and toddlers with disabilities: a research review. *Augment Altern. Commun.* 2009;25(4):274-86.

[98] Sandlund M, McDonough S, Häger-Ross C. Interactive computer play in rehabilitation of children with sensorimotor disorders: a systematic review. *Dev. Med. Child Neurol.* 2009;51(3):173-9.

[99] Pennington L, Miller N, Robson S. Speech therapy for children with dysarthria acquired before three years of age. *Cochrane Database Syst. Rev.* 2009;(4):CD006937.

[100] Guzzetta A, Mercuri E, Cioni G. Visual disorders in children with brain lesions: 2. Visual impairment associated with cerebral palsy. *Eur. J. Paediatr. Neurol.* 2001;5(3):115-9.

[101] Prasad R, Verma N, Srivastava A, Das BK, Mishra OP. Magnetic resonance imaging, risk factors and co-morbidities in children with cerebral palsy. *J. Neurol.* 2011;258(3):471-8.

[102] Holmström GE, Källen K, Hellström A, Jakobsson PG, Serenius F, Stjernqvist K, Tornqvist K. Ophthalmologic outcome at 30 months' corrected age of a prospective Swedish cohort of children born before 27 weeks of gestation: the extremely preterm infants in sweden study. *JAMA Ophthalmol.* 2014;132(2):182-9.

[103] Cupples L, Ching TY, Crowe K, Seeto M, Leigh G, Street L, Day J, Marnane V, Thomson J. Outcomes of 3-year-old children with hearing loss and different types of additional disabilities. *J. Deaf Stud. Deaf Educ.* 2014;19(1):20-39.

[104] Özdemir S, Tuncer Ü, Tarkan Ö, Kıroğlu M, Çetik F, Akar F. Factors contributing to limited or non-use in the cochlear implant systems in children: 11 years experience. *Int. J. Pediatr. Otorhinolaryngol.* 2013;77(3):407-9.

[105] Delgado MR, Hirtz D, Aisen M, Ashwal S, Fehlings DL, McLaughlin J, Morrison LA, Shrader MW, Tilton A, Vargus-Adams J. Practice parameter: pharmacologic treatment of spasticity in children and adolescents with cerebral palsy (an evidence-based review): report of the Quality Standards Subcommittee of the American Academy of Neurology and the Practice Committee of the Child Neurology Society. *Neurology.* 2010;74(4):336-43.

[106] Carr LJ. The expanding role of botulinum toxin type A injections in the management of children with cerebral palsy. *Dev. Med. Child Neurol.* 2009;51(9):687-8.

[107] Sakzewski L, Ziviani J, Boyd R. Systematic review and meta-analysis of therapeutic management of upper-limb dysfunction in children with congenital hemiplegia. *Pediatrics.* 2009;123(6):e1111-22.

[108] Boyd RN, Morris ME, Graham HK. Management of upper limb dysfunction in children with cerebral palsy: a systematic review. *Eur J Neurol.* 2001;8 Suppl 5:150-66.

[109] Patel DR. Therapeutic interventions in cerebral palsy. *Indian J. Pediatr.* 2005;72(11):979-83.

[110] Effgen SK, Chan L. Occurrence of gross motor behaviors and attainment of motor objectives in children with cerebral palsy participating in conductive education. *Physiother. Theory Pract.* 2010;26(1):22-39.

[111] Blank R, von Kries R, Hesse S, von Voss H. Conductive education for children with cerebral palsy: effects on hand motor functions relevant to activities of daily living. *Arch. Phys. Med. Rehabil.* 2008;89(2):251-9.

[112] Bourke-Taylor H, O'Shea R, Gaebler-Spira D. Conductive education: a functional skills program for children with cerebral palsy. *Phys. Occup. Ther. Pediatr.* 2007;27(1):45-62.

[113] Boyd RN, Sakzewski L, Ziviani J, Abbott DF, Badawy R, Gilmore R, Provan K, Tournier JD, Macdonnell RA, Jackson GD. INCITE: A randomised trial comparing constraint induced movement therapy and bimanual training in children with congenital hemiplegia. *BMC Neurol.* 2010;10(1):4.

[114] Huang HH, Fetters L, Hale J, McBride A. Bound for success: a systematic review of constraint-induced movement therapy in children with cerebral palsy supports improved arm and hand use. *Phys. Ther.* 2009;89(11):1126-41.

[115] Stearns GE, Burtner P, Keenan KM, Qualls C, Phillips J. Effects of constraint-induced movement therapy on hand skills and muscle recruitment of children with spastic hemiplegic cerebral palsy. *NeuroRehabilitation*. 2009;24(2):95-108.

[116] Cope SM, Forst HC, Bibis D, Liu XC. Modified constraint-induced movement therapy for a 12-month-old child with hemiplegia: a case report. *Am. J. Occup. Ther*. 2008;62(4):430-7.

[117] Charles JR, Gordon AM. A repeated course of constraint-induced movement therapy results in further improvement. *Dev. Med. Child Neurol*. 2007;49(10):770-3.

[118] Papavasiliou AS. Management of motor problems in cerebral palsy: a critical update for the clinician. *Eur. J. Paediatr. Neurol*. 2009;13(5):387-96.

[119] Garvey MA, Giannetti ML, Alter KE, Lum PS. Cerebral palsy: new approaches to therapy. *Curr. Neurol. Neurosci. Rep*. 2007;7(2):147-55.

[120] Novak I, Cusick A, Lannin N. Occupational therapy home programs for cerebral palsy: double-blind, randomized, controlled trial. *Pediatrics*. 2009;124(4):e606-14.

[121] Esdaile SA. Valuing difference: caregiving by mothers of children with disabilities. *Occup. Ther. Int*. 2009;16(2):122-33.

[122] Anttila H, Autti-Rämö I, Suoranta J, Mäkelä M, Malmivaara A. Effectiveness of physical therapy interventions for children with cerebral palsy: a systematic review. *BMC Pediatr*. 2008;8:14.

[123] Barry MJ. Physical therapy interventions for patients with movement disorders due to cerebral palsy. *J. Child Neurol*. 1996;11 Suppl 1:S51-60.

[124] Vaz DV, Mancini MC, da Fonseca ST, Arantes NF, Pinto TP, de Araújo PA. Effects of strength training aided by electrical stimulation on wrist muscle characteristics and hand function of children with hemiplegic cerebral palsy. *Phys. Occup. Ther. Pediatr*. 2008;28(4):309-25.

[125] Mockford M, Caulton JM. Systematic review of progressive strength training in children and adolescents with cerebral palsy who are ambulatory. *Pediatr. Phys. Ther*. 2008;20(4):318-33.

[126] Unnithan VB, Katsimanis G, Evangelinou C, Kosmas C, Kandrali I, Kellis E. Effect of strength and aerobic training in children with cerebral palsy. *Med. Sci. Sports Exerc*. 2007;39(11):1902-9.

[127] Wilton J. Casting, splinting, and physical and occupational therapy of hand deformity and dysfunction in cerebral palsy. *Hand Clin*. 2003;19(4):573-84.

[128] Rigby PJ, Ryan SE, Campbell KA. Effect of adaptive seating devices on the activity performance of children with cerebral palsy. *Arch. Phys. Med. Rehabil*. 2009;90(8):1389-95.

[129] Ryan SE, Campbell KA, Rigby PJ, Fishbein-Germon B, Hubley D, Chan B. The impact of adaptive seating devices on the lives of young children with cerebral palsy and their families. *Arch. Phys. Med. Rehabil*. 2009;90(1):27-33.

[130] Vekerdy Z. Management of seating posture of children with cerebral palsy by using thoracic-lumbar-sacral orthosis with non-rigid SIDO frame. *Disabil. Rehabil*. 2007;29(18):1434-41.

[131] Boldingh EJ, Jacobs-van der Bruggen MA, Bos CF, Lankhorst GJ, Bouter LM. Radiographic hip disorders and associated complications in severe cerebral palsy. *J. Pediatr. Orthop. B*. 2007;16(1):31-4.

[132] Holmes KJ, Michael SM, Thorpe SL, Solomonidis SE. Management of scoliosis with special seating for the non-ambulant spastic cerebral palsy population--a biomechanical study. *Clin. Biomech. (Bristol, Avon).* 2003;18(6):480-7.

[133] Merrill DR. Review of electrical stimulation in cerebral palsy and recommendations for future directions. *Dev. Med. Child Neurol.* 2009;51 Suppl 4:154-65.

[134] Kerr C, McDowell B, Cosgrove A, Walsh D, Bradbury I, McDonough S. Electrical stimulation in cerebral palsy: a randomized controlled trial. *Dev. Med. Child Neurol.* 2006;48(11):870-6.

[135] Ozer K, Chesher SP, Scheker LR. Neuromuscular electrical stimulation and dynamic bracing for the management of upper-extremity spasticity in children with cerebral palsy. *Dev. Med. Child Neurol.* 2006;48(7):559-63.

[136] Bolek JE. Use of multiple-site performance-contingent SEMG reward programming in pediatric rehabilitation: a retrospective review. *Appl. Psychophysiol. Biofeedback.* 2006;31(3):263-72.

[137] Colborne GR, Wright FV, Naumann S. Feedback of triceps surae EMG in gait of children with cerebral palsy: a controlled study. *Arch. Phys. Med. Rehabil.* 1994;75(1):40-5.

[138] Verrotti A, Greco R, Spalice A, Chiarelli F, Iannetti P. Pharmacotherapy of spasticity in children with cerebral palsy. *Pediatr. Neurol.* 2006;34(1):1-6.

[139] Khot A, Sloan S, Desai S, Harvey A, Wolfe R, Graham HK. Adductor release and chemodenervation in children with cerebral palsy: a pilot study in 16 children. *J. Child Orthop.* 2008;2(4):293-9.

[140] Ianieri G, Saggini R, Marvulli R, Tondi G, Aprile A, Ranieri M, Di Teo L, Altini S, Lancioni GE, Goffredo L, Megna M, Megna G. Botulinum toxin in cerebral child palsy. *Int. J. Immunopathol. Pharmacol.* 2009;22(3 Suppl):9-11.

[141] Motta F, Antonello CE, Stignani C. Upper limbs function after intrathecal baclofen therapy in children with secondary dystonia. *J. Pediatr. Orthop.* 2009;29(7):817-21.

[142] Lynn AK, Turner M, Chambers HG. Surgical management of spasticity in persons with cerebral palsy. *PM R.* 2009;1(9):834-8.

[143] Nordmark E, Josenby AL, Lagergren J, Andersson G, Strömblad LG, Westbom L. Long-term outcomes five years after selective dorsal rhizotomy. *BMC Pediatr.* 2008;8:54.

[144] Shikako-Thomas K, Lach L, Majnemer A, Nimigon J, Cameron K, Shevell M. Quality of life from the perspective of adolescents with cerebral palsy: "I just think I'm a normal kid, I just happen to have a disability". *Qual. Life Res.* 2009;18(7):825-32.

[145] Odman PE, Oberg BE. Effectiveness and expectations of intensive training: a comparison between child and youth rehabilitation and conductive education. *Disabil. Rehabil.* 2006;28(9):561-70.

[146] Law M, Darrah J, Pollock N, Rosenbaum P, Russell D, Walter SD, Petrenchik T, Wilson B, Wright V. Focus on Function - a randomized controlled trial comparing two rehabilitation interventions for young children with cerebral palsy. *BMC Pediatr.* 2007;7:31.

[147] Hoving MA, van Raak EP, Spincemaille GH, Palmans LJ, Becher JG, Vles JS; Dutch Study Group on Child Spasticity. Efficacy of intrathecal baclofen therapy in children with intractable spastic cerebral palsy: a randomised controlled trial. *Eur. J. Paediatr. Neurol.* 2009;13(3):240-6.

[148] Russman BS. Continuous intrathecal baclofen infusion for intractable spastic cerebral palsy--is it worth it? *Nat. Clin. Pract. Neurol.* 2008;4(9):476-7.

[149] Kanellopoulos AD, Mavrogenis AF, Mitsiokapa EA, Panagopoulos D, Skouteli H, Vrettos SG, Tzanos G, Papagelopoulos PJ. Long lasting benefits following the combination of static night upper extremity splinting with botulinum toxin A injections in cerebral palsy children. *Eur. J. Phys. Rehabil. Med.* 2009;45(4):501-6.

[150] Bradley LJ, Huntley JS. Question 2: is there any long-term benefit from injecting botulinum toxin-A into children with cerebral palsy? *Arch. Dis. Child.* 2014;99(4):392-4.

[151] Hawamdeh ZM1, Ibrahim AI, Al-Qudah AA. Long-term effect of botulinum toxin (A) in the management of calf spasticity in children with diplegic cerebral palsy. *Eura Medicophys.* 2007;43(3):311-8.

[152] Graham HK, Boyd R, Carlin JB, Dobson F, Lowe K, Nattrass G, Thomason P, Wolfe R, Reddihough D. Does botulinum toxin a combined with bracing prevent hip displacement in children with cerebral palsy and "hips at risk"? A randomized, controlled trial. *J. Bone Joint. Surg. Am.* 2008;90(1):23-33.

[153] Moore AP, Ade-Hall RA, Smith CT, Rosenbloom L, Walsh HP, Mohamed K, Williamson PR. Two-year placebo-controlled trial of botulinum toxin A for leg spasticity in cerebral palsy. *Neurology.* 2008;71(2):122-8.

[154] Tedroff K, Löwing K, Haglund-Akerlind Y, Gutierrez-Farewik E, Forssberg H. Botulinum toxin A treatment in toddlers with cerebral palsy. *Acta Paediatr.* 2010;99(8):1156-62.

[155] Willoughby K, Ang SG, Thomason P, Graham HK. The impact of botulinum toxin A and abduction bracing on long-term hip development in children with cerebral palsy. *Dev. Med. Child Neurol.* 2012;54(8):743-7.

[156] Ramachandran M, Eastwood DM. Botulinum toxin and its orthopaedic applications. *J. Bone Joint Surg. Br.* 2006;88(8):981-7.

[157] Tedroff K, Granath F, Forssberg H, Haglund-Akerlind Y. Long-term effects of botulinum toxin A in children with cerebral palsy. *Dev. Med. Child Neurol.* 2009;51(2):120-7.

[158] Alhusaini AA, Crosbie J, Shepherd RB, Dean CM, Scheinberg A. No change in calf muscle passive stiffness after botulinum toxin injection in children with cerebral palsy. *Dev. Med. Child Neurol.* 2011;53(6):553-8.

[159] Gough M, Fairhurst C, Shortland AP. Botulinum toxin and cerebral palsy: time for reflection? *Dev. Med. Child Neurol.* 2005;47(10):709-12.

[160] Fortuna R, Vaz MA, Youssef AR, Longino D, Herzog W. Changes in contractile properties of muscles receiving repeat injections of botulinum toxin (Botox). *J. Biomech.* 2011;44(1):39-44.

[161] Papadopoulos KI, Low SS, Aw TC, Chantarojanasiri T. Safety and feasibility of autologous umbilical cord blood transfusion in 2 toddlers with cerebral palsy and the role of low dose granulocyte-colony stimulating factor injections. *Restor. Neurol. Neurosci.* 2011;29(1):17-22.

[162] Lee YH, Choi KV, Moon JH, Jun HJ, Kang HR, Oh SI, Kim HS, Um JS, Kim MJ, Choi YY, Lee YJ, Kim HJ, Lee JH, Son SM, Choi SJ, Oh W, Yang YS. Safety and feasibility of countering neurological impairment by intravenous administration of autologous cord blood in cerebral palsy. *J. Transl. Med.* 2012;10:58.

[163] Jensen A, Hamelmann E. First autologous cell therapy of cerebral palsy caused by hypoxic-ischemic brain damage in a child after cardiac arrest-individual treatment with cord blood. *Case Rep. Transplant.* 2013;2013:951827.

[164] Jensen A. Autologous Cord Blood Therapy for Infantile Cerebral Palsy: From Bench to Bedside. *Obstet. Gynecol. Int.* 2014;2014:976321.

[165] Borowski A, Littleton AG, Borkhuu B, Presedo A, Shah S, Dabney KW, Lyons S, McMannus M, Miller F. Complications of intrathecal baclofen pump therapy in pediatric patients. *J. Pediatr. Orthop.* 2010;30(1):76-81.

[166] Autti-Rämo I, Anttila H, Mäkelä M. Are current practices in the treatment of children with cerebral palsy research-based? *Dev. Med. Child Neurol.* 2007;49(2):155-6.

[167] Sakzewski L, Gordon A, Eliasson AC. The State of the Evidence for Intensive Upper Limb Therapy Approaches for Children With Unilateral Cerebral Palsy. *J. Child Neurol.* 2014;Epub ahead of print.

[168] Tarkka IM, Könönen M. Methods to improve constraint-induced movement therapy. *NeuroRehabilitation.* 2009;25(1):59-68.

[169] Taub E, Uswatte G, Mark VW, Morris DM. The learned nonuse phenomenon: implications for rehabilitation. *Eura Medicophys.* 2006;42(3):241-56.

[170] Sunderland A, Tuke A. Neuroplasticity, learning and recovery after stroke: a critical evaluation of constraint induced therapy. *Neuropsychol. Rehabil.* 2005;15:81–98.

[171] You SH, Jang SH, Kim YH, Hallett M, Ahn SH, Kwon YH, Kim JH, Lee MY. Virtual reality-induced cortical reorganization and associated locomotor recovery in chronic stroke: an experimenter-blind randomized study. *Stroke.* 2005;36(6):1166-71.

[172] Sutcliffe TL, Gaetz WC, Logan WJ, Cheyne DO, Fehlings DL. Cortical reorganization after modified constraint-induced movement therapy in pediatric hemiplegic cerebral palsy. *J. Child Neurol.* 2007; 22(11):1281-7.

[173] Kuhnke N, Juenger H, Walther M, Berweck S, Mall V, Staudt M. Do patients with congenital hemiparesis and ipsilateral corticospinal projections respond differently to constraint induced movement therapy? *Dev. Med. Child Neurol.* 2008; 50:898-903.

[174] Staudt M, Grodd W, Gerloff C, Erb M, Stitz J, Krägeloh-Mann I. Two types of ipsilateral reorganization in congenital hemiparesis: a TMS and fMRI study. *Brain.* 2002;125(Pt 10):2222-37.

[175] Islam M, Nordstrand L, Holmström L, Kits A, Forssberg H, Eliasson AC. Is outcome of constraint-induced movement therapy in unilateral cerebral palsy dependent on corticomotor projection pattern and brain lesion characteristics? *Dev. Med. Child Neurol.* 2014;56(3):252-8.

[176] Kwon JY, Chang WH, Chang HJ, Yi SH, Kim MY, Kim EH, Kim YH. Changes in diffusion tensor tractographic findings associated with constraint-induced movement therapy in young children with cerebral palsy. Clin Neurophysiol. 2014; Epub ahead of print.

[177] Sirtori V, Corbetta D, Moja L, Gatti R. Constraint-induced movement therapy for upper extremities in stroke patients (Review). *Cochrane Database Syst. Rev.* 2009;Cd004433.

[178] Hoare BJ, Wasiak J, Imms C, Carey L. Constraint-induced movement therapy in the treatment of the upper limb in children with hemiplegic cerebral palsy. *Cochrane Database Syst. Rev.* 2007;(2):CD004149.

[179] Eliasson AC, Krumlinde-sundholm L, Shaw K, Wang C. Effects of constraint-induced movement therapy in young children with hemiplegic cerebral palsy: an adapted model. *Dev. Med. Child Neurol.* 2005;47(4):266-75.

[180] Charles J, Lavinder G, Gordon AM. Effects of constraint-induced therapy on hand function in children with hemiplegic cerebral palsy. *Pediatr. Phys. Ther.* 2001;13(2):68-76.

[181] Gordon AM, Charles J, Wolf SL. Methods of constraint-induced movement therapy for children with hemiplegic cerebral palsy: development of a child-friendly intervention for improving upper-extremity function. *Arch. Phys. Med. Rehabil.* 2005;86(4):837-44.

[182] Sung IY, Ryu JS, Pyun SB, Yoo SD, Song WH, Park MJ. Efficacy of forced-use therapy in hemiplegic cerebral palsy. *Arch. Phys. Med. Rehabil.* 2005;86(11):2195-8.

[183] Taub E, Ramey SL, DeLuca S, Echols K. Efficacy of constraint-induced movement therapy for children with cerebral palsy with asymmetric motor impairment. *Pediatrics.* 2004;113(2):305-12.

[184] Glover JE, Mateer CA, Yoell C, Speed S. The effectiveness of constraint induced movement therapy in two young children with hemiplegia. *Pediatr. Rehabil.* 2002;5(3):125-31.

[185] DeLuca SC, Echols R, Ramey SL, Taub E. Pediatric constraint induced movement therapy for a young child with cerebral palsy: Two episodes care. *Phys. Ther.* 2003;83:1003-13.

[186] Eliasson AC, Bonnier B, Krumlinde-Sundholm L. Clinical experience of constraint induced movement therapy in small children with hemiplegic cerebral palsy - a day camp model. *Dev. Med. Child Neurol.* 2003;45:357-60.

[187] Taub E, Wolf SL. Constraint Induction techniques to facilitate upper extremity use in stroke patients. *Top Stroke Rehabil.* 1997;3(4):1-24.

[188] Charles JR, Wolf SL, Schneider JA, Gordon AM. Efficacy of a child-friendly form of constraint-induced movement therapy in hemiplegic cerebral palsy: a randomized control trial. *Dev. Med. Child Neurol.* 2006;48(8):635-42.

[189] Gordon AM, Schneider JA, Chinnan A, Charles JR. Efficacy of a hand-arm bimanual intensive therapy (HABIT) in children with hemiplegic cerebral palsy: a randomized control trial. *Dev. Med Child Neurol.* 2007;49(11):830-8.

[190] Aarts P, Jongerius P, Geerdink Y, Van Limbeek J, Geurts A. Effectiveness of modified constraint-induced movement therapy in children with unilateral spastic cerebral palsy: a randomized controlled trial. *Neurorehabil. Neural. Repair.* 2010; 24 (6): 509–18.

[191] Al-Oraibi S, Eliasson A-C. Implementation of constraint-induced movement therapy for young children with unilateral cerebral palsy in Jordan: a home-based model. *Disabil. Rehabil.* 2011; 33(21-22): 2006–12.

[192] Case-Smith J, DeLuca SC, Stevenson R, Ramey SL. Multicenter randomized controlled trial of pediatric constraint-induced movement therapy: 6-month follow-up. *Am. J. Occup. Ther.* 2011; 66(1): 15–23.

[193] de Brito Brandao M, Mancini MC, Vaz DV, Pereira de Melo AP, Fonseca ST. Adapted version of constraint-induced movement therapy promotes functioning in children with cerebral palsy: a randomized controlled trial. *Clin. Rehabil.* 2010; 24(7): 639–47.

[194] Eliasson A-C, Shaw K, Berg E, Krumlinde Sundholm L. An ecological approach of constraint induced movement therapy for 2–3-year-old children: a randomized control trial. *Res. Dev. Disabil.* 2011; 32(6): 2820–8.

[195] Facchin P, Rosa-Rizzotto M, Visonà Dalla Pozza L, Turconi AC, Pagliano E, Signorini S, Tornetta L, Trabacca A, Fedrizzi E; GIPCI Study Group. Multisite trial comparing the efficacy of constraint-induced movement therapy with that of bimanual intensive training in children with hemiplegic cerebral palsy postintervention results. *Am. J. Phys. Med. Rehabil.* 2011; 90(7): 539–53.

[196] Gordon AM, Chinnan A, Gill S, Petra E, Hung Y-C, Charles J. Both constraint-induced movement therapy and bimanual training lead to improved performance of upper extremity function in children with hemiplegia. *Dev. Med. Child. Neurol.* 2008; 50(12): 957–8.

[197] Gordon AM, Hung YC, Brandao M, Ferre CL, Kuo HC, Friel K, Petra E, Chinnan A, Charles JR. Bimanual training and constraint-induced movement therapy in children with hemiplegic cerebral palsy: a randomized trial. *Neurorehabil. Neural. Repair.* 2011; 25(8): 692–702.

[198] Hoare B, Imms C, Villanueva E, Rawicki HB, Matyas T, Carey L. Intensive therapy following upper limb botulinum toxin A injection in young children with unilateral cerebral palsy: a randomized trial. *Dev. Med. Child Neurol.* 2013; 55(3): 238–47.

[199] Hsin YJ, Chen FC, Lin KC, Kang LJ, Chen CL, Chen CY. Efficacy of constraint-induced therapy on functional performance and health-related quality of life for children with cerebral palsy: a randomized controlled trial. *J. Child Neurol.* 2012; 27(8): 992–9.

[200] Lin KC, Wang TN, Wu CY, Chen CL, Chang KC, Lin YC, Chen YJ. Effects of home-based constraint-induced therapy versus dose-matched control intervention on functional outcomes and caregiver well-being in children with cerebral palsy. *Res. Dev. Disabil.* 2011; 32(5): 1483–91.

[201] Park ES, Rha DW, Lee JD, Yoo JK, Chang WH. The short-term effects of combined modified constraint-induced movement therapy and botulinum toxin injection for children with spastic hemiplegic cerebral palsy. *Neuropediatrics.* 2009; 40(6): 269–74.

[202] Rostami HR, Malamiri RA. Effect of treatment environment on modified constraint-induced movement therapy results in children with spastic hemiplegic cerebral palsy: a randomized controlled trial. *Disabil. Rehabil.* 2012; 34(1): 40–4.

[203] Sakzewski L, Ziviani J, Abbott DF, Macdonell RAL, Jackson GD, Boyd RN. Randomized trial of constraint-induced movement therapy and bimanual training on activity outcomes for children with congenital hemiplegia. *Dev. Med. Child Neurol.* 2011; 53(4): 313–20.

[204] Smania N, Aglioti SM, Cosentino A, Camin M, Gandolfi M, Tinazzi M, Fiaschi A, Faccioli S. A modified constraint-induced movement therapy (CIT) program improves paretic arm use and function in children with cerebral palsy. *Eur. J. Phys. Rehabil. Med.* 2009; 45(4): 493–500.

[205] Taub E, Griffin A, Uswatte G, Gammons K, Nick J, Law CR. Treatment of congenital hemiparesis with pediatric constraint-induced movement therapy. *J. Child Neurol.* 2011; 26(9): 1163–73.

[206] Wallen M, Ziviani J, Naylor O, Evans R, Novak I, Herbert RD. Modified constraint-induced therapy for children with hemiplegic cerebral palsy: a randomized trial. *Dev. Med. Child Neurol.* 2011; 53(12): 1091–9.

[207] Xu K, Wang L, Mai J, He L. Efficacy of constraint-induced movement therapy and electrical stimulation on hand function of children with hemiplegic cerebral palsy: a controlled clinical trial. *Disabil. Rehabil.* 2011; 34(4): 337–46.

[208] Chen HC, Chen CL, Kang LJ, Wu CY, Chen FC, Hong WH. Improvement of Upper Extremity Motor Control and Function After Home-Based Constraint Induced Therapy in Children With Unilateral Cerebral Palsy: Immediate and Long-Term Effects. *Arch. Phys. Med Rehabil.* 2014; Epub ahead of print.

[209] Brandão MB, Ferre C, Kuo HC, Rameckers EA, Bleyenheuft Y, Hung YC, Friel K, Gordon AM. Comparison of Structured Skill and Unstructured Practice During Intensive Bimanual Training in Children With Unilateral Spastic Cerebral Palsy. *Neurorehabil. Neural Repair.* 2013;28(5):452-461.

[210] Fedrizzi E, Rosa-Rizzotto M, Turconi AC, Pagliano E, Fazzi E, Pozza LV, Facchin P; GIPCI Study Group. Unimanual and bimanual intensive training in children with hemiplegic cerebral palsy and persistence in time of hand function improvement: 6-month follow-up results of a multisite clinical trial. *J. Child Neurol.* 2013;28(2):161-75.

[211] Hung YC, Casertano L, Hillman A, Gordon AM. The effect of intensive bimanual training on coordination of the hands in children with congenital hemiplegia. *Res. Dev. Disabil.* 2011;32(6):2724-31.

[212] Boyd RN, Ziviani J, Sakzewski L, Miller L, Bowden J, Cunnington R, Ware R, Guzzetta A, Al Macdonell R, Jackson GD, Abbott DF, Rose S. COMBIT: protocol of a randomised comparison trial of COMbined modified constraint induced movement therapy and bimanual intensive training with distributed model of standard upper limb rehabilitation in children with congenital hemiplegia. *BMC Neurol.* 2013;13:68.

[213] Eliasson AC, Krumlinde-Sundholm L, Gordon AM, Feys H, Klingels K, Aarts PB, Rameckers E, Autti-Rämö I, Hoare B; European network for Health Technology Assessment (EUnetHTA). Guidelines for future research in constraint-induced movement therapy for children with unilateral cerebral palsy: an expert consensus. *Dev. Med. Child Neurol.* 2014;56(2):125-37.

In: Handbook on Cerebral Palsy
Editor: Harold Yates

ISBN: 978-1-63321-852-9
© 2014 Nova Science Publishers, Inc.

Chapter 6

Assessment of Postural Control and Functionality in Children with Cerebral Palsy: Possibilities and Relevance

Cristina dos Santos Cardoso de Sá[*]
and Raquel de Paula Carvalho
Department of Human Movement Sciences,
Federal University of São Paulo, UNIFESP, SP, Brazil

Abstract

Cerebral palsy (CP) is one of the most common causes of chronic disability in childhood, with an incidence of 2 to 2.5 in 1000 live births in developed countries. In Brazil, 24.5 million people have some kind of disability, including CP. Cerebral palsy is group of permanent disorders related to mobility and postural development due to a non-progressive disturbance in immature brain during fetal period or childhood. Brain abnormalities associated with CP may also contribute to sensory, cognitive, communication and behavioral disorders including motor disabilities and spasticity. Children and adolescents with CP have lower level of physical activity than those with typical development. Problems in motor control can reduce the amount of movements performed by children resulting in a lack of experience with motor activities, which would delay concept formation about sensation and motor activity, sociality. The capability of maintaining postural control is essential for performing Activities of Daily Living (ADL's). In accordance with the level of motor function, children with CP have different degrees of trunk control and level of functionality that affect their performance in ADL's mainly when the upper limbs are affected. Therefore, CP can impose many limitations on social activity and participation. There is an ongoing effort to develop assessment methods that are suitable for people with CP to provide relevant information about their postural control and level of functionality to clinical and research proposes.

---

[*] E-mail: cristina.sa@uol.com.br.

The proposal of this chapter is to introduce the relevant aspects and evaluation protocols about postural control and functionality in children with CP.

Introduction

Cerebral palsy (CP) is one of the most common causes of chronic disability in childhood, with an incidence of 2 to 2.5 in 1000 live births in developed countries (Richards; Malouin, 2013). In Brazil, 24.5 million people have some kind of disability, including CP (Alves et al., 2004).

According to Rosenbaum et al. (2007), "Cerebral Palsy describes a group of permanent disorders of the development of movement and posture, causing activity limitations that are attributed to non-progressive disturbances that occurred in the developing fetal or infant brain. The motor disorders of CP are often accompanied by disturbances of sensation, perception, cognition, comunication and behavior; by epilepsy and by secondary musculoskeletal problems". It is considered the most recent definition of CP (Richards; Malouin, 2013) and it was outcome of an International Workshop in Bethesda, MD (USA) in 2004.

The complex nature of the control system induces vulnerability for dysfunctions in adverse conditions during early life, such as a pre or perinatally acquired lesions of the brain or preterm birth (Fallang; Hadders-Algra, 2005; Van der Heide; Hadders Algra, 2005; Woollacott, 2005). However, the consequences of a lesion for developing brain depend on developmental stage of the infant at time of insult, site and size of the lesion, animal species, exposure to chemical substances before and after the insult, and environmentally induced experience. It transpired that each stage, each neural system, has specific vulnerabilities and resources of resilience to cope with the effects of an early lesion (Hadders-Algra, 2011).

In cerebral palsy, the lesion occurs the period in which the child has rapid pace of development, compromising the process of skill acquisition. This lesion in the brain reduced the motor repertorie and it may interfere with the function, impairing the performance of activities commonly performed by children with normal development. In the children with CP the best motor solutions may differ from those of typicall developing child.

The classification of the CP can be done in several ways. Classifications may include different types, distribution and severity of motor impairments and associated impairments, and further the time and location of the lesion, etiology, and symptomatology. Although there are many types of classification, Rosenbaum et al. (2007) propose four major dimensions to classify CP: (1) motor abnormalities, (2) accompanying impairments, (3) anatomical and neuro-imaging findings, and (4) causations and timing of the lesion.

The motor disorders consist the nature and predominant motor disorder and functional motor skills. In relation to nature and type of predominant motor disorder, CP children are classified according to muscle tone and / or presence of involuntary movements such as spastic CP, dyskinetic CP (with the following subtypes: dystonic, athetoid and choreoathetosis), and ataxic CP. When more than one disorder is present, the recommendation is to classify the type of tone or prevailing movement and report other secondary disorders (Cans, 2000; Rethlefsen; Ryan; Kay, 2010).

In CP spastic there is increased tone, characterized as spasticity, which is defined as the increase in muscular resistence during passive movement which is speed dependent. This type of CP results from a lesion in the motor cortex, showing symptoms of pyramidal lesion, and it is a constituent of the upper motor neuron syndrome. Other signs and symptoms such as hyperreflexia, clonus, positive Babinski sign, and muscle weakness are also present (Rosenbaum et al., 2007).

Child with dyskinetic CP shows involuntary features that overlap with voluntary motor acts, and abnormal postures secondary automatic motor incoordination and impaired regulation of muscle tone resulting from the simultaneous activation of agonist and antagonist musculature. The motor impairment is characterized by the presence of extrapyramidal symptoms and associated with lesions in the basal ganglia. The most commonly seen dyskinetic movements are: dystonia, chorea and athetosis (Sanger et al., 2010). In dystonia, there are involuntary muscle contractions that cause repetitive movements and abnormal postures that characterize a fluctuation of extensor tone of the trunk (axial). In chorea there is a continuous and discrete random sequence or fragmented movements of motion. In athetosis there are slow and continuous involuntary movements that prevent the maintenance of a stable posture; these movements predominate in distal segments and face.

Ataxic CP is the rarest form and it is resulted from lesions in the cerebellum. There are changes in balance and motor coordination with muscular hypotonia (Rosenbaum et al., 2007).

In relation to the functional motor ability, which refers to gravity of neuromotor impairment, CP can be classified as mild, moderate or severe (O'Shea, 2008). However, it is considered a subjective classification and researchers recommend another way to classify the functional level in CP that is the Gross Motor Function Classification System (GMFCS) (Palisano et al., 1997). The GMFCS is a standardized, clinically applicable system that was valid and reliable. It is based on voluntary movement initiated, particularly emphasizing sitting (trunk control) and ambulatory abilities (Palisano et al., 1997). Levels of motor function encompass functional limitations, the need for assistive technology, including assistive mobility devices (walkers, crutches and canes) and wheelchair accessible, and quality of movement that is considered a lesser extent. GMFCS classifies gross motor function in five levels according to the age and defines the most severe, levels IV-V, and the mildest, levels I-II levels, with level III being intermediate. The level I is the one with greater freedom of movement and level V shows the greater severity and degree of dependency. The GMFCS has been translated into many languages and widely adopted internationally and it has been expanded and revised to include an age band from 12 to 18 years. This GMFCS version emphasizes the impact that environmental and personal factors may have on methods of mobility (Palisano et al., 2008).

It is also recommended to apply The Manual Ability Classification Systems (MACS), similar method to GMFCS that has been developed to classify the ability of children with CP to handle objects (Eliasson et al., 2006). In MACS, regardless of age, children who are able to easily manipulate objects are classified into level I and those that manipulate objects with lower quality belong to II. Children in level III manipulate objects with difficulty needing aid or adaptation of activity and the IV are those that perform manual tasks with limited success, requiring continuous supervision. At level V children are classified as severely compromised in manual skills, requiring total assistance.

The results of applying the function-based classification systems is that GMFCS and MACS have helped change the mind of the rehabilitation team, leading them to focus on what the individual child can do. GMFCS and MACS can help direct rehabilitation team to ensure care appropriate to the level of function and age.

In relation to classification based on accompanying impairments, it is described impairments that affect daily life activities and produce great activities limitations, such as epilepsy, hearing and visual problems, cognitive and attentional deficits, musculoskeletal disorders and emotional issues (Rosenbaum et al., 2007; Haslam et al., 2013).

In anatomical and neuro-imaging findings classification, CP is usually classified into topography-based sutypes: quadriparesis, diparesis, hemiparesis, which often result from various insults to different areas within the developing nervous system, occurring in uteri, during childbirth, or after birth during the first 3 years of life (Marret; Vanhulle; Laquerriere, 2013). However, it is adopt by Surveillance of Cerebral Palsy in Europe (SCPE) a differentiation between unilateral (hemiparesis) and bilateral (quadriparesis, diparesis) motor involvement. It is also recommended to apply this classification in association with GMFCS and MACS (Rosenbaum et al., 2007).

Causations and timing of the lesion refer to adverse events in the prenatal, perinatal and postnatal life that cause CP. There are many factors including intrauterine infection, abnormal intrauterine growth, chromosome abnormalities, central nervous system malformations, alcohol, tobacco, or drug use by pregmant, maternal infections, as some prenatal factors. Cerebral hypoxia and ischemia, prematurity, childbirth complications, and intracranial hemorrhage are examples of perinatal facts. During postnatal life, infant may have periventricular leukomalacia, hyperbilirubinemia, stoke, brain infection, prolonged mechanical ventilation, and metabolic disorders (Blitz et al., 1997; Neville et al., 2013).

Postural Control: Typical Child

To facilitate understanding of the control of posture and balance, imagine a child throwing the ball to his father in the garden of his house. The child is performing this task in a standing position, picks up the ball on the ground, holds it at head height with the shoulder abducted and elbow flexed at 90°, and propels the ball toward his father. Apparently, throwing the ball is a simple task to be performed, but it involves both the ability to recover stability as the ability to anticipate and move in a way that would avoid the instability.

From the foregoing, tasks performance change in accordance with an active organism, the environment, and action possibilities. From a constraint-led perspective, the development of action is generally brought about by changes within and between the constraints imposed upon the organism–environment system (Newell, 1986). Therefore, it is important to know the task and environment specificitiy to understand the human postural control during a task performance. Postural control also requires the coupling between perception (integration of sensory information to analyze the body position and movement in space) and action (ability to produce forces to control positioning systems of the body) resulted from a complex interaction between neural and musculoskeletal systems.

Postural control involves controlling the position of the body in space to achieve the twin goals of orientation and stability (Hadders-Algra, 2005; Shumway-Cook; Woollacott, 2007).

Postural orientation is defined as the ability to maintain an appropriate relationship between body segments and between body and the environment to perform a particular task. Postural stability is the ability to keep the balance, i.e., the ability to maintain the body center of mass within the limits of stability. When the body is stable balanced, it is called static equilibrium; when it is in steady motion, it is called dynamic equilibrium.

It is important to know how and why postural control develops to understanding it. How postural control develops in children?

Postural control is an essential part of motor development. In the first years of life the child develops an incredible repertoire of skills, learning to control head, sit, crawl, walk, jump, run, climb stairs and handle objects in many ways. The acquisition of these skills requires the maturation of postural activity, aiming to sustain the primary movement. This is the first step to determine the most appropriate therapeutic approach to achieve and / or improve the skills associated (Hadders-Algra, 2005; Shumway-Cook; Woollacott, 2007; Van Balen et al., 2012).

According to Forssber and Hirschfeld (1994), there are two leves of postural control. The first level (basic level) deals with the generation of direction-specific adjustments meaning that dorsal muscles are primarily activated when the body sways forward, whereas ventral muscles are primarily activated when the body sways backward. In the basic level, the nervous system explores its repertoires of possibilities, characterizing primary variability. The borders of the repertoires are determined by genetic instructions. Exploration of the repertoires results in abundant variation in motor behaviour and in a wealth of self-produced afferent information. Therefore, the afferent information is used to explore the motor repertoire and is not used for adaptation of motor behavior to specific situations (Van Balen et al., 2012).

The ability to recruit directionally appropriate muscle is an essential factor for balance. One month infants already show direct-specific postural adjustments (Forssber; Hirschfeld, 1994) and postural control changes systematically during first six months of life when early behaviors are emergent, decreasing complexity (Dusing et al., 2013). At 1 month of age direction-specific postural adjustments in sitting are present in 70 to 85% of the time when a sudden perturbation was applied, and at 6 month of age is over 90% (Herdberg et al., 2004; Herdberg et al., 2005). However, 1-month-old infants respond only 10% of the time with the complete pattern while 6-month-old infants respond in 50% (Graff-Peters et al., 2007), showing great variation in postural control during early development. There is a functional transition period around 3 months of age when minimum recruitment of postural muscles was found; after that, there is an improvement on postural control which it was related to the acquision of spontaneous motor behavior, such as reaching movements (Herdberg et al., 2005).

The second level involves the adaptation of the direction-specific adjustments according to postural task (Hadders-Algra, 2005; van Balen et al., 2012). In young children, the direction-specific muscles adjustments is characterized by variantion, that involve temporal ordering of muscle activity, recruitment of antagonist muscles and degree of muscle contraction (Graaf-Peters et al., 2007). In relation to recruitment ordering of muscles involved in postural control, in early development infants show preference for a top-down recruitment (Graaf-Peters et al., 2007). This preference is evident at 4 months when head stabilization is important for successful reaching (Hadders-Algra, 2008). Therefore, head control is an important frame of reference for postural control in young children (van Balen et al., 2012).

At 8-10 months of age, the preference is a bottom-up recruitment indicating that the focus of control moves towards the lower trunk (Hadders-Algra, 2008). Nevertheless, the main characteristic of recruitment order is variation with a mixture of top-down, bottom-up and mixed recruitment (Graaf-Peters et al. 2007; Van Balen et al., 2012). The co-activity of antagonistic muscle is present only between 6 and 24 months in specific situations, such as external perturbation to backwards or reaching (Hadders-Algra et al., 1998; Van der Heide et al., 2003). In relation to degree of muscle contraction, the ability to modulate postural adjustments in simple tasks, such as during reaching movements in different velocities, emerges around 8 months of age (Van der Fits et al., 1999).

On the second level, infants develop the ability to adapt postural activity to the specifics of the situation (Forssber; Hirschfeld, 1994). The afferent information is involved in exploration and trial-and-error experiences, which are used in the selection of appropriate movement strategies to each situation. The selection of appropriate strategies implies in mapping individual senses that precedes the mapping of multiple senses creating internal representations necessary for the coordinated postural ability. The motor strategies involve the combination of independent muscles, although associated in units called muscle synergies (Horak; Nashner, 1986; Graaf-Peters et al. 2007; Van Balen et al., 2012).

In order to maintain balance, the body performs continuous postural adjustments. During a voluntary movement, the body tends to destabilize, and therefore changes of posture (adjustments) before the execution of the movement itself, in order to minimize and anticipate the consequences of actions occur, and thereby avoid the loss of balance. Beside, the body is able to recover balance if it was lost in consequence of actions. These adjustments are characterized as anticipatory and compensatory postural adjustments.

Anticipatory postural adjustment (APA) can be defined as the activation or inhibition of the musculature of the trunk and lower limbs to minimize the negative consequences of an expected postural imbalance (Santos et al., 2010). It is pre-programmed actions voluntarily initiated and centrally triggered. APA depends on the potential of the expected disturbance of intrinsic properties for the performance of voluntary action and fear of falling, and the integration between the visual, vestibular and somatosensory systems to anticipate the outcome of the action and act on possible fixes (Aruin, 2003).

In the APA, there is a pre-activation of muscle synergies associated with disturbance. This type of adjustment is characterized by its adaptability to task conditions. The more complex the task, the more APA lantency, or the complexity of the task influence on latency of postural response. Another characteristic of this type of adjustment is to reduce the latency of the postural muscles associated with adjustment repetition of the movement (Nashner et al., 1979).

The emergence of APA is at 12-14 months of age (Hadders-Algra, 2010). Anticipatory visiomotor behavior increases at 15-18 months when dorsal and ventral postural muscles activion were analysed 200ms before the onset of deltoid during a reaching task; however, it was not observed when a window of 100ms before the onset was analysed (Van der Fits et al., 1999; van Balen et al., 2012). The development of strategies of movement is noticeable from 6 months of life, and it is more striking at about of 9-12 months. However, similar to the pattern reaches an adult at about 7 - 10 years of age (Shumway-Cook; Woollacott, 2007).

During locomotion, infants under two years of age present pattern different from that shown by adults, characterized by increased variability in this pattern of anticipatory adjustment setting (Schmitz, 2006). The observation of postural responses in children from 4 to 9 years revealed that anticipatory adjustments increase with age, and this increase is accompanied by increased consistency in the kinematic pattern of postural responses.

Compensatory postural adjustment (CPA) is another strategy that the postural control system employs to maintain system stability. It is triggered by a sensory stimulus available and unpredictable and depends on environmental conditions. In other words, the CPA restores postural control after an imbalance happened (Montgomery; Connoly, 2002). CPA responses depends on the direction, magnitiude and preditability of the perturbation, involvement in a second task, instruction that something is going to happen and dimensions of base of support (Santos et al., 2010).

There are three basic coordination patterns of CPA to remain postural stability in standing, called equilibrium strategies. For displacements in the anteroposterior direction, three strategies are known: hip, ankle and stepping strategies. In the medial-lateral direction, there is the strategy of shifting weight (Shumway-Cook; Woollacott, 2007). Chidren aged between 5 and 13 years used all strategies to maintain balance control in a quiet stance with opened and closed eyes. However, they used hip protraction/retraction and body transverse synergies, with minimal use of ankle control, to recover balance when it was lost in excessive sway (Ferdjallah et al., 2002).

A major difference between CPAs and APAs is the temporal patterns of postural muscle activities. Postural muscle activities in CPA are observed after postural perturbations. On the other hand, postural muscles in APA are activated before postural perturbations, suggesting that APAs associated with voluntary movements are controlled by centrally preprogrammed motor commands (Friedli et al., 1984; Horak et al., 1984, Horak; Macpherson, 1996).

Summarizing, the development of postural control is a fundamental part of the development of essential skills, such as handling and locomotion. This is best characterized as a continuous development of sensory systems and multiple motor systems manifested the behavioral point of view in a broken and sequential progression of motor milestones. Strategies acquired for the sensation of movement can be associated with an apparent regression in behavior, as the child enters new strategies to their motor repertoire.

It is worth remembering, that not all systems that contribute to the emergence of postural control simultaneously develop, and at the same pace. The components that limit the development restrict the speed in which an independent behavior arises. Thus, the emergence of postural control waits for the slower development of the essential component.

Postural Control: Child with Cerebral Palsy

Postural control develops differently in children with and without CP. In typical children, the development of postural control improves with age; in children with CP, it depends on the severity of the condition. (Rose et al., 2002).

In typical children, the development of functional skills tends to follow a gradual linearity; in children with CP this sequence of acquisitions tends to be less uniform. Probably the difficulties in motor control influence the functional performance of children with CP differently the pattern shown by typical children (Mancini et al., 2002). Primary impairments in CP include loss of selective mucles control, abnormal muscle tone, balance impairment and motor weakness (Gross et al., 2013). Because postural control depends on interaction between neural and musculoskeletal systems, it is clear that these children will have problems in development of postural control. There are several changes in postural control of children with CP. For example, during reaching, children with CP show direction-specific postural djustments (Van der Heide et al., 2004) and during standing they show abnormalities in muscle timing and increased levels of coativation (Woollacott et al., 1998).

Children with CP may have different levels of functionality, clinical presentation, such as tonus and unilateral or bilateral impairment, and profile of brain injury. The higher level of GMFCS, the worse postural control (Rosenbaum et al., 2007). Infants with spastic hemiplegia, with mild motor impairment, showed direction-specific adjustments since 15 months during reaching task but they were not able to modulate EMG-amplitude until 18 months when the velocity of reaching was changed (Hadders-Algra et al.; 1999). Nevertheless, in severe bilateral spastic CP with high level in GMFCS, the infant was not able to adjust postural activity to task-specific conditions neither to show direct-specific postural adjustment (Hadders-Algra et al.; 1999). However, Bigongiari et al. (2011) did not find linear relationship between GMFCS and postural adjustments when it was analysed trunk control during a reaching task in sitting in children with CP aged between 7 and 11 years. Additionally, hemiparetic spastic children with CP may have underestimated their lower extremity skill if their motor prognosis is based only on GMFCS level; diparectir spastic children may have their lower extremity skill overestimated (Damiano et al., 2006).

According to two leves of postural control proposed by Forssber and Hirschfeld (1994), CP children with mild impairment are able to generate direction-specific adjustments, i.e., they show the first level of postural control (Graaf-Peters et al., 2007; Girolami et al., 2011). However, CP children with severe impairments show problems to recruit direction-specific adjustments (Hadders-Algra et al.; 1999; Graaf-Peters et al., 2007).

In relation to the second level, children with CP have not the same performance than their peers with typical development. Atypical development is characterized by reduced variation (Hadders-Algra, 2010). Infants with disabilities have consistently reduced complexity or increased repeatability in postural control strategies (Dusing; Harbourne, 2010) that may result in reduced ability to alter postural control strategies under different conditions (Dusing et al., 2012). Multiple forms of disorganization of postural control were found in CP. Children with CP showed preference for a top-down recruitment in different conditions as sitting and standing (Neshner; McCollum, 1985; Woollacott et al., 1998; Van der Heide et al., 2004). There is high amount of antagonistic co-ativiations when an external perturbation is imposed in sitting and standing positions (Woollacott et al., 1998; 2005). These children have reduced or absent capacity to module the degree of muscle contractions according to specifics situations (Bigongiari et al., 2011; Girolami et al., 2011; Woollacott et al., 2005).

Typical development of postural adjustments is characterized by variation and an increasing ability to adapt the variable repertoire to the specifics of the situation. The latter is facilitated by an increasing role of anticipatory mechanisms in the second half of infancy. Atypically developing infants may have a reduced repertoire and usually have difficulties in adapting postural adjustments (Hadders-Algra, 2013).

Children with CP in general have the ability to generate direction-specific adjustments, but they show a delayed development in the capacity to recruit direction-specific adjustments in tasks with a mild postural challenge (Graaf-Peters et al., 2007)

The APA during reaching in sitting posture in typically developing children is consistently present from 15 months of age onwords. In children with CP, the APA during reaching while sitting is variable in their development. Children level IV and V of GMFCS outcome due to CP show visible deficits in postural control. Their motor and functional capacities need to be improved for the maintenance of standing and sitting position through the head and trunk stabilization and aligment (Liao et al., 2003). Another study with CP spastic diparetic suggests that lower leg muscles play a minor role in APAs in individuals with spastic diparesis. In addition, it is likely that these individuals have difficulty modulating anticipatory postural muscle activity with changes in the degree of postural perturbation. In the individuals with CP spastic diparetic both of these abilities are impaired (Tomita et al., 2011).

In standing position, Girolami et al. (2011) verified that diparetic and hemiparetic spastic children are able to generate direction-specific APA in trunk and lower limbs muscle when performing bilateral shoulder flexion or extension. Diparetic children had higher baseline muscle activity and lower amplitude of APA than hemiparetic and typical developing peers.

Studies reporting CPA in children with CP suggest that CPA is reduced in children with both spastic hemiparesis and diparesis. This reduction includes a longer time to stabilize balance and more movement of the center of pressure during balance recovery. The neuromuscular response characteristics contribuing to these balance constraints include a delayed onset of muscle contractions, a desorganized timing of muscle response (proximal muscles activated before distal muscles) and an increased coactivation the antagonist muscles with agonists (Donker et al., 2008; Tomita et al., 2011), confirming problems in adaptation of postural control under different situations.

Atypical alignment and tonus in plantiflexor ankle muscles is a commum characteristic in children with spastic CP and result in a poor control at the ankle. It is also commom to find children with contractures of the hip, knee, and ankle muscles that may contribute to atypical postures in sitting and standing. Because ankle and hip control synergies are altered in children with CP, they may prefere to use the mechanism of hip protraction/retraction that requires less muscular effort than ankle control to remain the balance (Ferdjallah et al., 2002). Therefore, children with CP can not use properly equilibrium strategies to maintain balance.

Children with CP encounter problems during static upright standing in altered sensory environments and when rapid weight shifts during standing are required, either in gait initiation or in reaction to external perturbations (Nashner et al. 1983; Woollacott; Burtner 1996; Rose et al. 2002; Stackhouse et al. 2007). Postural control is the result of interection between sensory information and motor action and children with CP have motor impairments that may be accomplish by sensorial disorders. To verify sensory and motor coopling in children with CP, Barela et al. (2011) analysed the balance in 8 to 16-year-old children with spastic hemiplegia during stand upright position in a moving room, i. e., in a room where walls moving independent of the floor in specific velocities and amplitude. Individuals with CP were able to coopling body sway with visual information provided by moving room. However, they showed higher amplitude and more variable body sway in relation to tipically developmental participants when visual information was manipulated by moving room. In CP, they also demonstrate adaptive sensory motor coopling properties by down-weighting body sway when room amplitude and velocity increased but with lower magnitude than their typical developing peers.

Summarizing, a variety of problems can contribute to changes in postural control in children with CP. These changes may occur due to impairment of motor and / or sensory components of postural control resulting from brain injury, and even worsen due to secondary brain injury musculoskeletal problems. Thus, the differences in the changes in postural control may result from variability in the type, location, extent of brain injury, and when the injury occurred.

Clinical Assessment of the Postural Control

To determine the ability of balance in children with neuromotor disabilities and to assess the effectiveness of therapeutic approaches in rehabilitation processes there are a number of evaluation systems. These assessment tools measure a wide range of balance functions, from sitting through walking abilities, and incorporate evaluation of trunk control as one of the subtests within the assessment (Butler et al., 2010).

Gross Motor Function Measure (GMFM)

The GMFM is a measure designed to assess change in gross motor function for children aged 5 months to 16 years with CP. There are two versions of the GMFM - the original 88-item measure (GMFM-88) and the more recent 66-item GMFM (GMFM-66). Items on the GMFM-88 span the spectrum from activities in lying and rolling up to walking, running and jumping skills. The GMFM-66 is comprised of a subset of the 88 items identified (through Rasch analysis) as contributing to the measure of gross motor function in children with CP. The GMFM-66 provides detailed information on the level of difficulty of each item thereby providing much more information to assist with realistic goal setting (Rusell et al., 1993; Finch et al., 2002).

GMFM scores of a sample of over 650 Ontario children with CP with varying GMFCS levels have been used to create five Motor Growth Curves. These curves describe the patterns of motor development of this sample of children, grouped by GMFCS level, and are similar to the growth charts that are used to follow the height and weight of children as they grow.

The GMFM include items for quiet sitting which include measures of trunk control but do not differentiate between different levels of trunk control. The dimensions do GMFM are: a) lying and rolling; b) sitting; c) crawling and kneeling; d) standing; and e) walking, running and jumping.

Chailey Levels of Ability

The Chailey Levels of Ability was established to assess motor ability in children and young adults with low levels of physical ability. The instrument provides a means of recording change in postural ability in children with movement disorders, and it is a validated assessment tool. The method assesses a child's posture in each of five positions – lying supine (face up), lying prone (face down), floor sitting, box sitting and standing. Each of these postures has between six and eight descriptors with Level 1 being greatest abnormality and asymmetry and the top level or score representing normal. A child must achieve all of the components for a level before he or she is said to have reached that level. Thus, a child with one body area that is resistant to change will not progress to the next level (Pountney et al., 1999).

The Chailey levels of ability as the GMFM include measures of trunk control but do not differentiate between different levels of trunk control.

Seated Postural Control Measure (SPCM)

The Seated Postural Control Measure (SPCM) has been created as an outcome measure of adaptive seating interventions. It is designed to measure change in postural control as a result of adaptive seating intervention. As this research version of the SPCM is not validated, its responsiveness to detect clinically significant change has not yet been determined. It is available as a research edition for use by investigators interested in its measurement capabilities (Fife et al., 1991).

The two domains of sitting behaviours measured are static postural alignment and functional movement. The alignment section consists of 22 graphically depicted items that measure the alignment of each body segment. Deviation away from neutral alignment is scored on a 4 point ordinal scale. The function section is comprised of 12 functional movement items which examine the achievement of seated functions. Items are scored on a 4 point ordinal scale reflecting increasing task achievement.

The SPCM includes assessment of pelvic, trunk and head inclination, but does not examine subunits of trunk control.

Spinal Alignment and Range of Motion Measure (SAROMM)

The Spinal Alignment and Range of Motion Measure (SAROMM) is intended to be administered to people with a diagnosis of CP. The SAROMM has two following sections: 1) spinal alignment and 2) range of motion and muscle extensibility. In both of these sections, the protocol begins with observation of the person's alignment and posture. If "normal" or "optimal" spinal alignment is not observed (i.e., the first picture for each of the first four items), the person is given up to three opportunities to actively correct to assume these positions. If these positions are assumed, a score of "zero" is given for these items. If the person cannot attain normal alignment through active movement, passive correction is conducted and the severity of the limitation is scored according to specific criteria which are subsequently described. For the range of motion items, if a person demonstrates posturing, passive range of motion is conducted and severity of limitation is also rated according to criteria that follow: determination of "End Range" (if the person is unable to actively correct or demonstrates characteristic posturing) (Chen et al., 2013).

The SAROMM evaluates the child's ability to actively or passively achieve alignment of the cervical, thoracic or lumbar spine, but tests only assess static (steady state) and active (APA) balance control, through evaluation measures of ability to hold a particular posture or to reach for an object while in that posture, and do not include the ability to recover balance (CPA).

Segmental Assessment of Trunk Control (SATCo)

The Segmental Assessment of Trunk Control (SATCo) provides a systematic method of assessing discrete levels of trunk control in children with motor disabilities (Butler et al., 2010). This assessment include tests of (1) static or steady state balance, examining the child's ability to maintain a steady posture without support, (2) active or anticipatory balance adjustments, examining the child's ability to balance while reaching, and (3) reactive balance, examining the child's ability to maintain or regain balance following a brief perturbation, such as a translation of the base of support. The SATCO allows determining the different levels of trunk control (Head Control, Upper Thoracic Control, Mild Thoracic Control, Lower Thoracic Control, Upper Lumbar Control, Lower Lumbar Control or Full Trunk Control).

This systhematic method of assessing is important beause the children with neuromotor disability development of sitting balance is delayed and, depending on the level of disability, children may continue to show constraints on sitting balance throughout their lives with some never gaining independent control of the trunk and head (Brogren et al., 2001; Carlberg; Hadders-Algra, 2005).

The study of Carvalho et al. (2014) aimed to identify the relation between level of trunk control and upper limb function of children with CP in different GMFCS levels. Twelve children with CP aged between 5 and 13 years were classified using GMFCS and evaluated using Segmental Assessment of Trunk Control (SATCo) and Quality of Upper Extremity Skills Test (QUEST). The QUEST objectively evaluate movement patterns and hand function in children with cerebral palsy. This instrument is a reliable and valid measure for assessing the quality of upper limb movements in children with CP within the functional context (DeMatteo et al., 1993). The results indicated that there were moderate-strong correlation between GMFCS level and total score of Quest, and trunk control level and total score of QUEST, and strong correlation between GMFCS and trunk control levels. Therefore, total score of QUEST and trunk control levels tend to increase when GMFCS level decrease and total score of QUEST tend to increase when trunk control level increases. The authors concluded the function of upper limbs depends on trunk control level and the level of impairment has influence on trunk control and upper limbs function in children with CP (Carvalho et al., 2014).

It is noteworthy, the development of evaluation protocols to children with CP to measure their ability, and the degree of independence that they can achieve, is clearly important, for children with CP have predominant motor impairment, with different degrees of trunk control and level of functionality that affect their performance in Activities of Daily Living (ADL's) mainly when the upper limbs are affected.

Instrumentation for Assessment of Postural Control

Evaluation of postural control can be done in various ways. We do not intend to write a review about biomechanics instrumentation to assess postural control. We are going to describe the methods used more often in researchs about postural control in children.

The measuring of body center of mass (CoM) and center of pressure (CoP) has been extensively used to assess postural sway. The CoP is an indirect measure of postural sway and it is evaluated through force platform. It is defined as location of a single resultant force exerced at the point where the resultant moment is zero. The net of CoP is a result of both antero-posterior and medio-lateral planes (Roberson et al., 2004; Barela; Duarte, 2011). Amplitude, area, length, velocity and frequency of CoP sway and its components antero-posterios and medial-lateral are examples of effective parameters for monitoring body sway. CoM is defined as a balance point of humans' mass. It is a point where the distributed mass sums zero. The estimation of CoM requires inverse dynamic analysis of a computerized multi-joint modern by kinematic measurements using an integrated motion analysis system (Ferdjallah et al., 2002).

To assess postural adjustments is an important way to understand postural development and control. Electromyography (EMG) is an evaluating tool to measure and record the electrical activity of muscles. Frequency and amplitude of EMG are important parameters that indicate firing rate and magnitude of muscle activity (Roberson et al., 2004). EMG amplitudes are scaled to activation levels recorded either during an isometric maximal voluntary contraction (MVC) or a specified steady-state sub maximal contraction (Felthman et al., 2010). Performing maximal contraction may be very difficult for children with CP because of their motor and sensorial impairments, invalidating the method of recording MVC. Sub-maximal contraction does not provide a valid solution (Felthman et al., 2010). A suggestion to solve this problem is to analyse EMG with kinematic data in children com CP to determine the beginng and ending of movement (Felthman et al., 2010; Girolami et al., 2011; van der Heide et al., 2005).

Kinematics is concern about describing and quantifying linear and angular positions of body and their time derivations (Roberson et al., 2004). It is a useful tool to analyse body sway trough a marked positioned at 8th thoracic vertebra to provide information about the participants' trunk sway (Godoi; Barela, 2008) in specific situations, such as in standing with opened and closed eyes and in a moving room.

Final Considerations

Cerebral palsy is group of permanent disorders related to mobility and postural development due to a non-progressive disturbance in immature brain during fetal period or childhood. Brain abnormalities associated with CP may also contribute to sensory, cognitive, communication and behavioral disorders including motor disabilities and spasticity. Assessment of postural adjustments is an important way to understand the postural development and control in typical and atypical children.

There are many evaluation systems to determine the ability of balance in children with neuromotor disabilities and to assess the effectiveness of therapeutic approaches in rehabilitation processes. These assessment tools measure a wide range of balance functions and control, from sitting through walking abilities, and some of them incorporate evaluation of trunk control.

References

Alves ACM, Coelho ZAC, Figueiredo EM, Mancini MC, Sampaio RF, Schaper C, Tirado MGA, et al. Classification of motor function and functional performance in children with cerebral palsy. *Braz. J. Phys. Ther.* 2004, 8:253-260.

Aruin AS. The effect of changes in the body configuration on anticipatory postural adjustments. *Mot. Contr.* 2003; 7:264-277.

Barela AMF, Duarte M. Use of force plate for acquisition of kinetic data during human gait. *Braz. J. Mot. Beh.* 2011; 6:56-61.

Barela JA, Focks GMJ, Hilgeholt T, Barela AMF, Carvalho RP, Salvesbergh GJP. Perception-action and adaptation in postural control of children and adolescents with cerebral palsy. *Res. Dev. Disabil.* 2011; 32:2075-2083.

Bigongiari A, Souza FA, Franciulli PM, Neto SER, Araujo RC, Mochizuki L. Anticipatory and compensatory postural adjustments in sitting in children with cerebral palsy. *Hum. Mov. Sc.* 2011; 30:648-657.

Blitz RK, Wechtel RC, Blackmon I. Neurodevelopmental outcome of extremely low birth weight infants in Maryland. *Md. Med. J.* 1997; 46:18-24.

Brogren E, Forssberg H, Hadders-Algra M. Influence of two different sitting positions on postural adjustments in children with spastic diplegia. *Dev. Med. Child Neurol.* 2001;43:534–546.

Butler P, Saavedra S, Sofranac M, Jarvis S, Woollacott M. Refinement, Reliability and Validity of the Segmental Assessment of Trunk Control (SATCo). *Pediatr. Phys. Ther.* 2010 ; 22(3): 246–257.

Cans C. Surveillance of cerebral palsy in Europe: a collaboration of cerebral palsy surveys and registers. Surveillance of Cerebral Palsy in Europe (SCPE). *Dev. Med. Child Neurol.* 2000, 42:816-824.

Carlberg EB, Hadders-Algra M. Postural dysfunction in children with cerebral palsy: some implications for therapeutic guidance. *Neural Plast.* 2005;12:221–228.

Carvalho RP, Gomes CS, Sá CSC. Relation between trunk control, upper limbs function and GMFCS level in children with cerebral palsy. *Inspiring Infancy conference* 2014: 31-32.

Chen CL, Wu KP, Liu WY, Cheng HY, Shen IH, Lin KC Validity and clinimetric properties of the Spinal Alignment and Range of Motion Measure in children with cerebral palsy. *Dev. Med. Child Neurol.* 2013; 55:745-50.

Damiano D, Abel M, Romness M, Oeffinger D, Tylkowski C, Gorton G, Bagley A, Nicholson D, Barnes D, Calmes J, Kryscio R, Rogers S. Comparing functional profiles of children with hemiplegic and diplegic cerebral palsy in GMFCS Levels I and II: Are separate classifications needed? *Dev. Med. Child Neurol.* 2006; 48:797-803.

Dematteo C, Law MC, Russell DJ, Pollock N, Rosenbaum PL, Walter SD. The reliability and validity of the quality of upper extremity skills test. *Phys. Occup. Ther. Pediatr.* 1993; 13:1–18.

Donker SF, Ledebt A, Roerdink M, Savelsbergh GJ, Beek PJ. Children with cerebral palsy exhibit greater and more regular postural sway than typically developing children. *Ex. Brain Res.* 2008; 184:363-70.

Dusing SC, Harbourne RT. Variability in postural control during infancy: implications for development, assessment, and intervention. *Phys. Ther.* 2010; 90:1838-49.

Dusing SC, Thacker LR, Stergiou N, Galloway JC. Early complexity supports development of motor behaviors in the first months of life. *Dev. Psychobiol.* 2013; 55:404-14.

Eliasson AC, Krumlinde-Sundholm L, Rösblad B, Beckung E, Arner M, Ohrvall AM, Rosenbaum P. The Manual Ability Classification System (MACS) for children with cerebral palsy: scale development and evidence of validity and reliability. *Dev. Med. Child Neurol.* 2006; 48:549-54.

Fallang B, Hadders-Algra M. Postural behavior in children born preterm. *Neural Plast.* 2005,12: 103-110.

Feltham MG, Ledebt A, Deconinck FJa, Savelsbergh GJP. Assessment of neuromuscular activation of the upper limbs in children with spastic hemiparectic cerebral palsy during dynamical task. *J. Eletromyogr. Kinesiol.* 2010; 20:448-456.

Ferdjallah M, Harris GF, Smith P, Wertsch JJ. Analysis of postural control synergies during quiet standing in healthy children and children with cerebral palsy. *Clin. Biomech.* 2002; 17:203-210.

Fife SE, Roxborough LA, Armstrong RW, Harris SR, Gregson JL, Field D. Development of a Clinical Measure of Postural Control for Assessment of Adaptive Seating in Children with Neuromotor Disabilities. *Phys. Ther.* 1991; 71:981-993.

Forssberg H, Hirschfeld H. Postural adjustments in sitting humans following external perturbations: muscle activity and kinematics. *Exp. Brain Res.* 1994; 97:515-27.

Friedli WG, Hallet M, Simon SR. Postural adjustments associated with rapid arm movement 1. Electromyographic data. *J. Neurol Neurosurg. Psychiatry* 47: 611–622, 1984.

Graaf-Peters VB, Bakker H, van Eykern LA, Otten B, Hadders-Algra M. Postural adjustments and reaching in 4- and 6-month-old infants: an EMG and kinematical study. *Exp. Brain Res.* 2007; 181:647-56.

Graaf-Peters VB, Blauw-Hospers CH, Dirks T, Bakker J, Bos AF, Hadders-Algra M, Development of postural control in typically developing children and children with cerebral palsy: Possibilities for intervention? *Neurosci. Biobeh. Rev.* 2007, 141-174.

Godoi D; Barela JA. Body Sway and Sensory Motor Coupling Adaptation in Children: Effects of Distance Manipulation *Dev. Psychobiol.* 2008; 50: 77–87.

Gross R, Leboeuf F, Hardouin JB, Lempereur M, Perrouin-Verbe B, Remy-Neris O, Brochard S. The influence of gait speed on co-activation in unilateral spastic cerebral palsy children. *Clin. Biomech.* 2013; 28:312-7.

Hadders-Algra M. Development of Postural Control During the First 18 Months of Life. *Neural Plasticity* 2005, 12:99-108.

Hadders-Algra M. Variation and variability: key words in human motor development. *Phys. Ther.* 2010; 90:1823-37

Hadders-Algra M. Challenges and limitations in early interventio. *Dev. Med. Child Neurol.* 2011, 53 (Suppl 4) 52-55.

Hadders-Algra, Brogren E, Forssberg H. Postural adjustments during sitting at preschool age: presence of a transient toddling phase. *Dev. Med. Child Neurol.* 1998; 40:436-47.

Hadders-Algra M, Carlberg EB. Postural control: A key issue in developmental disorders. London: Mac Keith 2008.

Hadders-Algra, M., Van Der Fits, I. B. M., Stremmelaar, E. F. and Touwen, B. C. L. Development of postural adjustments during reaching in infants with CP. *Dev. Med. Child Neurol.* 1999; 41:766–776.

Hadders-Algra M. Typical and atypical development of reaching and postural control in infancy. *Dev. Med. Child Neurol.* 2013; 55 Suppl 4:5-8.

Haslam RHA. Clinical neurological examination of infants and children. *Handb. Clin. Neurol.* 2013; 111:18-25.

Hedberg Å, Carlberg EB, Forssberg H, Algra MH. Development of postural adjustments in sitting position during the first half year of life. *Dev. Med. Child Neurol.* 2005; 47: 312–320.

Hedberg A, Forssberg H, Hadders-ALgra M. Early development of postural adjustments in sitting position: evidence for the innate origin of direction specificity. *Exp. Brain Res.* 2004;157:10-7.

Horak FB, Esselman P, Anderson ME, Lynch MK. The effects of movement velocity, mass displaced, and task certainty on associated postural adjustments made by normal and hemiplegic individuals. *J. Neurol. Neurosurg. Psychiatry* 1984; 47:1020–1028.

Horak FB, Nashner LM. Central programming of postural movements: adaptation to altered support-surface configurations. *J. Neurophysiol.* 1986; 55:1369-81.

Horak FB, Macpherson JM. Postural orientation and equilibrium. In: Handbook of Physiology. Exercise: Regulation and Integration of MultipleSystems. Neural Control of Movement. Bethesda, MD: *Am. Physiol. Soc.* 1996: 255–290.

Liao SF, Yang TF, Hsu TC, Chan RC, Wei TS. Differences in seated postural control in children with spastic cerebral palsy and children who are typically developing. *Am. J. Phys. Med. Rehabil.* 2003; 82:622-626.

Mancini MC, Fiúza PM, Rebelo JM, Magalhães LM, Coelho ZAC, Paixão ML, Gontijo APB, Fonseca ST. Comparação do desempenho de atividades funcionais em crianças com desenvolvimento normal e crianças com paralisia cerebral. *Arq. Neuropsiquiatr.* 2002; 60:446-452.

Marret S, Vanhulle C, Laquerriere A. Pathophysiology of cerebral palsy. *Handb. Clin. Neurol.* 2013; 111:169-176.

Montgomery PC, Connoly BH (eds). Clinical applications for motor control. SLACK Incorporated, New Jersey: 2002.

Nashner L, Woollacott M, Tuma G. Organizations of rapid responses to postural and locomotor-like perturbations of standing man. *Experimental Brain Res.* 1979; 36:463-476.

Nashner LM, Shumway-Cook A, Marin O. Stance posture control in select groups of children with cerebral palsy: déficits in sensory organization and muscular coordination. *Exp. Brain Res.* 1983; 49:393–409.

Nashner LM, McCollum G. The organization of human postural movements: a formal basis and experimental synthesis. *Behav. Brain Sci.* 1985; 8: 135-172.

Neville BGR. Pediatric neurology: the diagnostic process. *Handb. Clin. Neurol.* 2013; 111:27-33.

Newell KM. Constrains on the development of coordination. In M. Wade & H. T. A. Whitng (Eds.), Motor development in children: Aspects of coordination and contro. Boston: Martin Jhoff 1986: 351–360.

O'Shea TM. Diagnosis, treatment, and prevention of cerebral palsy in near-term/term infants. *Clin. Obstet. Gynecol.* 2008; 51:816-828.

Palisano RJ, Rosenbaum PL, Walter SD, Russell DJ., Wood EP, Galuppi, BE. Development and reliability of a system to classify gross motor function in children with cerebral palsy. *Dev. Med. Child Neurol.* 1997; 39:214-23.

Palisano RJ, Rosenbaum PL, Barlett D, Livingston MH. Content validity of the expanded and revised Gross Motor Function Classification System. *Dev. Med. Child Neurol.* 2008 50;744-750.

Pountney TE, Cheek L, Green E, Mulcahy C, Nelham R Content and Criterion Validation of the Chailey Levels of Ability Physiotherapy 1999; 85:410-416.

Rethlefsen SA, Ryan DD, Kay RM., Classification systems in cerebral palsy. *Orthop. Clin. North Am.* 2010; 41:457-67.

Richards Cl, Malouin F. Cerebral palsy: definition, assessment and rehabilitation. *Handb. Clin. Neurol.* 2013; 111:183-195.

Robertson DGE, Caldwell GE, Hamill J, Kamen G, Whittlesey SN. Research methods in Biomechanics. Human Kinetics, 2004.

Rose J, Wolff DR, Jones VK, Bloch DA, Oehlert JW, Gamble JG. Postural balance in children with cerebral palsy. *Dev. Med. Child Neurol.* 2002; 44:58-63.

Rosenbaum P, Paneth N, Leviton A, Goldstein M, Bax M. The definition and classification of cerebral Palsy. *Dev. Med. Child Neurol.* 2007;8-14.

Sanger TD, Chen D, Fehlings DL, Hallet M, Lang AE. Definition and Classification of hyperkinetic movements in childhood. *Mov. Disord.* 2010; 25:1538-49.

Santos MJ, Kanekar N, Aruin AS. The role anticipatory postural adjustments in compensatory control of posture: 1. electromyographic analysis. *J. Electromyogr. Kinesiol.* 2010; 20:388-397.

Schumway-Cook A, Woollacott MH. Control Motor: Translating Research into Clinical Practice. Lippincott William & Wilkins Inc. 2006.

Schmitz TJ. Gait training with assistive devices. In: O'Sullivan S, Schmitz TJ, eds. Physical rehabilitation, ed. Hardcover 2007.

Stackhouse C, Shewokis PA, Pierce SR, Smith B, McCarthy J, Tucker C. Gait initiation in children with cerebral palsy. *Gait Post* 2007, 26:301–308.

Tomita H, Fukaya Y, Ueda T, Honma S, Yamashita E. Deficits in task-specific modulation of anticipatory postural adjustments in individuals with spastic diplegic cerebral palsy. *J. Neurophysiol.* 2011; 105: 2157–2168.

Van Balen LC, Dijkstra LJ, Hadders-Algra M. Development of postural adjustments during reaching in typically developing infants from 4 to 18 months. *Exp. Brain Res.* 2012, 220:109–119.

Van der Heide JC, Otten B, van Eykern LA, Hadders-Algra M. Development of postural adjustments during reaching in sitting children. *Exp. Brain Res.* 2003; 151:32-45.

Van der Heide JC, Begger C, Fock A, Otten B, Stremmelaar EF, Van Eykern LA, Hadders-Algra M. Postural control during reaching in preterm children with cerebral palsy. *Dev. Med. Child Neurol.* 2004; 46:253-266.

Van der Heide JC, Hadders-Algra M. Postural muscle dyscoordination in children with cerebral palsy. *Neural Plast.* 2005, 12:125-132.

Van der Fits IB, Otten E, Klip AW, Van Eykern LA, Hadders-Algra M. The development of postural adjustments during reaching in 6- to 18-month-old infants. Evidence for two transitions. *Exp. Brain Res.* 1999; 126:517-28.

Woollacott MH, Burtner P. Neural and musculoskeletal contributions to the development of stance balance control in typical children and in children with cerebral palsy. *Acta Paediatr. Suppl.* 1996, 416:58–62.

Woollacott MH, Burtner P, Jensen J, Jasiewicz J, Roncesvalles N, Sveistrup H. Development of postural responses during standing in healthy children and children with spastic diplegia. *Neurosci. Biobehav. Rev.* 1998; 22:583-589.

Woollacott M. Postural dysfunction during standing and walking in children with cerebral palsy. *Neural Plast.* 2005, 12:139-148.

In: Handbook on Cerebral Palsy
Editor: Harold Yates

ISBN: 978-1-63321-852-9
© 2014 Nova Science Publishers, Inc.

Chapter 7

Improving Gait in Individuals with Cerebral Palsy: Novel Treatment Options

Luanda André Collange Grecco[1-3,*], *Natália de Almeida Carvalho Duarte*[1-2] *and Alejandra Malavera*[3]

[1]Department of Physiotherapy, Pediatric Neurosurgery Center (CENEPE) – Rehabilitation, Sao Paulo, SP, Brazil
[2]Department of Rehabilitation Sciences, Universidade Nove de Julho, Sao Paulo, SP, Brazil
[3]Laboratory of Neuromodulation, Center of Clinical Research Learning Spaulding Rehabilitation Hospital, Harvard Medical School, Boston, Massachusetts, US

Abstract

Independently of the size of the brain lesion in individuals with cerebral palsy (CP), a global reduction occurs in the activation of the central nervous system during the execution of movements[1] with changes in the excitability of the primary motor cortex and a reduction in the processing of corticospinal and somatosensory circuits. Thus, approximately 90% of individuals with CP have some degree of gait impairment stemming from neurological abnormalities that result in muscle weakness, reductions in selective motor control and postural reactions as well as changes in joint kinematics.[5] Gait pattern and independent locomotion are closely associated with the topography of the motor impairment (hemiparesis, diparesis or quadriparesis) and the level of gross motor function determined by the Gross Motor Function Classification System (GMFCS, Levels I to V).

---

[*] Corresponding author: Luanda A. C. Grecco, e-mail: luandacollange@hotmail.com, Adress: Pediatric Neurosurgery Center – Rehabilitation. Rua Diogo de Faria 775, Vila Mariana, CEP 04037-000, Sao Paulo, SP, Brazil.

A number of methods and resources are currently employed in the rehabilitation process of children and adults with CP, such as stretching and muscle strengthening exercises, spasticity control through muscle relaxant drugs (e.g., botulinum toxin) and gait training methods (treadmill training with or without body weight support). More recently, encouraging preliminary results have been achieved with noninvasive cerebral stimulation, specifically transcranial direct current stimulation, which has been used to facilitate the excitability of the primary motor cortex during gait and balance training.

In the last five years, a large number of studies have demonstrated and discussed the effects of treadmill training with body weight support. Despite the divergences, the findings suggest benefits mainly in gait velocity and gross motor function in children classified on Levels II to IV of the GMFCS. The most important results are achieved with training protocols that involve a gradual reduction in body weight support and sessions with a frequency of two or three times a week. Papers published in the last two years report positive results with treadmill training without body weight support and training velocity performed at the aerobic threshold in children classified on Levels I to III of the GMFCS. Besides an increase in gait velocity, these studies also report important improvements in balance and cardiopulmonary fitness, which favors the independence of the child.

Introduction

Walk with or without assistance is an important motor function for independence and quality of life. The independent movement permits the individual to be able to perform daily activities with greater ease. In cases of children and adolescents with cerebral palsy, gait is committed to approximately 90% of cases. [1] According to the degree of neurological impairment and topography of this commitment we can observe different abnormal patterns of gait. Over the years many studies have described in detail the patterns of gait, especially of individuals with hemiparesis and diparesis. [2] It is known that the child with cerebral palsy type hemiparesis presents an asymmetry of movement, with the paretic lower limb usually presenting a pattern of external rotation of the hip, knee extension and equinus foot. [2] However, the children with spastic diparesis tend to show a pattern of motion in squats, with significant flexion of the hips and knees, besides equinus foot. [3] Different patterns can be observed in cases of extrapyramidal lesion, but overall the standards have an important incoordination.

Currently, the system of classification of gross motor function (GMFCS) offers guidance on the prognosis of the gait. It is known that children with level I or II tend to walk independently without the use of auxiliary resources gait, but with restrictions on more complex activities. Generally, children with level III show a motor commitment compatible with the gait, but with the utilization of auxiliary resources and limitations in gait speed and independence. Levels IV and V are related with important gait commitments, with the level IV compatible, in some cases, with the gait for short distances, with adapted auxiliary resources and not functional way. The children at level IV use the wheelchair as a functional locomotion. The level V does not present a gait prognosis and usually refers to children who will depended on a wheelchair adaptations. [4]

Cerebral palsy reverberate in decreased activation of the central nervous system during the execution of movements. [5] The impairment of gait may be due to changes in cortical excitability, excessive muscle weakness, spasticity, joint kinematic changes and decreased postural reactions. [1] The sum of these alterations reflects an important dysfunctional pattern, with global impairment of gait, involving the injury of space-temporal parameters, kinematic and kinetic.

The improved performance during gait is an important functional target in the rehabilitation of children with CP. [6] Many interventions have been studied over the years. In the last five years, many randomized controlled trials were done involving children and adolescents with cerebral palsy. The improvement of gait presents an important emphasis in recent studies, where it is possible to observe the fall of some paradigms, for example, not effectiveness of muscle strengthening exercises.

This chapter aims to present an update on the potential effects of interventions related to neurorehabilitation of children and adolescents with cerebral palsy. Besides presenting a critical analysis on important issues facing the motor therapies focus on improving performance during gait.

Motor Training

The motor training, specifically physiotherapy, can be regarded as an established feature in the literature to improve gait in children with cerebral palsy and adolescents. Several evidences demonstrate that performing physical therapy appropriately, with trained professionals and with regular frequency can result in significant improvement in acquisition (depending on the prognosis of each child) and improved of gait pattern. [7, 8]

There are important aspects to be discussed on the motor training in cerebral palsy. The first aspect to be discussed in the opinion of the authors refers to the proper frequency. There is not a consensus on the ideal number of weekly sessions of physiotherapy to get a good result engine. Typically, physical therapy sessions are conducted with a frequency of two or three sessions per week. However, clinicians and researchers are beginning to focus on the role of intensive and repetitive protocols, involving a frequency of five sessions per week and in some cases more than one session per day. It is observed that these intensive protocols may provide potential benefits, with a major peak improvement, especially in quantitative parameters of gait. The great difficulty is to convey the findings of research protocols for clinical practice. Often patients do not have easy access to rehabilitation centers, limiting the implementation of intensive intervention protocols. Another aspect related to engine intensive training protocols that should be discussed is related to the duration. In clinical practice, we observe a significant improvement in the first weeks of intensive intervention, often followed by a period of poor results. We believe that intensive protocols should have a relatively short duration, not exceeding three or four weeks. Especially in younger children, extremely lengthy protocols eventually result in fatigue and low motivation, which negatively interfere with the final result of the intervention. Apparently, the trend in the coming year will be to perform interleaved intensive protocols with conventional dictates of the frequency (physical therapy two or three times per week).

There are an extremely large variety of types of motor training. The Bobath concept [9, 10] can be considered the most sacred in research. Neurorehabilitation professionals around the world often use and believe in this concept. Over the years the Bobath concept has gained important space in the main centers of rehabilitation, demonstrating effectiveness in treating motor children diagnosed with cerebral palsy. It is not a sequence of exercises, but a concept that involves the inhibition of abnormal reflex patterns and facilitation of the nearest physiological movements. Although there are not many randomized controlled trials comparing physical therapy based on the Bobath concept with other methods of motor therapy, the results demonstrated that the available motor training to improve gait based on this concept can result in improved overall gait pattern of the child. Through specific handlings or key points, therapists are able to direct the movement and promote a repetitive workout activity with appropriate proprioceptive stimulation, providing for patient gait training with a more harmonic pattern.

However, we believe that exercises based on concepts of biomechanics and classical cinesiotherapy can result in excellent outcomes for children with cerebral palsy. To draw a proper strategy physiotherapy is important to have complete knowledge of the biomechanics of the movement that aims to change or facilitate. The unique knowledge of the pathophysiological mechanism of injury related to cerebral palsy allows the organization of a suitable motor training. Proven crucial that professionals understand the biomechanics of movement, being able to identify muscle imbalances and then intervene appropriately. Overall, the children with spastic cerebral palsy have spastic agonist muscles and weak antagonist muscles. Based on this principle is important to consider exercises engines that promote the reduction of spasticity of the agonist muscle, such as muscle stretching exercises, joint mobilizations, exercises with body weight unloading and others. Aiming the antagonist muscle, the main focus will be building muscle, which will be discussed later below. This makes it possible to minimize muscle imbalance, preventing the development of severe deformities and improving the quality of gait.

The selective motor control is important for quality of joint motion, the accuracy of the motor execution and independence at finer activities. In the case of the gait, the important thing is to perform a motor training that involves two important phases. First it is important to work the muscles specifically, with the focus on reducing spasticity and strengthen weak muscles. However, one of the most important stages in our opinion refers to the practice of selective motor control during gait. There is the importance of directing the muscles facilitating execution of the most close to physiological motion, respecting the different phases of gait. The improvement in gait pattern is related to the approximation of the movements with the expected phases of gait, such as having a proper extension of the hips and knees during the stance phase, adequate peak flexion during the swing phase and / or contact the calcaneus during the initial contact of gait.

Muscle Strengthening

Over the years the muscle strength was considered inappropriate for patients with cerebral palsy. It was believed that muscle strengthening could increase spasticity and worsen motor impairment. Currently, it is known that muscular strengthening programs properly planned can offer the patient an improved functionality. Several aspects must be considered in planning exercises, especially when we use external load during the free movement of the individual. [11]

The first aspect to be considered by the professional is the target muscle strengthening. In clinical practice it is observed that the strengthening of the antagonistic muscles to spastic muscles may reflect improvement in active motion. The orthopedic deformities in cerebral palsy are developed by a biomechanical imbalance, with the spastic muscle agonist and weak antagonist. The higher the spasticity of the lower agonist will be the joint range of motion and muscle strength as a result of the antagonist.

The first aspect to be considered by the professional is the target muscle strengthening. In clinical practice it is observed that the strengthening of the spastic muscles antagonistic muscles may reflect improvement in active motion. The orthopedic deformities in cerebral palsy are developed by a biomechanical imbalance, with the spastic muscle agonist and weak antagonist. The higher spasticity agonist, less the joint range of motion, and hence muscle strength antagonist.

One of the clearest examples is the squat gait in patients with spastic diparesis caused by this type of muscle imbalance. In this pathological gait pattern stands out in spasticity of isquiostibais and weakness of the quadriceps femoris, resulting in knee flexion constantly during the gait cycle. The reasoning in these cases is to promote the strengthening of knee extensors (Figure 1), so that this muscle group can perform its function, increasing the extension, especially during the stance phase of gait. Besides enhancing motor function, strengthening the antagonist may assist in the prevention of orthopedic deformities.

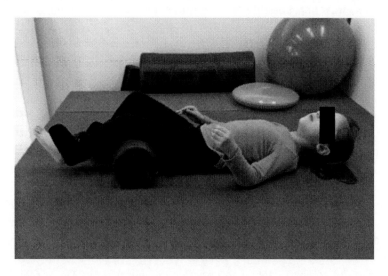

Figure 1.

After selecting the target muscle strengthening is important to consider which is the most appropriate method for promoting the gain in muscle strength. It is believed that the most important is to undertake muscle strengthening, involving greater joint range of motion possible without significant postural compensations. For this, there are many resources cited in the literature. The protocols muscle building can be achieved using sophisticated equipment or just the active-resisted movement. The benefits can be seen with different protocols strengthening, if well planned. Positive results are evident; it is known the importance of quantifying the degree of muscle strength. It is important to understand the best approach for different degrees of muscle strength. For example, in muscles with muscle strength grade two, the own force of gravity is an extra charge and is able to promote strengthening. However, in children with degree of muscle strength equal to or greater than three is necessary to impose an external resistance, whether made with manual resistance with a therapist or (properly determined) external load. Although there is not a consensus on how to determine the maximum load, as is done in orthopedic patients, we believe that a good method refers to the use of a percentage (60-80%) literature of lifting the child is able to perform the desired movement, but with greater range of motion and lower postural compensations. The standardization of methods of evaluation and determination of the target load appears necessary; it may properly determine the intervention and the increasing intervention, besides being a standard for comparing scientific results.

Specifically, in the case of children who are able to walk but have alterations in gait pattern due to muscle weakness seems valid to implement strategies for functional strengthening. In this case it is important to promote the strengthening during the act of walking. Since the child does not perform postural compensations or display discomfort, it is believed that applies the use of external load during gait, for example, during gait training on the treadmill.

In the meta-analysis published in 2014, [12] it was observed that in general the strengthening protocols involving 40-50 minute exercises with frequency of three times a week were able to generate positive effects. This meta-analysis also demonstrated the effects of strengthening for improved gait pattern in ambulatory individuals with cerebral palsy. Unfortunately, it was not possible to determine effects on non-ambulatory individuals. Another limitation is related to the number of studies involving patients with not spastic cerebral palsy. Even today you can not say that there are benefits of muscle strengthening for patients with dyskinesia or ataxia. Although in clinical practice we can observe positive effects, there is no evidence able to base this assertion.

Another aspect to be considered is the strengthening of the spastic muscles. We believe there is an important limitation to strengthen the extremely spastic muscle. However after interventions aiming to reduce spasticity, for example, after the use of Botulinum toxin, we believe that building muscle can be considered. It is known that the spastic muscle is also weak. With reduced spasticity becomes easier strengthen the antagonist muscle and also the agonist muscle, seeking an improved selective muscle control. Knowing neurolitic blocks present results in the short and medium term in reducing spasticity, probably improved selective motor control offered by specific training can optimize these long-term results.

The children and adolescents with cerebral palsy in the course of their lives will require several orthopedic surgeries. A major goal of subjecting a child to an orthopedic surgical procedure in cases of cerebral palsy is to optimize the gait pattern. The surgeries are arguably necessary, but are followed by long periods of immobilization. These periods may vary according to the type and complexity of surgical procedures involving weeks or months. Muscle weakness after surgery and immobilization are of concern among professionals in physical rehabilitation. During the physical rehabilitation in orthopedic postoperative protocols strengthening should have a prominent role. Always initiated after medication with adequate support release may promote recovery, reduce the time to restore the gait and optimize the improvement of gait pattern.

Like any resource intervention is important that professionals understand that muscle building can offer benefits for children and adolescents with cerebral palsy. For these benefits are observed planning of the intervention is necessary, determining the target muscle, method of strengthening (resistance manual, external load, functional exercises, etc.), frequency and duration of the intervention, in addition to functional objective to be achieved. Like any intervention, the lack of planning can have negative effects. For example, conducting an exercise with heavy loads can cause orthopedic injuries, in addition to reinforcing the use of postural compensations.

Treadmill Training

Several approaches have been used to promote cortical activation, selective motor control, coordination of muscle action in the realization of gait. [1] Among the approaches currently under study highlights the gait training on a treadmill. The gait training on a treadmill can be done with or without body weight support and is intended to provide specific task training with multiple repetitions of the steps of gait. [13] Facilitates motor learning from repetitive training on function, with resulting sensorimotor stimulation and corticospinal.

The majority of studies involving the body weight supported treadmill training. There are a variety of conflicting results on the use of body weight support in cerebral palsy. [14, 15] Studies have shown good effects or the absence of effects. We believe that the use of support of body weight treadmill training using the resources of robotics are particularly important for patients with motor impairment more pronounced, as in the cases of levels IV and V of the GMFCS. In these cases the realization of treadmill training without body weight support is limited by the difficulty to control and execute the movement of the lower limbs. The weight support refers to the mechanisms that provide the partial removal of the weight, the percent body weight taken according to the therapeutic purposes and in order to facilitate the execution of the movement.

Studies analyzing the treadmill training with weight support have varying protocols, relationship with the percentage of body weight withdrawal patterns to increase the body weight, number of sessions per week and number of weeks of training. [16, 17] The main results are presented in protocols with at least three training sessions per week, demonstrating effect mainly in gait velocity. It is observed that in general about 20% of body weight is taken in the beginning of protocols, with a gradual increase in weight during the evolution of this protocol. It is not yet possible to say that this feature is a significant impact on motor function and specifically on the gait. The final systematic revisions show that there is insufficient evidence for a conclusion about the benefits.

For children with mild motor (levels I and II of the GMFCS) and moderate (some cases without orthopedic deformities installed), the treadmill training can be done without the use of body weight support. Some studies point to the benefits of treadmill training performed in conventional treadmill, but with proper support for the upper limbs. [6, 18] Conventional electric treadmills have a lower and easier access cost, allowing the treadmill training can be performed in simple physical spaces and not necessarily large.

There is the importance of adjusting the workout according to the objectives and characteristics of the child. Besides thinking about the frequency of training, the therapist needs to identify what is the optimum speed for your workout and this speed will be increased or not during sessions. We believe that a good tool is the use of stress tests on the treadmill. There is a limitation of exercise tests for children, especially for children with neurological impairment. With this goal Grecco et al. (2013) proposed in their study that the speed of training is determined by a stress test limited by symptoms, an increase of 0.5 km/h per minute (Figure 2). Thus, the training can be performed using between 60 - 80% of the maximum speed tolerated by the child. The use of a standardized test can assist in the quality of training and especially in the evaluation of the effects obtained, since it can be performed before and after the training protocol.

Overall, the main results reported in the literature demonstrate that treadmill training can improve walking speed, [6, 16, 19] stride length, [20] gross motor function related to orthostatic and gait, [6, 16, 20] functional performance and functional and static balance. [18] When the treadmill training is conducted based on an exercise test, i.e., at a rate that promotes a workout on cardio above the threshold results in gait training conducted on the floor, functional mobility test (six-minute walk and timed effects up and go), thick in motor function (walking, running and jumping), the functional balance, static balance and cardiorespiratory fitness.

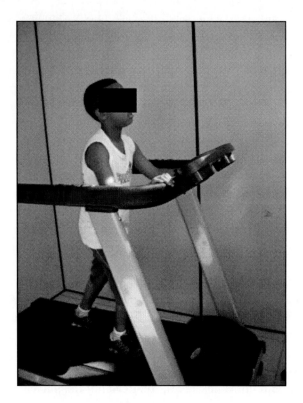

Figure 2.

Virtual Reality

New rehabilitation techniques have been studied in the pediatric population as an attempt to innovate therapy and encourage the child to make proposals in a playful way and therapeutic activities. In this context, the use of virtual reality as adjunctive therapy in this population have shown to be a great ally to the success of the rehabilitation process. [21, 22]

The game of virtual reality generated by the interaction of people from different age groups with the video game, allowing their use in children because of some limitation of motion or not. In the case of children with cerebral palsy, we work with focus and dedication to promote immersion in the activity, with visual and audio feedback in real time.

Virtual reality can be used as a specific form of therapy for rehabilitation of upper or lower limbs, depending on the therapeutic goal. It is for the therapist to indicate what activity to accomplish, because through different games could give focus will target the therapy area and generate a motivational component to treatment. Games must be chosen according to each patient's physical ability to succeed in therapy.

The fact that children interact with the game and receive visual information about it is performance, brings a personal incentive to overcome their answers in the game and thus potentiate the activity where we managed to get almost 100% of success.

Order to reach the goal of therapy should consider the integration of diverse systems for compiling the activity and performance of the movement required in the game. The integration of visual, proprioceptive and vestibular systems is critical for success in the proposed activity.

Neuromodulation

In recent years neuromodulation, specifically the techniques of non-invasive brain stimulation, has occupied an important space in the scientific literature on neurological rehabilitation. [23] The transcranial direct-current stimulation refers to the use of a low current intensity on the scalp which has the ability to achieve cortical areas by facilitating or hindering the cortical excitability depending on the used current hub. Specifically, the anode electrode has the ability to facilitate and the cathode has the ability to hinder cortical excitability. The effects are obtained due to the polarity and displacement of ions that can make the region below the most positive or negative electrode, inhibiting or facilitating cortical excitability respectively. This feature has few adverse effects, but requires adequate knowledge of the technique and anatomy and physiology of the central nervous system properties. [24]

Although the results of this technique are shown in different clinical conditions and there is an extensive scientific literature on the subject, yet there is not a consensus or sufficient studies to guide the use in the pediatric population. In the last two years, some published studies have shown that apparently is a safe method for use in children. The few professionals who investigate this feature in children show good results. In stroke there is evidence that the association of transcranial direct current stimulation on motor cortex with motor therapies can enhance the results, both on the gait or on the function of the upper limbs.

Specifically about cerebral palsy, the first literature report was released in 2014. [25] Refers to the case of a child with developmental delay, not with the functional gait walker who made ten sessions of anodal stimulation on the motor cortex during treadmill training. Besides getting effects on balance and gait speed, the child was able to swap the walker steps without support after the end of the protocol (10 sessions). After this promising result, the same research group developed a cross-sectional study involving a session of stimulation in children with cerebral palsy levels I, II and III of the GMFCS. The results showed that a session can deliver positive but short duration on static balance (reducing fluctuations of the center of pressure with and without visual restriction) and increased gait speed and cadence changes.

It is shown that further studies involving rational use of this resource, especially randomized controlled trials. The partial results demonstrate that disclosed positive results are identified, particularly with regard to increasing the size of the effect obtained from the therapy. We believe that this tool can enhance the results achieved with different motor therapies available. Another important aspect is still under investigation the effect of optimization of motor learning. Once learned or relearned a new motor task, probably the effect will be not lost since the job continues to run. This can be observed in studies involving anodic stimulation demonstrating the maintenance of the results on assessments of follow-up after completion of the intervention.

We believe that the association of non-invasive brain stimulation with motor training may result in potentiated and faster results in improved gait. However, studies should be conducted testing this hypothesis.

Final Considerations

Several resources are used in physical rehabilitation of children and adolescents with cerebral palsy in order to maximize the march. Regardless of whether or not the prognosis involves the necessity of auxiliary resources gait is important to promote a well-planned intervention and quality, so that patients are able to achieve their maximum potential. Currently, the major features discussed in the literature and used in clinical practice involve conventional training since the said motor, with sequential exercises and planned, until activities with treadmill training, training using virtual reality. More recently, the resources of neuromodulation, such as the transcranial direct-current stimulation begin to occupy space in the literature. In contrast, the peripherals exercises aimed at promoting activation of cortical areas in order afferent noninvasive stimulation can be performed for facilitation of cortical excitability in specific areas of the cortex, depending on the therapeutic purpose. Probably the future of motor rehabilitation to improve gait in cerebral palsy cases will involve the association of physical therapy with the resources of non-invasive brain stimulation. Thus, interventions will involve central and peripheral stimuli, probably enhancing learning or relearning motor, reflecting improvements in motor function and gait.

References

[1] Chagas PSC, Mancini MC, Barbosa A, Silva. Analysis of the interventions used for gait promotion in children with cerebral palsy: a systematic review of the literature. *Brazilian Journal of Physical Therapya.* 2004;8(2):155 - 63.

[2] Szopa A, Domagalska-Szopa M, Czamara A. Gait pattern differences in children with unilateral cerebral palsy. *Research in developmental disabilities.* 2014;35(10):2261-6.

[3] Hägglund G, Lauge-Pedersen H, Wagner P. Characteristics of children with hip displacement in cerebral palsy. *BMC musculoskeletal disorders.* 2007;8(1):101.

[4] Russell DJ, Avery LM, Rosenbaum PL, Raina PS, Walter SD, Palisano RJ. Improved scaling of the gross motor function measure for children with cerebral palsy: evidence of reliability and validity. *Physical Therapy.* 2000;80(9):873-85.

[5] Shin YK, Lee DR, Hwang HJ, You SH, Im CH. A novel EEG-based brain mapping to determine cortical activation patterns in normal children and children with cerebral palsy during motor imagery tasks. *NeuroRehabilitation.* 2012;31(4):349-55.

[6] Grecco LAC, Zanon N, Sampaio LMM, Oliveira CS. A comparison of treadmill training and overground walking in ambulant children with cerebral palsy: randomized controlled clinical trial. *Clinical Rehabilitation.* 2013;27(8):686 - 96.

[7] Anttila H, Autti-Rämö I, Suoranta J, Mäkelä M, Malmivaara A. Effectiveness of physical therapy interventions for children with cerebral palsy: a systematic review. *BMC pediatrics.* 2008;8(1):14.

[8] Palmer FB, Shapiro BK, Wachtel RC, Allen MC, Hiller JE, Harryman SE, et al. The effects of physical therapy on cerebral palsy. *New England Journal of Medicine.* 1988;318(13):803-8.

[9] Bobath K. A neurophysiological basis for the treatment of cerebral palsy: Cambridge University Press; 1991.

[10] Bobath K, Bobath B. The facilitation of normal postural reactions and movements in the treatment of cerebral palsy. *Physiotherapy.* 1964;50:246.

[11] Verschuren O, Ada L, Maltais DB, Gorter JW, Scianni A, Ketelaar M. Muscle strengthening in children and adolescents with spastic cerebral palsy: considerations for future resistance training protocols. *Physical Therapy.* 2011;91(7):1130-9.

[12] Park E-Y, Kim W-H. Meta-analysis of the effect of strengthening interventions in individuals with cerebral palsy. *Research in developmental disabilities.* 2014;35(2):239-49.

[13] Mattern-Baxter K. Locomotor treadmill training for children with cerebral palsy. *Orthopaedic Nursing.* 2010;29(3):169-73.

[14] Willoughby KL, Dodd KJ, Shields N. A systematic review of the effectiveness of treadmill training for children with cerebral palsy. *Disability & Rehabilitation.* 2009;31(24):1971-9.

[15] Zwicker JG, Mayson TA. Effectiveness of treadmill training in children with motor impairments: An overview of systematic reviews. *Pediatric Physical Therapy.* 2010;22(4):361-77.

[16] Smania N, Bonetti P, Gandolfi M, Cosentino A, Waldner A, Hesse S, et al. Improved gait after repetitive locomotor training in children with cerebral palsy. *American Journal of Physical Medicine & Rehabilitation.* 2011;90(2):137-49.

[17] Mutlu A, Krosschell K, Spira DG. Treadmill training with partial body-weight support in children with cerebral palsy: a systematic review. *Developmental Medicine & Child Neurology.* 2009;51(4):268-75.

[18] Grecco LAC, Tomita SM, Christovão TCL, Pasini H, Sampaio LMM, Oliveira CS. Effect of treadmill gait training on static and functional balance in children with cerebral palsy: a randomized controlled trial. *Brazilian Journal of Physical Therapy.* 2013;17(1):17-23.

[19] Dodd KJ, Foley S. Partial body-weight-supported treadmill training can improve walking in children with cerebral palsy: a clinical controlled trial. *Developmental Medicine & Child Neurology*. 2007;49(2):101-5.

[20] Cherng R-J, Liu C-F, Lau T-W, Hong R-B. Effect of treadmill training with body weight support on gait and gross motor function in children with spastic cerebral palsy. *American journal of physical medicine & rehabilitation*. 2007;86(7):548-55.

[21] Bryanton C, Bosse J, Brien M, Mclean J, McCormick A, Sveistrup H. Feasibility, motivation, and selective motor control: virtual reality compared to conventional home exercise in children with cerebral palsy. *Cyberpsychology & behavior*. 2006;9(2):123-8.

[22] You SH, Jang SH, Kim Y-H, Kwon Y-H, Barrow I, Hallett M. Cortical reorganization induced by virtual reality therapy in a child with hemiparetic cerebral palsy. *Developmental Medicine & Child Neurology*. 2005;47(09):628-35.

[23] Liew S-L, Santarnecchi E, Buch E, Cohen L. Noninvasive brain stimulation in neurorehabilitation: Local and distant effects for motor recovery. *Frontiers in Human Neuroscience*. 2014;8:378.

[24] Brunoni AR, Nitsche MA, Bolognini N, Bikson M, Wagner T, Merabet L, et al. Clinical research with transcranial direct current stimulation (tDCS): challenges and future directions. *Brain stimulation*. 2012;5(3):175-95.

[25] Grecco LAC, Mendonça ME, Duarte NA, Zanon N, Fregni F, Oliveira CS. Transcranial Direct Current Stimulation Combined with Treadmill Gait Training in Delayed Neuro-psychomotor Development. *Journal of physical therapy science*. 2014;26(6):945.

In: Handbook on Cerebral Palsy
Editor: Harold Yates

ISBN: 978-1-63321-852-9
© 2014 Nova Science Publishers, Inc.

Chapter 8

Fine Motor Performance of Children with Ataxic Cerebral Palsy during Tracing Activity: A Case Report

Maraísa Fonseca Machado[1], Rita de Cássia Tibério Araújo[2]
and Lígia Maria Presumido Braccialli[3,*]

[1]Occupational Therapy of APAE, Universidade Estadual Paulista Júlio de Mesquista
Filho - UNESP – Marília, São Paulo, Brazil
[2]Department of Physical Therapy and Occupational Therapy,
Universidade Estadual Paulista Júlio de Mesquista Filho -
UNESP – Marília, São Paulo, Brazil
[3]Department of Special Education, Universidade Estadual Paulista
Júlio de Mesquita Filho - UNESP – Marília, São Paulo, Brazil

Abstract

The aim of this study was to test the effect of weight bracelet and adapted pen on fine motor graphic activity performance. Two patients with a diagnosis of ataxic cerebral palsy from the Occupational Therapy service participated in the study. The effect of these adaptations was tested during tracing activities on a tablet, with records related to time, jerk, pressure and strokes. The data represent four experimental situations: a) without adaptation, b) with weight bracelet, c) with weight bracelet and weight on an adapted pen, and d) with weight on an adapted pen. Participant P1 showed less tremor and execution time in situation "d", and less stroke and pressure in situation "c". Participant P2 had a shorter execution time, tremor and pen force in situation "d", and less stroke incidence in situation "c". This study suggests that the prescription of weight using weight bracelet in addition to weight on an adapted a pen to cerebral palsy patients would be suitable to perform graphic tasks with higher quality.

---

* Email: bracci@marilia.unesp.br.

Keywords: Motor performance, cerebral palsy, motor learning

1. Introduction

Children with cerebral palsy (CP) often have difficulties in executing activities of reaching, grasping and handling objects due to motor disorders. The damage in the function of the upper limbs depend on several factors, including the severity of paresis, the extent of sensory loss, muscle tone, and whether associated dyskinesia is present or not (Fedrizzi, Pagliano, Andreucci, & Oleari, 2003) which will result in slower motion and deficient coordination (Coluccini, Maini, Martelloni, Sgandurra, & Cioni, 2007; Gonçalves, Braccialli, & Carvalho, 2013).

To facilitate functionality and participation of children with cerebral palsy in the activities carried out in different environments, especially school and at home, therapists usually prescribe assistive devices that configure assistive technology resources.

The elaboration and use of assistive technology can improve social interaction, motor skills and child's quality of life. However, studies have indicated that over 30% of all purchased devices are abandoned by the user between the first and the fifth year of use, and some are not even used (Goodman, Tiene, & Luft, 2002; Huang, Sugden, & Beveridge, 2009; Phillips & Zhao, 1993; Scherer, 2002; Verza, Carvalho, Battaglia, & Uccelli, 2006). To decrease abandonment of the prescribed resource, greater attention should be given to the user's opinion and understand that a device must be made to meet the specific needs of a user (Huang, Sugden, & Beveridge, 2009; Scherer, 2002).

Considering that the development of a child's movement of reach and grasp depends on intrinsic and extrinsic factors to the organism (Sugden, 2000), during the prescription process and elaboration of a resource to a child with CP, manipulation of some of these factors can be suggested to facilitate handling and mobility of upper limbs while performing activities at school and home environment.

Studies have shown that among the extrinsic factors that may interfere with the reach and grasp of objects include: the position of the body in space (Carvalho, Tudella, Caljouw, & Savelsbergh, 2008), the physical properties of objects (de Campos, Rocha, & Savelsbergh, 2009; Gonçalves, Braccialli & Carvalho, 2013; Mason & Bruyn, 2009), the additional weight on the child's arm (Audi, 2006; de Campos et al., 2009; Lucareli et al., 2010) and the spatial orientation of objects (Mason & Bruyn, 2009).

Familiarity with the object and its physical characteristics can also facilitate the adjustment of the strength required to perform the task, allowing a better control of the activity by the individual (Duff & Gordon, 2003; Eliasson & Gordon, 2000). In this context, the adaptation of the objects in their physical aspects such as shape, weight, size and texture can minimize the functional, sensory and motor limitations of the child with cerebral palsy, facilitating handling and grasping of objects (Paiva & Braccialli, 2009).

In relation to the person with dyskinetic cerebral palsy, Lucareli et al. (2010) and Audi (2006) found that the use of stabilizing straps have improved the quality of movement during the activity of reaching. However, Gonçalves, Braccialli and Carvalho (2013) in a study with a child with dyskinetic cerebral palsy found that the time taken to carry out the removal and placement of an object is shorter when the object is small, light and smooth. Van Vliet &

Sheridan (2007) have shown that people with hemiparesis took longer to move a bigger glass because of the limitation that these individuals have to extend the fingers.

In this scenario, this study investigated how adding weight, weight bracelet and adapted pen can interfere with fine motor skills while performing an activity of tracing, by children with ataxic cerebral palsy, valuing the motivational aspects of assistive devices for improving motor performance.

2. Method

2.1. Participants

The study included two children diagnosed with ataxic cerebral palsy classified at levels I and II of Gross Motor Function Classification System (GMFCS) (Palisano et al., 1997) and Manual Ability Classification System (MACS) (Eliasson et al., 2006), participants on an intervention program of physiotherapy and occupational therapy to support the participation and school performance in regular school (Table 1).

Table 1. Characteristics of participants

	Age (years)	School grade	Gender	Diagnosis	GMFCS	MACS
P1	8	3rd grade	Female	Ataxic Cerebral Palsy	Level II	Level II
P2	10	5th grade	Female	Ataxic Cerebral Palsy	Level I	Level I

2.2. Location

The research was conducted in the Laboratory of Motor Performance Analysis (LADEMO) of a Brazilian public university that provides occupational therapy and physiotherapy care for patients with neuromuscular disorders.

2.3. Materials and Data Collection Procedures

For data collection, a Wacom Intuos3 tablet, PTZ-930 model with a total height of 25.5 centimeters (cm) and total length of 34 cm was used. For collection and subsequent data analysis, the tablet was connected to a computer, having been set up according to the manufacturer's instructions so that the computer could record the data for pen pressure. The limit of pen sensitivity and other data were set on the tablet program installed on the computer. The limit of sensitivity was left in neutral position so that data were recorded correctly. An A4 sheet of paper was placed on the surface of the tablet; the paper contained the activity of tracing that should be performed by the study participant using an Ink Pen ZP-130 model. For collection and analysis, the software MovAlyseR 6.1 was used.

2.4. Experimental Situations

Data were collected in four consecutive experimental situations: a) use of the tablet's pen (Ink Pen with ink), ZP-130 Model with conventional design (situation 1: without adaptation); b) use of the tablet's pen (Ink Pen with ink), ZP-130 Model with conventional design and weight bracelet (situation 2: weight bracelet); c) use of the tablet's pen (Ink Pen with ink), ZP-130 Model with adaptation and weight bracelet (situation 3: weight bracelet and adapted pen); d) use of the tablet's pen (Ink Pen with ink), ZP-130 Model with adaptation (situation 4: adapted pen) (Figure 1).

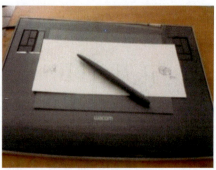
Without adaptation

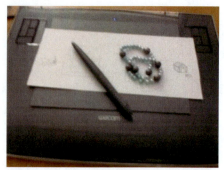
Weight bracelet

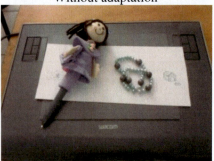
Weight bracelet and adapted pen

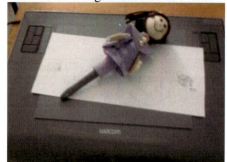
Adapted pen

Figure 1. Trials.

Each of the four situations represented one experimental situation, per participant, requiring a new software configuration. The tablet has been resized four times per participant so that there were no spatial errors in the positioning of the activity. The MovAlyseR software was also programmed with a specific time for each experimental situation.

Data from five trials for each experimental situation were collected so that each participant brought together a total of 20 tested episodes. In each experiment, the participants were given some resting time between one trial and the other. This time was determined by MovAlyseR software set to 15 second rest.

Throughout the collection period, the researcher remained in front of the participants, providing the necessary information for executing the activity and holding the sheet of paper, at the ideal location for that activity.

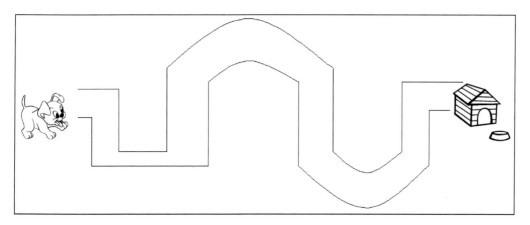

Figure 2. Tracing Activity used for data collection.

2.5. Adaptation of the Pen and Definition of the Activity to be Performed to Assess Motor Performance

The definition of the weight to be added in the pen Ink Pen, ZP-130 Model with ink, with conventional design was based on: a) the intervention history of patient P2 who was already using a 50g weight bracelet, b) the weight of the pen in its conventional design, and c) the users' interests aiming their motivation for its use.

The design of the adapted pen was aimed to support a total weight of 50g: a) a doll built in EVA material weighing 5.8 g, b) the pen Ink Pen ZP-130 model with ink with 11, 8g, and c) a copper tube with silver nitrate bath with a weight of 32.4 g, resulting in a total weight of 50g. The doll was built using EVA, for the body, and styrofoam ball for the head. After several experiments, for the purpose of better defining the position of silver nitrate tube in the pen, it was concluded that the tube should be at the center of the pen, for a more even weight distribution across the length of the object.

An activity of maze was proposed, with the path signaled in the dimensional picture. This activity brought straight lines and curves, and was chosen because MovAlyseR software provide a more accurate analysis with this type of activities (Codogno, 2011). The graphic activity occupied the dimensions of an A4 sheet of paper measuring 16.1 cm by 21 cm, and was proposed in landscape (Figure 2).

2.5. Procedures for Data Analysis

Graphs were used to evaluate the records concerning the time, Jerk, Pressure and Strokes, for each experimental situation. Statistical analysis was performed through analysis of mean and dispersion values.

3. Results and Discussion

The results were presented through the analysis of variables: (1) time taken to carry out the activities; (2) disfluency in fine motor skills while performing the activity; (3) pressure of the pen on the paper while performing the activity; (4) fluency in writing.

3.1. Time Taken to Carry out the Activity

The time taken for the participant to perform the activity was calculated from the first touch of the pen tip on the tablet until the final suspension, as recommended by the literature (Calvo, 2007).

Participant P1 showed no significant variation in time taken to perform the activity without the use of adaptation and with weight bracelet. In these two situations, participant P1 spent on average 16 seconds to perform them, observing similarity in the variation of the time spent on the five trials. However, with the concomitant use of weight bracelet and adapted pen, time spent, on average, was slightly shorter (15.34s), and the variation interval for the five trials also decreased, registering an interval between 14.25s and 16.03s. In the situation using only the adapted pen, participant P1 performed the activity in a shorter mean time (13.74s) and interval between 11.64s and 16.26s (Graph 1).

Participant P2 showed a gradual reduction in the average time taken to perform the activities in the course of the four tested situations. There was greater variation between the minimum and maximum time in the situation with the weight bracelet. In the situation with the adapted pen, participant P2 could perform the activity in shorter time (6.41s) and smaller variation (between 5.46s to 7.09s) during the 5 trials.

The result of performance, following the tested situations, suggests a trend of gradual decrease in time to perform the activity, being able to hypothesize the influence of motor learning following the experiments.

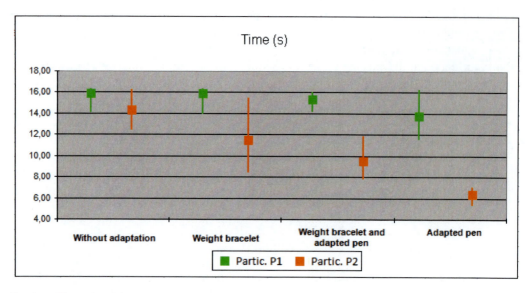

Graph 1. Time of activity performance.

Bandeira et al. (2010) argued that motor learning is related to the ability of the individual, during the process of performing an activity, to acquire skills that favor the performance of specific tasks due to practice or experience on the motor act.

The practice of fine motor coordination influences the speed, acceleration and fluency of manual activities such as writing (Calvo, 2007; Codogno, 2011).

Another important datum relates to gain on stability in acquisition of skill for improving competence, afterwards. In the third tested situation, there was a trend for greater stability and in the fourth situation, there was an improvement in the performance time.

A study by Schwellnus et al. (2013), which investigated the impact of pencil grip on the speed and legibility of handwriting before and after a 10-minute copy task, the occupational therapist noted that eligibility decreased after the 10-minute copy task, whereas the speed increased.

However, if on one hand, the data presented in Graph 1 can be attributed to motor learning, on the other hand, taking into account that the second and fourth situations showed the same additional weight (50g), one can consider that participant P2 responded better when the weight was placed in the most distal region of the arm.

Audi (2006) and Lucareli et al. (2010) noted that the best motor performance with the use of weight bracelet would be related to the load imposed by the weight bracelet on the upper limb of participants, favoring the slower movement and allowing a better planning to achieve the final goal.

According to Cruz (2003), experimentation is an important factor for the construction of motor memory, for it reduces the need for constant correction as it automates the learned and regularly practiced movements, thus leading to motor learning.

4.2. Disfluency in Fine Motor Coordination during the Execution of the Activity

Disfluency in fine motor coordination, i.e., the amount of tremor while performing the activity was measured by the variable jerk (Caligiuri, Teulings, Dean, & Alexander, 2010).

Participant P1 showed, on average, greater tremor and greater variation while performing the activity with the weight bracelet, noting an average acceleration of 10996.06 cm/s ^{3} and a variation between 2518.45 cm/s^3 and 33500.61 cm/s^3. In the situation with the concomitant use of weight bracelet and adapted pen, tremor decreased yielding an average acceleration of 6032.341 cm/s^3, and a variation between 1994.86 cm/s^3 and 9485.56 cm/s^3. The lowest acceleration average of 5218.209 cm/s^3 was observed in the situation using only the adapted pen (Graph 2).

Participant P2 showed a progressive fall of representative values of tremor following the experiment, recording the worst result without adaptation (2424.93 cm/s^3) and the best result using only the adapted pen (460.26 cm/s^3), observing also smaller variation (between 298.94 cm/s^3 and 611.27 cm/s^3) in the fourth situation of the experiment (Graph 2).

The results found in this study, according to Graph 2 suggests benefits in adding weight to control tremor. In the study by Santos (1998) weight was also found to decrease involuntary movements by the use of weight bracelet. Zerbinato, Makita and Zerloti (2003) reported that adjustments with weight could reduce involuntary movements and thus facilitate hand-mouth coordination, suggesting the use of weight bracelets with different weights for training this skill. Galvão and Damasceno (2003) employed the weight bracelet in students with athetoid cerebral palsy and observed that typing became faster and more efficient.

Taking into consideration the responses of P1 during the four tested situations, it can be inferred that the introduction of weight caused instability in controlling the tremor, which was controlled in the course of the tested situations, with the resumption of the initial pattern, suggesting interference in learning to master this motor skill.

In the study by Teulings and Romero (2003), jerk increased according to the performed activities. The more curves and complex the activities were, the greater the observed jerk value.

In this study, there was a better fine motor coordination through the use of weight on a body region more distal to the user.

4.3. Pressure of the Pen on Paper while Performing the Activity

Graph 3 shows the results obtained regarding to the amount of pressure (in Newtons) exerted by the participants to the paper during the execution of the activity.

Regarding the motor behavior of participant P1, the highest mean values of the pressure exerted on the paper occurred in the situation with the use of weight bracelet and the situation using the adapted pen. The lowest mean values occurred in the situation without adaptation and in the situation with the concomitant use of weight bracelet and adapted pen. The dispersion of values was lower in the situation with the use of adapted pen.

Regarding participant P2, there was a greater mean value of the pressure exerted on the paper in the situation with the use of weight bracelet (796.10 N). In the situation using the adapted pen, it was observed a mean pressure of 625.25N, similar to the situation without adaptation (641.66N), but the dispersion was smaller in the latter situation (Graph 3).

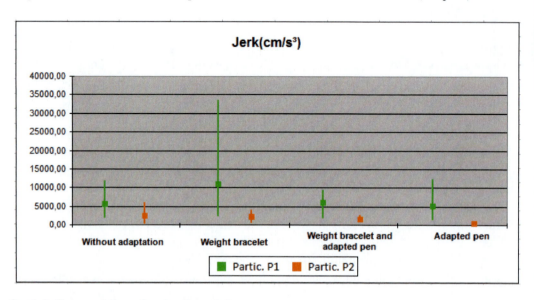

Graph 2. Tremor while performing the activity.

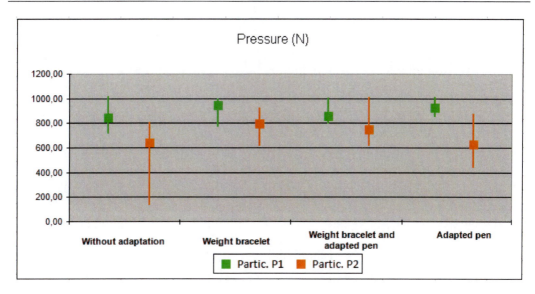

Graph 3. Pressure of the pen on paper while performing the activity.

The study by Codogno (2011) observed that the higher the pressure, the greater the physical wear of the student to perform the tracing activity, because it requires greater coordination and dissociation of fingers of the students with cerebral palsy. In this direction, although the mean values may suggest that the weight did not favor the improvement of tested skills, on the other hand, the results suggest its influence on a lower dispersion.

4.4. Fluency in Writing

Stroke is a measure that indicates fluency in writing so that the more strokes in the activity, the lower the fluency. When there is little fluency, the quality of drawing or writing is impaired (Van Doorn & Keuss, 1991; Calvo, 2007).

The records on the number of times that P1 and P2 took the pen from the paper while performing the tracing activity enabled the analysis of motor skills quality in the four tested situations (Graph 4).

It is verified that when participant P1 used the weight bracelet, she fragmented the graphic pattern fewer times when compared to the pattern obtained by using the pen without adaptation. In the situation with the use of adapted pen, the pattern was better when compared to the situation with the use of weight bracelet, but it was with the concomitant use of weight bracelet and adapted pen that she showed smaller stroke and smaller variation. It was also observed that in the last two situations there was a trend of motor pattern stability.

Participant P2 showed fewer strokes (5.4 u) and smaller variation in the situation with concomitant use of weight bracelet and adapted pen. In the situation with the use of adapted pen, stroke (6.4 u) was fewer compared to the situation using weight bracelet (7.0u).

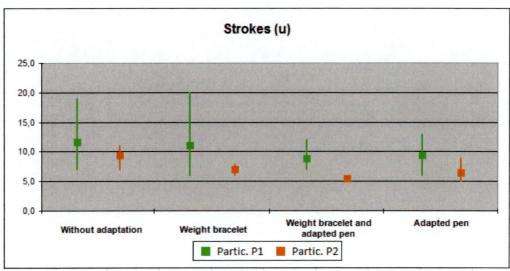

Source: Authors' production.

Graph 4. Strokes while performing the activity.

It is evident, therefore, that the two participants had better motor pattern in the situation with the concomitant use of weight bracelet and adapted pen. These results suggest that the addition of more weight resulted in better domain of the skill related to continuous movement of the upper limb.

Children with cerebral palsy have poor motion control and coordination of the upper limbs (Volman, 2005) which explains the greater number of strokes during the activities (Codogno, 2011). The results of this study show that the strategy of concomitant use of weight bracelet and adapted pen can reduce the occurrence of strokes while conducting activities with fine motor demand.

Final Considerations

The literature has pointed to a lack of consensus regarding the use of weight bracelet, depending on the demands of motor activity. The study by Sankako (2013), which aimed to determine the efficacy of weight bracelet and the sloped plane on motor performance of the upper limbs of students with dyskinetic cerebral palsy during sharpening activity, found that the use of the sloped plane seemed to have been positive for two participants, while the weight bracelet was not effective for all participants. Conversely, Audi (2006) found that the weight bracelet favored the performance of sharpening activity in adults with involuntary movements. Lucareli et al. (2010) also observed better movements with the use of weight bracelet in a study carried out with a child with cerebral palsy and choreoathetoid movements.

In this study, the concomitant use of adapted pen and weight bracelet produced the best results of motor ability for both participants.

The addition of weight on the pen enabled less time and less tremor while performing the task of tracing for both participants.

Regarding stroke, both participants had better performance in the situation with the concomitant use of weight bracelet and adapted pen.

In relation to the pressure, the adaptation in the pen provided a better result for participant P2, and concomitant use of weight in the pen and weight bracelet provided better performance for participant P1.

Even though motor learning following the examined situations is an important aspect to be considered as a possibility of interference, the results suggest that adding weight to the pen favored fine motor performance for both participants, with the advantage of adaptation prescription being close to the real object used in the school environment.

References

Audi, M. (2006). Estudo comparativo do comportamento motor de membro superior em encefalopatas que fazem uso de pulseira estabilizadora. Universidade Estadual Paulista.

Bandeira, C., Monteiro, D. M., Jakabi, C. M., Carla, G., Torriani-pasin, C., Miranda, C. De, & Junior, M. (2010). Motor Learning in Children With. *Journal of Human Growth and Development*, 20(3), 11–23.

Caligiuri, M. P., Teulings, H., Dean, C. E., & Alexander, B. N. (2010). Handwriting movement kinematics for quantifying EPS in patients treated with atypical antipsychotics. Psychiatry Res, 177(1-2), 77–83. doi:10.1016/j.psychres.2009.07.005. Handwriting

Calvo, A. P. (2007). A produção gráfica e escrita: focalizando a variação da produção de força. Universidade Estadual Paulista.

Carvalho, R. P., Tudella, E., Caljouw, S. R., & Savelsbergh, G. J. P. (2008). Early control of reaching: effects of experience and body orientation. *Infant Behavior & Development*, 31(1), 23–33. doi:10.1016/j.infbeh.2007.06.001

Codogno, F. T. de O. (2011). Influência do mobiliário na coordenação motora fina e no controle postural de alunos com paralisia cerebral. Universidade Estadual Paulista.

Coluccini, M., Maini, E. S., Martelloni, C., Sgandurra, G., & Cioni, G. (2007). Kinematic characterization of functional reach to grasp in normal and in motor disabled children. Gait & Posture, 25(4), 493–501. doi:10.1016/j.gaitpost.2006.12.015

Cruz, C. F. (2003). SISTEMA DE BIOFEEDBACK PARA OTIMIZAÇÃO DE MOVIMENTO DE MEMBROS SUPERIORES DE CORREDORES COM PARALISIA CEREBRAL. Universidade Estadual de Campinas.

De Campos, A. C., Rocha, N. A. C. F., & Savelsbergh, G. J. P. (2009). Reaching and grasping movements in infants at risk: a review. *Research in Developmental Disabilities*, 30(5), 819–26. doi:10.1016/j.ridd.2009.01.004

Duff, S. V, & Gordon, A. M. (2003). Learning of grasp control in children with hemiplegic cerebral palsy. Developmental Medicine and Child Neurology, 45(11), 746–57. Retrieved from http://www.ncbi.nlm.nih.gov/pubmed/14580130

Eliasson, a C., & Gordon, a M. (2000). Impaired force coordination during object release in children with hemiplegic cerebral palsy. Developmental Medicine and Child Neurology, 42(4), 228–34. Retrieved from http://www.ncbi.nlm.nih.gov/pubmed/10795560

Eliasson, A.-C., Krumlinde-Sundholm, L., Rösblad, B., Beckung, E., Arner, M., Ohrvall, A.-M., & Rosenbaum, P. (2006). The Manual Ability Classification System (MACS) for children with cerebral palsy: scale development and evidence of validity and reliability. *Developmental Medicine and Child Neurology*, 48(7), 549–54. doi:10.1017/S0012162206001162

Fedrizzi, E., Pagliano, E., Andreucci, E., & Oleari, G. (2003). Hand function in children with hemiplegic cerebral palsy: prospective follow-up and functional outcome in adolescence. *Developmental Medicine and Child Neurology*, 45(2), 85–91. Retrieved from http://www.ncbi.nlm.nih.gov/pubmed/12578233

Gonçalves, A., Braccialli, L. M. P., & Carvalho, S. M. R. (2013). Desempenho motor de aluno com paralisia cerebral discinética frente à adaptação das propriedades fisicas de recurso pedagogico. *Rev. Bras. Educ.*, 19(2), 257–272. Retrieved from http://www.scielo.br/pdf/rbee/v19n2/a09v19n2.pdf

Goodman, G., Tiene, D., & Luft, P. (2002). Adoption of assistive technology for computer access among college students with disabilities. *Disability and Rehabilitation*, 24(1-3), 80–92. Retrieved from http://www.ncbi.nlm.nih.gov/pubmed/11827158

Huang, I.-C., Sugden, D., & Beveridge, S. (2009). Assistive devices and cerebral palsy: factors influencing the use of assistive devices at home by children with cerebral palsy. *Child: Care, Health and Development*, 35(1), 130–9. doi:10.1111/j.1365-2214.2008.00898.x

Lucareli, P. R. G., Oliveira, D., Lima, M., Lima, F., Artilheiro, M., Braccialli, L., … Correa, J. C. F. (2010). The influence of the use of stabilizer bracelet in a child with choreoathetoid cerebral palsy. *Terapia Manual*, 40, 101–104.

Paiva, P., & Braccialli, L. M. P. (2009). TEXTURA DO RECURSO PEDAGÓGICO E IMPLICAÇÕES EM ATIVIDADE DE ENCAIXE REALIZADA POR INDIVÍDUOS COM PARALISIA CEREBRAL. *Revista Brasileira de Educação Especial*, 15(2), 307–318.

Palisano, R., Rosenbaum, P., Walter, S. D., Russell, D. J., Wood, E., & Galuppi, B. E. (1997). Development and reliability of a system to classify gross motor function in children with cerebral palsy. *Develop*, 39(2), 214–223. Retrieved from http://onlinelibrary.wiley.com/doi/10.1111/j.1469-8749.1997.tb07414.x/full

Phillips, B., & Zhao, H. (1993). Predictors of assistive technology abandonment. *Assistive Technology*, 5(1), 36–45. Retrieved from http://www.tandfonline.com/doi/abs/10.1080/10400435.1993.10132205

Sankako, A. N. (2013). Tecnologia assistiva das salas de recursos multifuncionais: avaliação de dispositivos para adequação postural. Universidade Estadual Paulista.

Scherer, M. J. (2002). The change in emphasis from people to person: introduction to the special issue on assistive technology. *Disability and Rehabilitation*, 24(1-3), 1–4. Retrieved from http://www.ncbi.nlm.nih.gov/pubmed/11827143

Sugden, D. (2000). Dynamic coupling: intrinsic and extrinsic influences on reaching and grasping in children wirh hemiplegic cerebral palsy. Revista Paulista de Educação Física, (3), 24–28.

Teulings, H., & Romero, D. H. (2003). Submovement analysis in learning cursive handwriting or block print. Proceedings of the 11th Conference of the International Graphonomics Society, (November), 2–5.

Van Vliet, P. M., & Sheridan, M. R. (2007). Coordination between reaching and grasping in patients with hemiparesis and healthy subjects. *Archives of Physical Medicine and Rehabilitation*, 88(10), 1325–31. doi:10.1016/j.apmr.2007.06.769

Verza, R., Carvalho, M. L. L., Battaglia, M. a, & Uccelli, M. M. (2006). An interdisciplinary approach to evaluating the need for assistive technology reduces equipment abandonment. *Multiple Sclerosis* (Houndmills, Basingstoke, England), 12(1), 88–93. Retrieved from http://www.ncbi.nlm.nih.gov/pubmed/16459724

Volman, M. J. M. (2005). Spatial coupling in children with hemiplegic cerebral palsy during bimanual circle and line drawing. *Motor Control*. 9 (4), 395-416.

Zerbinato, L.; Makita, L. M.; Zerloti, P. (2003). Paralisia cerebral. In: Teixeira, E.; Sauron, F. N.; Santos, L. S. B.; Oliveira, M. C. Terapia ocupacional na reabilitação física. São Paulo: Roca, 503-534.

In: Handbook on Cerebral Palsy
Editor: Harold Yates

ISBN: 978-1-63321-852-9
© 2014 Nova Science Publishers, Inc.

Chapter 9

The Value of Providing Cerebral Palsy Children and Caregivers an Oral Health Program

Renata Oliveira Guaré, D.D.S., Ph.D.[*1],
Daniel Cividanis Gomes Nogueira Fernandes, M.D.[2],
Ana Lídia Ciamponi, Ph.D.[3]
and Maria Teresa Botti Rodrigues Santos, D.D.S., Ph.D.[1]

[1]The Discipline of Dentistry, Persons with Disabilities Division,
Universidade Cruzeiro do Sul, São Paulo, Brazil
[2]Department of Integrated Clinic, School of Dentistry
University of São Paulo, São Paulo, Brazil
[3]Department of Orthodontics and Pediatric Dentistry;
School of Dentistry, University of São Paulo, São Paulo, Brazil

Abstract

Purpose: The purpose was to evaluate the effect of an education program on the oral health of individuals with cerebral palsy (CP) and their caregivers. Methods: 67 individuals with CP (8.87±3.91) of both sexes were evaluated, together with their caregivers (38.43±9.78) by a single examiner (kappa=0.88). Oral hygiene was evaluated using the Simplified Oral Hygiene Index (OHI-S) and the Gingival Index (GI). The general linear model for repeated measures was used to compare the effect of the intervention. Multivariate linear regression models were used to identify predictor variables. Results: The intervention achieved through the oral health program managed to reduce the OHI-S and GI in both the individuals with CP and their caregivers. The study also revealed that the only significant predictor for periodontal disease in individuals with

---

[*] Address for correspondence: Renata de Oliveira Guaré[1,] Rua Jorge Tibiriçá, n°74, apto 113, ZIP CODE:04126-000 São Paulo (SP), Brazil, e-mail:renataguare@uol.com.br.

CP was age. Conclusion: This research highlights the importance of early preventive guidelines through an oral health program that is also directed toward the caregivers.

Keywords: Cerebral palsy, oral health, oral hygiene training, special needs

Introduction

Cerebral palsy (CP) describes a group of movement and posture development disorders, which are attributed to nonprogressive disturbances that occur in the developing fetal or infant brain that cause activity limitation and may be accompanied by disturbances of sensation, cognition, communication and seizure disorders. [1] CP is the most common cause of severe physical disability in childhood [2], with an estimated prevalence of 2.4 per 1000 children. [3]

The severity of CP motor impairment and presence of associated conditions lead to reduced self-cleaning function of the oral cavity, identified as a negative factor for oral health. [4] The consumption of a soft diet, rich in carbohydrates, mastication by pressure at the back of the tongue and palate, incoordination of the mastication muscles, food remaining in the oral cavity and decreased salivary flow, are some of the factors responsible for the increased prevalence of dental caries in individuals with CP. [5-8]

Moreover, the fact that an expressive part of caregivers show difficulties in performing proper oral hygiene on CP individuals [9-11], and that most of these individuals are fed on a semi-solid diet, means dental biofilm tends to accumulate and becomes a risk factor for periodontal disease in these individuals [12-14].

Maintaining the oral health of CP individuals requires adequate systematic hygiene practices, demanding supervision or even the realization of their oral hygiene by the caregivers. However, when CP individuals are considered, this process of participation, involvement and support is not restricted to the development period. The task of taking care of a child with complex disabilities at home might be somewhat daunting for caregivers [15,16] and may sometimes reflect in the way these individuals are cared for. [17]

Since dental caries and periodontal disease are still widespread in CP children, it is important to recognize the caregiver's perception regarding the real condition of the oral health of children with CP and their own. Engaging the caregiver and the participant in their own oral hygiene will reflect in the oral cavity of the individual being cared for, i.e., the child with CP, and could lead to reduced periodontal indices in both the child and the caregiver following the intervention. Thus, the aim of this study was to evaluate the effect of the intervention of an education program on oral health in individuals with cerebral palsy and their caregivers.

Methods

This study was approved by the Ethics Committee on Human Research of the Cruzeiro do Sul University under protocol number 136/2009. After being informed of the aim of the investigation, written informed consent for participation and publication was obtained from the adult responsible for each child who agreed to participate in this study.

Population

Eighty-six noninstitutionalized individuals with a medical diagnosis of CP attending the Rehabilitation Center Lar Escola São Francisco, São Paulo, Brazil, were invited to participate in this study; 67 of these responded to the invitation. The inclusion criteria were individuals with a clinical medical diagnosis of cerebral palsy, aged 8 to 18 years-old, of both sexes, whose parents/caregivers provided informed consent and also agreed to participate in this study. Patient medical records were reviewed for demographic and clinical data, including sex, age, type of movement disorder (spasticity, dyskinesia or ataxia) and clinical patterns of involvement among the spastic individuals (quadriplegia, diplegia, hemiplegia).

Measurements

A single calibrated examiner (kappa=0.88) was responsible for all periodontal measurement (caregiver and CP child). The examiner observed and scored six teeth (four posterior and two anterior) for each child according to the Simplified Oral Hygiene Index (OHI-S). [18] For the posterior teeth, the first fully erupted tooth distal to the second premolar or primary molar was examined in each quadrant. For maxillary molars, the buccal surfaces were scored, and for mandibular molars, the lingual surfaces were scored. For anterior teeth, the labial surfaces of the maxillary right and mandibular left central incisors were scored. The OHI-S is a combination of visible plaque and oral calculus.

During the examinations, the amount of visible plaque on teeth was observed and scored using a four-point scale: 0= no debris or stain detectable; 1= soft debris covering no more than cervical one-third of tooth surface or extrinsic stains, with no other debris regardless of the surface area covered; 2= soft debris covering more than one-third, but no more than two-thirds of the exposed tooth surface; and 3= soft debris covering more than two-thirds of the exposed tooth surface.

For oral calculus, a four-point scale was also used: 0= no calculus present; 1= supragingival calculus covering no more than one third of the exposed tooth surface being examined; 2= supragingival calculus covering more than one-third, but no more than two-thirds of exposed tooth surface, or the presence of small portions of subgingival calculus around the cervical area of the tooth; and 3= supragingival calculus covering more than two-thirds of the exposed tooth surface or a continuous subgingival calculus along the cervical area of the tooth.

The gingival condition of the children was scored according to the Gingival Index (GI) [19], using a four-point scale: 0= absence of inflammation; 1= mild inflammation, with discrete change in color and texture; 2= moderate inflammation, with rubor, edema, and presence of bleeding on probing; and 3= severe inflammation, intense rubor and edema, and ulcerated tissue with a tendency for spontaneous bleeding. Each gingival unit (buccal, mesial, lingual, and distal) of the individual tooth was given a score from 0-3, called the GI for the area. The mean score of the four areas of the tooth provide the GI for the tooth. The scores of the individual teeth (maxillary right first molar, maxillary right lateral incisor, maxillary left primary molar or first bicuspid, mandibular left first molar, mandibular lateral incisor and mandibular right primary molar or first bicuspid) were added up and divided by six. The GI for the child was the mean score of all the areas examined.

Education Program on Oral Health

This program consisted of five stages involving a total of 67 individuals with CP and their caregivers. All five stages were performed by a single trained examiner over 3 months.

1st *Stage* - Initial clinical evaluation of the individuals with CP and their caregivers: All the caregivers and individuals with CP were evaluated clinically regarding their periodontal health (initial status of patient and caregiver).

2nd *Stage* - Professional instruction: Caregivers received instructions concerning the following: disability, principal diseases of the oral cavity, their etiological factors, forms of prevention and maintenance of oral health. The importance of oral health as part of overall health was emphasized, including information concerning frequent risk factors for systemic diseases.

3rd *Stage* - Hands-on: Oral hygiene practices in children with CP were performed by the primary caregiver, under the supervision of the examiner, including use of dental floss, individualization of oral hygiene, maintaining the mouth opening (use of mouth openers), brushing the tongue, desensitization of reflexes like vomiting and biting, and cleaning and storing a toothbrush.

4th *Stage* - Sensitization of individuals with CP: This was achieved through a playful approach, including interactive games, puzzles, puppet shows, and crafts based on issues strictly related to oral health education.

5th *Stage* - Final clinical evaluation of the individuals with CP and their caregivers: All the caregivers and individuals with CP were evaluated clinically regarding their periodontal health (final status of patient and caregiver), after the educational stages.

It should be emphasized that the interval between the initial and final stage was 90 days, such that for stages 2 through 4, the encounters with the examiner were weekly, lasting 30 min for both the child with CP and their caregiver.

Statistical Analyses

Analyses were performed using the Statistical Package for Social Sciences (SPSS v18.0). The Shapiro-Wilk test was used to test the normality of the quantitative variables. The general linear model (GLM) for repeated measures was used to compare the effect of intervention, the types of PC and their interaction on the OHI-S and GI in children and to compare the effect of intervention on the caregivers. Multivariate linear regression models were used to identify predictors of the difference (delta) between the initial and final OHI-S and between the initial and final GI, considering sex, age, type of PC and whether the individual was receiving dental care as independent variables of the model. A value of 5% was the criterion for significance.

Results

Sixty-seven children with a medical diagnosis of CP and their primary caregivers were enrolled in this study.

Thirty-six were males (53.7 %) and 31 were females (46.3%), ranging in age from 8 to 18 years-old (8.87±3.91 years-old), and 59 (88.1%) had spastic CP. The sample included 32 (47.8 %) children with a diplegic pattern of CP; 16 (23.4 %) were quadriplegic; 11 (16.4%) were hemiplegic, 5 athetoid (7.5%) and 3 ataxic (4.5%). The caregivers were mostly women (92.5 %), ranging in age from 18 to 68 years-old (38.43±9.78 years-old), and mostly mothers (92.5%).

Table 1. Simplified Oral Hygiene Index and Gingival Index in cerebral palsy children and their caregivers before (initial) and after (final) the implementation of an oral health program

Variable	Mean± SD (range)
Cerebral palsy children	
Age	8.87±3.91 (1-18.8)
Initial OHI-S	1.29±0.99 (0-3.3)
Final OHI-S	0.49±0.56 (0-2)
Initial GI	1.27±1.58(0-6)
Final GI	0.58±0.74(0-2)
Caregivers	
Age	38.43±9.78(18-69)
Initial OHI-S	1.75±1.84(0-6)
Final OHI-S	0.57±0.82(0-4)
Initial GI	1.42±1.46(0-6)
Final GI	0.59±0.76(0-3)

GI= Gingival Index; OHI-S= Simplified Oral Hygiene Index.

A significant effect of the program was verified on the OHI-S, independent of the type of CP ($p<0.05$).

Similarly, a significant effect of the program was verified on the GI ($p<0.05$). Following the intervention, the GI was reduced independent of the type of CP. No effect was determined for the type of CP, nor for the interaction between intervention and type of CP. A significant effect of the intervention was verified on the OHI-S and GI of the caregivers ($p<0.05$). Following the intervention, the OHI-S and GI of the caregivers was reduced.

Analysis of the linear regression models showed that the only variable that predicted significant variation in the OHI-S was the child's age (B=-0.068, p=0.009). An increase of 1 year in the child's age diminished the variation (final - initial) of the OHI-S by 0.068, i.e., the older the child, the less they improved. Similarly, the child's age (B=-0.092, p=0.020) was also able to significantly predict variation in the GI. Again, an increase of 1 year in the child's age diminished the variation (final - initial) of the GI by 0.092, i.e., the older the child, the less they improved.

Table 2. Results of the general linear model for repeated measures verifying the effect of the oral health program, types of PC and the interaction between them on the Simplified Oral Hygiene Index and Gingival Index of children with cerebral palsy and their caregivers

Variable	F	p
Cerebral palsy children		
OHI-S (Cerebral palsy children)		
Program	26.924	<0.001
CP type	1.487	0.217
GI (Cerebral palsy children)		
Program	11.523	0.001
CP type	1.916	0.119
Program and CP type interaction	1.873	0.126
Caregiver		
OHI-S (Caregivers)		
Program	46.438	<0.001
GI (Caregivers)		
Program	41.253	<0.001

GI= Gingival Index; OHI-S= Simplified Oral Hygiene Index.

Discussion

This study showed the importance of controlling the biofilm of the primary caregiver to achieve control of the biofilm of the CP patient and that over the three month evaluation period, an effect was verified for the education program on oral health aimed at children with cerebral palsy and their caregivers.

The severity of physical disability and mental problems associated with oral problems and socioeconomic factors may have an impact on the quality of life of individuals with CP. [20] Studies have shown that the more severe the neurological damage in children with CP, the greater the risk of oral diseases. [4,7] This is not only due to the consistency of their diet, but also to the increased difficulty that these individuals face when performing or receiving proper oral hygiene. [21] It should be highlighted that the majority of the patients evaluated attend a high complexity rehabilitation center and require care, because they are totally dependent on their caregivers.

This is the first study to suggest that a program of oral health aimed at the primary caregivers resulted in improvements in both their own oral health and that of the individual with cerebral palsy. However, these positive results must be interpreted within the limitations of a 90-day cross-sectional study. Regarding the OHI-S and GI, this study showed that significant effects were verified on the OHI-S ($p < 0.05$) and the IG ($p < 0.05$). Intervention through the implementation of an oral health program involving the caregiver was able to reduce the indices independent of the type of CP. In the caregivers, intervention also showed a significant effect on the two indices ($p < 0.001$). Magalhães et al. [22] submitted CP patients to a program of caries and periodontal disease prevention, based on awareness, stimulation and the search for new alternatives that would promote plaque control. The OHI-S was also applied before and after the onset of the program and the results showed a statistically significant reduction in plaque. However, in contrast to this study, the caregiver was not assessed and index of gingival bleeding was not determined.

In this study, the only variable able to predict significant variation in the OHI-S was the child's age (p=0.009). An increase of one year in the child's age diminished the variation (final - initial) of the OHI-S by 0.068, i.e., the older the child, the less they improved. This is because as the child's age increases, the number of teeth increases, together with associated factors, such as hormonal changes and the difficulty involved in modifying established behaviors, leading to an increased risk of periodontal disease. The mean initial OHI-S in individuals with CP was 1.2 and 1.8 for caregivers. These hygiene indices are considered "good" for individuals with CP and "regular" for caregivers. [18] At the end of the program, the mean value for both groups was approximately 0.5, indicating a significant improvement in the caregivers group.

Regarding the GI, an increase of one year in the child's age diminished the variation (final - initial) of the GI by 0.092, i.e., the older the child, the less they improved. In this case, it is important to highlight how a lack of early prevention programs in these high-risk individuals often leads to more invasive dental treatments and the need for emergency interventions, often resulting in negative experiences concerning dental treatment. The most effective way to resolve this issue is to provide preventive guidance from infancy onward.

Logistic regression, using the presence of periodontal disease as a dependent variable and age, the child's sex and type of PC as independent variables, determined that the only predictor of periodontal disease was age (p=0.049). In this case, an increase in age of one year increased the chances of the child presenting periodontal disease 1.176 times. The presence of periodontal disease in children with CP occurs due to the accumulation of biofilm and the inability to maintain adequate oral hygiene. Another predisposing factor that should be highlighted is the pasty consistency of the food these children ingest, which can aggravate periodontal problems. [11]

Patients with CP can present poor oral hygiene, since they often do not have the level of motor skills required to adequately clean the oral cavity. [23] In addition to these limitations in personal skills, caregivers of individuals with CP also experience difficulties in maintaining adequate oral hygiene in these patients. [8] Difficulty in maintaining the mouth opened due to muscle tone [24], hyperresponsivity to oral hygiene stimulus and oral manipulation [24], and non-cooperative behavior [25] contribute to food residues.

Important points of the oral health program included the use of low-cost mouth openers and the "hands-on" stage, when the difficulties involved in achieving individual oral hygiene for patients with CP were observed, and the positive benefits were highlighted. This stage, involving caregiver knowledge of oral hygiene habits, the use of open mouth devices to facilitate tooth-brushing, the use of fluoride dentifrice and diet control, was the most important and must be emphasized in CP children.

Other parameters investigated in this study related to the children's motor skills. The level of oral motor dysfunction in CP children is essential for determining peculiarities in the stomatognathic structures that could be correlated with periodontal diseases. Furthermore, compromised oral motor performance interferes with fluid intake, enhanced bacterial agglutination and the formation of an acquired pellicle and biofilm, which increase periodontal disease. [26]

It is well known that dental plaque is the principal cause of dental caries and periodontal disease. Also relevant to this discussion is the fact that the maintenance of adequate oral hygiene is a hard task for the caregivers [14]. Motor and intellectual disabilities [25], the presence of pathological oral reflexes of biting and vomiting [4]· the position of the child at the time of oral hygiene, and alterations in intraoral sensitivity, are some of the factors that influence both tooth brushing and biofilm control. [12] Implementing prevention programs is critical to the maintenance and promotion of oral health in individuals with CP. Dental professionals need to develop and implement educational tools to prepare caregivers to adequately control the biofilm of dependents with CP. It is equally important that the dental professional orients and prepares the primary caregiver, providing them with the capacity to orient and train other family caregivers. [12] The implementation of an education program on oral health directed toward the caregiver led to a change in behavior, particularly in the caregiver, who acquired knowledge concerning the principal diseases that affect the oral cavity of children with CP, emphasizing the importance of oral health as part of overall health.

Conclusion

The intervention achieved through the oral health program managed to reduce the OHI-S and GI in both the individuals with CP and their caregivers. The study also revealed that the only significant predictor for periodontal disease in individuals with CP was age. This research highlights the importance of early preventive guidelines through an oral health program that is also directed toward the caregivers.

Acknowledgments

This study was supported by AUX-PE-PROSUP-CAPE grants 2198/2010.

References

[1]   Bax M, Goldstein M, Rosenbaum P, et al. Executive Committee for the Definition of Cerebral Palsy. Proposed definition and classification of cerebral palsy. *Developmental Medicine and Child Neurology* 2005; 47: 571-6.

[2]   Kuban KC, Leviton A. Cerebral palsy. *The New England Journal of Medicine* 1994; 330:188-95.

[3]   Hirtz D, Thurman DJ, Gwinn-Hardy K, et al.How common are the "common" neurologic disorders? *Neurology* 2007; 68 : 326-37.

[4]   Dos Santos MT, Nogueira ML. Infantile reflexes and their effects on dental caries and oral hygiene in cerebral palsy individuals. *Journal of Oral Rehabilitation* 2005;32: 880-5.

[5] Dos Santos MT, Masiero D, Simionato MR. Risk factors for dental caries in children with cerebral palsy. *Spec. Care Dentist* 2002; 22: 103-7.

[6] Rodrigues dos Santos MT, Masiero D, Novo NF,et al. Oral conditions in children with cerebral palsy. *Journal of Dentistry for Children* 2003; 70: 40-6.

[7] Guaré RO, Ciamponi A. Dental caries prevalence in the primary dentition of cerebral palsied children. *The Journal of Clinical Pediatric Dentistry* 2003; 27:287-92.

[8] De Camargo MA, Antunes JL. Untreated dental caries in children with cerebral palsy in the Brazilian context. *Int. J. Paediatr. Dent.* 2007, 18:131-8.

[9] DU RY, McGrath C, Yiu CK, et al. Oral health in preschool children with cerebral palsy: a case-control community-based study. *Int. J. Paediatr. Dent.* 2010; 20:330-5.

[10] Chu CH, Lo EC. Oral health status of Chinese teenagers with cerebral palsy. *Community Dent. Health* 2010;27:222-6.

[11] Guare Rde O, Ciampioni AL. Prevalence of periodontal disease in the primary dentition of children with cerebral palsy. *J. Dent. Child* 2004;71:27-32.

[12] Rodrigues dos Santos MT, Bianccardi M, Celiberti P, et al. Dental caries in cerebral palsied individuals and their caregivers' quality of life. *Child Care Health Dev.* 2009;35: 475-81.

[13] Santos MT, Guare RO, Celiberti P, et al. Caries experience in individuals with cerebral palsy in relation to oromotor dysfunction and dietary consistency. *Spec. Care Dentist* 2009; 29:198-203.

[14] Santos MT, Biancardi M, Guare RO, et al. Caries prevalence in patients with cerebral palsy and the burden of caring for them. *Spec. Care Dentist* 2010; 30:206-10.

[15] Manuel J, Naughton MJ, Balkrishnan R, et al. Stress and adaptation in mothers of children with cerebral palsy. *Journal of Pediatric Psychology* 2003;28:297–301.

[16] Raina P, O'Donnell M, Rosenbaum P, et al. The health and well-being of caregivers of children with cerebral palsy. *Pediatrics* 2005; 115: 626–36.

[17] Benedict MI, Wulff LM, White RB. Current parental stress in maltreating and nonmal treating families of children with multiple disabilities. *Child Abuse and Neglect* 1992; 16:155–63.

[18] Greene JC, Vermillion JR. The Simplified Oral Hygiene Index. *J. Am. Dent. Assoc.* 1964;68:7-13.

[19] Loe H, Silness J. Periodontal Disease In Pregnancy. I. Prevalence and Severity. *Acta Odontol Scand.* 1963;21:533-51.

[20] Abanto J, Carvalho TS, Bönecker M, et al. Parental reports of the oral health-related quality of life of children with cerebral palsy. *BMC Oral Health* 2012; 12:15.

[21] Dickinson HO, Parkinson KN, Ravens-Sieberer U, et al. Self-reported quality of life of 8-12-year-old children with cerebral palsy: a cross-sectional. *European study Lancet* 2007; 369:2171–8.

[22] Magalhães MHCG, Becker MM, Ramos M. Aplicaçäo de um programa de higienização supervisionada em pacientes portadores de paralisia cerebral. *RPG* 1997; 4:109-13.

[23] Rao D, Amitha H, Munshi AK. Oral hygiene status of disabled children and adolescents attending special schools of South Canara, India. *Hong Kong Dent. J.* 2005; 2:107-13.

[24] Rosenbaum P, Paneth N, Leviton A, et al. A report: the definition and classification of cerebral palsy. *Dev. Med. Child Neurol. Suppl.* 2007; 109: 8-14.

[25] Moreira RN, Alcântara CE, Mota-Veloso I, et al. Does intellectual disability affect the development of dental caries in patients with cerebral palsy? *Res. Dev. Disabil.* 2012; 33: 1503-7.

[26] Ryu M, Ueda T, Saito T, et al. Oral environmental factors affecting number of microbes in saliva of complete denture wearers. *J. Oral. Rehabil.* 2010; 37:194-201.

In: Handbook on Cerebral Palsy
Editor: Harold Yates

ISBN: 978-1-63321-852-9
© 2014 Nova Science Publishers, Inc.

Chapter 10

The Use of Weight Bracelet in Individuals with Encephalopathy

*Mauro Audi[1], Andréia Naomi Sankako[2] and Lígia Maria Presumido Braccialli[2],**

[1]Marilia University, Marilia, Brazil
[2]Faculdade de Filosofia e Ciências, Unesp –
University Estadual Paulista, Marília, Brazil

Abstract

This study aimed to analyze the function of upper limbs, in the reach movement to a target, with and without a weight bracelet, in individuals with encephalopathy who had involuntary movements of upper limbs. 7 individuals with diagnosis of encephalopathy who had involuntary movements, 2 females, 5 males, aged 21 to 38 years (mean = 26) participated in this study. Significant statistical differences were found (p = 0.03) to the obtained results of the distance gone through upper limb and to straightness index values (p = 0.03), comparing the obtained results with and without weight bracelet. The use of weight bracelet on the wrist influenced the values of the traveled distance and the straightness index during the reach movement to a target, which were lesser when compared to the movement without weight bracelet. Results demonstrated a better motor performance of upper limbs from participants of this study with weight bracelet.

Keywords: Movement disorders, Encephalopathy, Motor skills, Upper extremity

---

* Corresponding author: Drª. Lígia Maria Presumido Braccialli, Department of Special Education, Faculdade de Filosofia e Ciências, Unesp - Univ Estadual Paulista, Avenida Hygino Muzzi Filho, 737, Caixa Postal: 181, C.E.P.: 17.525-900, Marília, São Paulo, Brazil. Telephone: 55 14 3402-1331, fax: 55 14 3402-1331. e-mail: bracci@marilia.unesp.br.

Introduction

Individuals with encephalopathy who present injuries in basal ganglia or cerebellum commonly have unwanted movements while performing their voluntary movements The presence of this movements can promote discomforts and postural disturbances, interfere in voluntary movements, limit the function of the affected limbs, and injure the performance in school and daily life activities (Chang, Wu, Wu and Su, 2005).

To perform daily life and school activities, the reach movement is essential, therefore it has widely been studied by many researchers (Nicholson, Morton, Attfield and Rennie, 2001; Chang et al., 2005; Coluccini, Maini, Martelloni, Sgandurra and Cioni, 2007; Utley, Sugden, Lawrence and Astill, 2007). Individuals with any type of motor impairment have difficulties to perform this movement (Volman, Wijnroks and Vermeer, 2002; Chang et al., 2005; Lang, Wagner, Edwards, Sarhmann and Dromerick, 2006; Chen, et al., 2007; Utley et al., 2007; Van Vliet and Sheridan, 2007), and for those who present athetosis, occur loss of fixation and the movement is performed in excessive amplitude (Nicholson et al., 2001).

Several studies have investigated the kinematical analysis of reach movements in individuals with hemiparesis (Chang et al., 2005; Lang et al., 2006; Reisman and Scholz, 2007; Chen, et al., 2007; Wu, Chen, Tang, Lin and Huang, 2007; Van Vliet and Sheridan, 2007), with Parkinson's disease (Ma; Trombly; Wagenaar and Tickle-Degnen, 2004; Maitra, 2007), and diskynetics (Nicholson et al., 2001; Coluccini et al., 2007).

Forsstrom and Von Hofsten (1982) studied individuals with athetoid cerebral palsy (CP) and found that they exhibit longer phases during object transport compared to individuals without disability, but can perform the reach and object prehension, even when the target was moved quickly. This suggests that when planning a reach movement, these individuals are able to compensate for the deficits that result in slow times of movement. The movement is directed sufficiently in advance of the target, so that they can maintain the acuity during the reach, even with their motors impairments.

Adults with dyskinetic cerebral palsy (DCP) performs the task of bringing a mug to the mouth more slowly than the control group, with significant difference in average speed, maximum speed, and the time required to reach peak velocity (Artilheiro et al., 2013).

Butler, Ladd, Lamont and Rose (2010) found that people with CP increased nearly two-fold increase in the total time required to reach for a glass, lift it to the mouth, and return it to its original position.

However, few studies analyze the reach movement in individuals with involuntary movements associated with the use of some type of instrument, in the attempt to verify if occurring or not motor performance improvement of upper limbs.

Nicholson et al. (2001) found that lycra garments in children with athetoid and ataxic cerebral palsy improved the proximal stability, and it results in a better performance of the reach movement.

Maitra (2007) observed a better performance in the reach movement in individuals with Parkinson's disease using his own voice as a command to start the movement.

In another study with individuals with Parkinson's disease, it was also observed performance improvement of the reach movement using a bell ring to start it (Ma et al., 2004).

The Use of Weight Bracelet in Individuals with Encephalopathy 153

Lucareli et al. (2010) in a study with CP choreoathetoid identified that the use of weight bracelet in forearm, with 25%, 50% and 75% load, decreased the error range of the target and showed a statistically significant difference ($p \leq 0.05$) when compared to control group.

Study with adults with DCP identified that a load of 10% during functional activity of taking a cup of 350ml to the mouth resulted in decreased run time (Lucareli et al., 2013).

Individuals with dyskinesia have some unusual movement patterns during the reach and prehension, as increasing the duration of the prehension phase, and significantly increased in head and trunk movements in all three planes (Coluccini, et al., 2007). In the attempt to minimize these difficulties presented by these individuals, and improve their performance, physiotherapists and occupational therapists have been suggested to use of weight bracelets in the arms to reduce these involuntary movements (Lucareli et al., 2010).

However, there are still doubts about the real functional benefits that weight bracelet could provide for individuals with involuntary movements. Thus, this study had as purpose to analyze the function of upper limbs, in the reach movement to a target, with and without the weight bracelet, in individuals with encephalopathy who presented involuntary movements of upper limbs.

Method

Participants

Seven individuals were selected, aged 21 to 38 years (mean = 26), 2 female and 5 male. The characteristics of the participants are demonstrated in Table 1. The inclusion criteria were: to present diagnosis of encephalopathy; to present involuntary movements in upper limbs; to reach a target against the gravity action; to maintain the seated posture, to comprehend the required task and to have parents or caregivers signed the Informal Consent Term. The exclusion criteria were: no diagnosis of encephalopathy; not to reach a target against the gravity action with the less affected upper limb and visual impairment that hindered to see the target. The participants were evaluated by two physiotherapists to verify if the subjects presented the characteristics necessary to participate in this study and classified according the motor scale Gross Motor Function Classification System – GMFCS (Russel, Rosenbaun, Avery and Lane, 2002). The 7 individuals presented all inclusion criteria.

This study was submitted to the Research Ethics Committee of the Faculty of Philosophy and Science – Professor Júlio de Mesquita Filho – UNESP, Marília, São Paulo, Brazil, and approved by the number 465/2005. The research was developed at the Laboratory of Motor Performance Analysis in Faculty of Philosophy and Science (FFC), Unesp, Marília.

Instruments and Materials

Camera to register the images; computer with video capture plate to catch the images registered by the camera; software Kavideo to analyze the movement; support to fix the camera; reflexive markers to be placed at the major joints that will be analyzed; load for the weight bracelet; bracelet with velcro on the wrist to fix load and adapted furniture.

Table 1. Characteristics of participants

Participants	Classification GMFCS	Skillfull upper limb	Gender	Age (years)
P1	degree V	Left	female	24
P2	degree IV	Right	male	38
P3	degree I	Right	female	25
P4	degree I	Left	male	29
P5	degree V	Left	male	24
P6	degree V	Left	male	25
P7	degree V	Right	male	21

Procedure

A pilot study was previously conducted with a child without neurological disorders to determine the space to perform the task and the position of the camera. This pilot study allowed to adjust the height, position and distance of the camera in relation to the space where the task was performed; to define the pole scale to be used and the distance between the targets that were fixed on the table. It was determined that the camera should be superior positioned to register the movement, because this is the better position to register all markers fixed on the participants' upper limb. It was also defined that the distance between the targets fixed on the table should correspond to maximum reach of the less affected upper limb of each individual.

Experimental Protocol

The participants wore clothes that allowed to see the entire upper limb. It was fixed reflexive markers at the joints of the less affected upper limb. For this study 4 anatomical points were chosen: prominence of the acromion, ulna styloid process, head of the radio and distal surface of the third metacarpal, because corresponded to the main joints axis of the upper limb and they are easily palpable.

After the participant was comfortably positioned in an adapted chair, that allowed adjustment, with the feet flat on the floor, knees and hip in 90° flexion and neutral position for abduction, adduction and rotation of hip. In front of the participant was positioned a table in semicircle and height adjustment, which was adjusted for each one. On this table two targets of different colors were fixed. The first target was fixed parallel to the anterior sternum axis, and was called initial point, from 0.15 m of each participant's trunk, because this distance maintained the elbow joint in flexion. The second target, called final point, was parallel to the first target at a variable distance for each participant (Figure 1).

The distance between the initial and final points varied according to the maximum transverse reach of each participant. The maximum transverse reach corresponds to the anthropometric measurement which determines the hypothetical axis of the upper limb centered in the shoulder joint, and from this point is drawn a radius that is the same to the upper limb length. The determination of maximum reach is used to define the necessary space for the work or activity (Nowak, 1996; Jaroz, 1996).

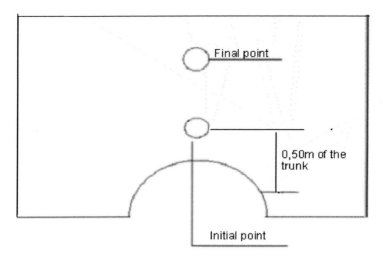

Figure 1. Illustration of the targets fixed on the table.

To the reconstruction of the points in the space was necessary to mark the pole scale on the table for each participant. The pole scale is required by software Kavideo of movement analysis to execute a conversion factor of orthogonal coordinates XY. The measurement of pole scale corresponds to extreme limits between maximum reach of the participant and the root of the shoulder joint of the upper limb used to perform the task.

The camera was positioned on a base, so the filming could be done from a superior view, and the height was adjusted for each participant.

The participant was instructed to put the upper limb, which would not be used to perform the task, resting on the table, and those who had no adequate control to keep the limb resting, were helped by another person. Then, this limb did not interfere in the less affected limb movement during the execution of the task.

The task consisted in the outward movement from initial to final points. This movement was repeated three times, with and without the use weight bracelet. The order to execute the task, with or without weight bracelet, was random, by draw.

The used loads were individually calculated for each participant by maximum resistance (MR) calculus prescribed by Macardle, Katch and Katch (2006). This calculus was made using a load which the individual could perform the total amplitude movement in ten repetitions. The load was gradually increased until the maximum resistance load was established. According to Mendoza, García, Pino, Martín and Ferrer (2003), strength training in children with CP should be performed between 50% and 60% of maximum load. In this study, the weight bracelet load corresponded to 50% of maximum load of each participant. The weight bracelet was distally put in the forearm of each one.

Kinematic Analysis

The images registered by the camera were captured by software Kavideo of movement analysis through a video plate. It was made the digitalization of each marker fixed on participant's skin for reconstruction of the performed movement. By kinematic analysis it was possible to obtain, for this study, data about distance gone through each participant's upper limb during the performed movement. From this distance gone through upper limb during the experiment, and minimum displacement that should be performed during the task, it was possible to calculate the straightness index.

The straightness index indicates how many times the participant had to travel a longer trajectory in relation to the shorter displacement performed by the upper limb. The calculus was made by ratio between distance gone through upper limb and the minimum displacement that could be performed in this trajectory. Straightness index equals 1 indicates that the movement was performed in a shorter possible distance. The straightness index more than 1 indicates how much the movement trajectory was longer than the minimum displacement that the upper limb could have traveled (Carvalho, Tudella, Caljouw and Savelsbergh, 2008).

Statistical Analysis

A statistical descriptive analysis was made by mean, standard deviation, maximum and minimum data from distance gone through each participant's upper limb during the performed movement and the straightness index, velocity and time execution. The comparison of the upper limb motor performance with and without weight bracelet was made by a non-parametric statistical test, Wilcoxon Test. The adopted value was $p \leq 0.05$.

Results

Table 2 presents data related to distance gone through participants' upper limb during the task with and without weight bracelet. It was found statistically significant difference ($p = 0.03$) by Wilcoxon test when compared the obtained results of the distance gone through upper limb without and with weight bracelet. This demonstrates that the distance gone through upper limb during the movement was influenced by the use of weight bracelet.

Table 3 demonstrates results referred to the straightness index during the movement performance with and without the use of weight bracelet.

It was observed statistically significant difference ($p = 0.03$) by Wilcoxon test for the straightness index, when compared the obtained results with and without weight bracelet. Thus, the use of weight bracelet also influenced the values of straightness index.

Table 2. Result from analysis of the distance gone through (m) upper limb during the task without and with weight bracelet

	Without weight bracelet	With weight bracelet
Mean	0,77	0,579
Standart Deviation	0,235	0,182
Minimum	0,503	0,425
Maximum	1,18	0,974
Variation of coeficient	0,305	0,315

Wilcoxon Test p = 0.03.

The Use of Weight Bracelet in Individuals with Encephalopathy

Table 3. Result of the straightness index analysis during the movement performance without and with the use of weight bracelet

	Without weight bracelet	With weight bracelet
Mean	2,781	2,082
Standart Deviation	0,978	0,709
Minimum	1,720	1,530
Maximum	4,540	3,590
Variation of coeficient	0,354	0,340

Wilcoxon Test p = 0.03.

Table 4. Result from analysis of the average velocity (m/s) during the task without and with weight bracelet

	Without weight bracelet	With weight bracelet
Mean	0.32	0.28
Standart Deviation	0.06	0.12
Minimum	0.23	0.10
Maximum	0.43	0.25
Variation of coeficient	0.19	0.45

Wilcoxon Test p = 0.05.

Table 5. Result from analysis of the time execution (s) during the task without and with weight bracelet

	Without weight bracelet	With weight bracelet
Mean	2.46	2.58
Standart Deviation	0.97	1.26
Minimum	1.33	1.35
Maximum	4.17	5.53
Variation of coeficient	0.39	0.49

Wilcoxon Test p = 0.08.

Table 4 indicates a statistical difference for the average velocity when comparing the movement performed with and without the weight bracelet. The use of weight bracelet decreased velocity. In Table 5 it can be see no statistical difference when comparing the movement execution time with and without use of weight bracelet.

Discussion

The use of weight bracelet in order to facilitate voluntary movement in individuals who present sequels of involuntary movement and thus, provide a better motor performance during daily life and school activities, is a common practice.

The use of weight bracelet on motor performance of upper limbs in patients with involuntary movements has been little investigated, researchers report different difficulties in evaluating: lack of protocol performance evaluation of upper limbs, presence of involuntary movements and difficulty in maintaining markers attached to the exact position (Artilheiro et al., 2013).

In the present study the weight bracelet was placed on the wrist, in other words, distally, and it was possible to observe a better motor performance with the use of weight bracelet by the analysis of straightness index and traveled distance for all participants, that were lower when compared to without weight bracelet. This demonstrates that the use of weight bracelet may have contributed to better coordination and movement precision. The results coincide with those found by Lucareli et al. (2010) who found that the use of additional load on the upper limbs in individual with choreoathetosis CP decreased the error range of a target. In another study Lucareli et al. (2013) found that the use of an additional load of 10% on a cup decreased the time and did not affect the execution velocity to perform the task of bringing the cup to the mouth.

Dyskinesia is characterized by uncontrolled movements, which generate inconsistent patterns, inharmonious and slow movements (Artilheiro et al., 2013). The movement segmentation is also a characteristic of the motor performance in individuals with involuntary movements, which results in inaccurate, uncoordinated and slow movements (Menegoni et al., 2009). The mechanisms of co-contraction of the involved muscles, can also be a factor responsible for these inaccurate, uncoordinated and slow movements (Coluccini et al., 2007; Malfait and Sanger, 2007). The execution of the movement more slowly seems to be a strategy to improve the motor performance, smoothness and accuracy in performing the task (Menegoni et al., 2009; Sanger, Kaiser and placek, 2005).

For a good motor control, proximal stability is essential, and so it has been the main focus during therapy in order to improve the quality of movements in individuals with motor disorders. Thus, the use of weight bracelet placed distally can have contributed to a better proximal stability and consequently for a better motor performance, as it was observed in all participants of this study.

This is just an initial research, but there is much to be investigated yet, for example, how would be the motor performance with the use of weight bracelet in proximal region and with other loads?; how would be the mechanism of co-contraction activation of the involved muscles in the movement with the use of weight bracelet?; and for what type of involuntary movement the weight bracelet would provide greater benefits?

The weight bracelet is of low cost, easy use, not interfering in individuals' independence and it is not uncomfortable, so it can be an important resource to help individuals with involuntary movements during the therapy, and performance of their daily life and school activities, in order to promote a better motor performance.

References

Artilheiro, M. C., Corrêa, J. C. F., Cimolin, V., Lima, M. O., Galli, M., Godoy, W., Lucareli, P. R. G. (2013). Three-dimensional analysis of performance of an upper limb functional task among adults with dyskinetic cerebral palsy. *Gait Posture*, GAIPOS-4098; No. of Pages 7.

Butler, E. E., Ladd, A. L., Lamont, L. E., Rose, J. (2010). Temporal-spatial parameters of the upper limb during a reach and grasp cycle for children. *Gait and Posture*, 32(3), 301-6.

Carvalho, R. P., Tudella, E., Caljouw, S. R., and Savelsbergh, G. J. P. (2008). Early control of reaching: effects of experience and body orientation. *Infant and Behavior development*, 31 (1), 23-33.

Chang, J. J., Wu, T. I., Wu, L. W., and Su, F. C. (2005). Kinematical measure for spastic reaching in children with derebral palsy. *Clinical Biomechanics*, 20, 381-388.

Chen, Y. P., Kang, L. J., Chuang, T. Y., Doong, J. L., Lee, S. J., Tsai, M. W... Sung, W. H. (2007). Use of virtual reality to improve upper-extremity control in children wuth cerebral palsy: A single subject design. *Physical Therapy*, 87 (11), 1441-1457.

Coluccini, M., Maini, E. S., Martelloni, S., Sgandurra, G., and Cioni, G. (2007). Kinematic characterization of functional reach to grasp in normal and in motor disabled children. *Gait and Posture*, 25, 493-501.

Forsstrom, A. and Von Hofsten, C. Visually directed reaching in children with motor impairments. *Dev. Med. Child Neuro.* 1982; 24: 653-661.

Jaroz, E. (1996). Detrmination of the workspace of wheelchair users. *International Journal of Industry Ergonomics*, 17, 123-133.

Lang, C. E., Wagner, J. M., Edwards, D. F., Sarhmann, S. A., and Dromerick, A. W. (2006). Recovery of grasp versus reach in people with hemiparesis poststroke. *Neurorehabilitation and Neural Repair*, 20 (4), 444-454.

Lucareli, P. R. G., Oliveira, D., Lima, M. O., Lima, F. P., Artilheiro, M., Braccialli, L. M. P., and Corrêa, J. C. (2010). The influence of the use of stabilizer bracelet in a child with choreoathetoid cerebral palsy. *Terapia Manual*, Londrina, 40, S101-S104.

Lucareli, P. R. G., Artilheiro, M., Cimolin, V., Galli, M., Garbelotti, S. A., and Correa, J. C. F. (2013). 3D quantitative analysis of upper limb movements by using weight bracelets in adults with dyskinetic cerebral palsy. *ESMAC 2012 abstract / Gait and Posture*, 38, S1-S116.

Ma, H. I., Trombly, C. A., Wagenaar, R. C., and Tickle-Degnen, L. (2004). Effect of one single auditory cueon movement kinematics in patients with Parkinson's disease. *American Journal of Physical and Medicine Rehabilitation*, 83 (7), 530-536.

Maitra, K. K. (2007). Enhancement of reaching performance via self-speech in people with Parkinson's disease. *Clinical Rehabilitation*, 21, 418-424.

Malfait, N. and Sanger, T. D. (2007). Does dystonia always include co-contraction? A study of unconstrained reaching in children with primary an secondary dystonia. *Experimental Brain Research*, 176, 206-216.

McArdle, W. D., Katch, F. I. and Katch, V. L. (2006). *Exercise physiology: Energy, Nutrition and Human Performance,* 6 ed. Lippincott Williams andWilkins.

Mendoza, N., García, J. M., Pino, J., Martín, O., and Ferrer, R. (2003) *Evaluation of maximal dynamic leg strength of soccer-7 players with cerebral palsy*. Available at: <ncbi.nlm. nhi.gov/entrez/query.fcgi>.

Menegoni, F., Milano, E., Trotti, C., Galli, M., Bigoni, M., Baudo, S., and Mauro, A. (2009). Quantitative evaluation of functional limitation of upper limb movements in subjects affected by ataxia. *European Journal of Neurology*, 16, 232-239.

Nicholson, J. H., Morton, R. E., Attfield, S., and Rennie, D. (2001). Assessment of upper-limb function and movement in children with cerebral palsy wearing lycra garments. *Development Medicine and Child Neurology,* 43, 384-391.

Nowak, E. (1996). The role of anthropometry in design of work and life environments of the disable population. *International Journal of Industryal Ergonomics*, 17, 113-121.

Reisman, D. S. and Scholz, J. P. (2007). Deficit in surface force production during seated reaching in people after stroke. *Physical Therapy*, 87 (3), 326-336.

Rennie, D. J., Attfield, S. F., Morton, R. E., Polak, F. J., and Nicholson, J. (2000). An evaluation of lycra garments in the lower limb using 3-D gait analysis and functional assessment (PEDI). *Gait and Posture*, 12, 1-6.

Russel, D. J., Rosenbaun, P. L., Avery, L. M., and Lane, M. (2002) *Gross motor function measure (GMFM66 and GMFM88) user's manual.* London: Mackeith Press.

Sanger, T. D., Kaiser, J. and Placek, B. (2005) Reaching movements in childhood dystonia contain signal-dependent noise. *Journal of Child Neurology*, 20(6):489-96.

Utley, A., Sugden, D. A., Lawrence, G., and Astill, S. (2007). The influence of perturbing the working surface during reaching and grasping in children with hemiplegic cerebral palsy. *Disability and Rehabilitation*, 29, 79-89.

Van Vliet, P. M. and Sheridan, M. R. (2007). Coordination between reaching and grasping in patients with hemiparesis and healthy subjects. *Archives of Physical Medicine and Rehabilitation*, 888, 1325-1331.

Volman, J. M., Wijnroks, A. and Vermeer, A. (2002). Effects of task context on reaching performance in children with spastic hemiparesis. *Clinical Rehabilitation*, 16, 684-692.

Wu, C., Chen, C. L., Tang, S. F., Lin, K. C., and Huang, Y. Y. (2007). Kinematic and clinical analyses of upper-extremity movements after constraint-induced movement therapy in patients with stroke: A randomized controlled trial. *Arch physical Med Rehabilitation*, 88, 964-970.

In: Handbook on Cerebral Palsy
Editor: Harold Yates

ISBN: 978-1-63321-852-9
© 2014 Nova Science Publishers, Inc.

Chapter 11

Is Cerebral Palsy Associated with Cardiac Changes?

Maria Cristina Duarte Ferreira[1]*, Jaqueline Wagenfuhr[3],
Renata de Oliveira Guaré[4], Sergio Tufik[5], Dalva Poyares[5],
Wercules Oliveira[5], Carlos Alberto Pastore[3]
and Maria Teresa Botti Rodrigues Santos[2]

[1]Pediatric Dentistry, Universidade Paulista, Sao Paulo, Brazil
[2]Individuals with Special Needs, Universidade Cruzeiro do Sul, Sao Paulo, Brazil
[3]Electrocardiology and Echocardiography Service, Instituto do Coração,
Hospital das Clínicas, Universidade de São Paulo, Sao Paulo, Brazil
[4]Pediatric Dentistry. Program,Ciências Biológicas e da Saúde,
Universidade Cruzeiro do Sul, Sao Paulo, Brazil
[5]Psychobiology Department, Universidade Federal de Sao Paulo, Brazil

Abstract

Background: Some studies have suggested that an autonomic abnormality is associated with cerebral palsy. The modulation effects on autonomic function might be disturbed resulting in unbalanced sympathovagal activity,

Aim: To investigate whether children with cerebral palsy (CP) present any cardiac abnormalities compared with healthy controls.

Methods: Thirty-three CP children aged 5-14 years and 22 sibling controls underwent echocardiography and heart rate variability evaluations. Snoring and body mass index were also assessed.

Results: The CP children presented lower values of body mass index (p=0.02), left ventricular mass index (p=0.03) and E/A ratio (p=0.01), as well as higher cardiac output (p=0.05), heart rate and blood pressure (p=0.01, both) compared with controls. With

---

* Corresponding author: Rua Cancioneiro de Évora, 24, ZIP CODE:04708-010 São Paulo (SP), Brazil, e-mail:duarteferreira@uol.com.br.

regard to heart rate variability, CP children presented higher values of High-frequency and Low-frequency and lower Low-frequency/High-frequency ratios (p=0.04, all) than controls

Conclusion: Children with CP present with chronic autonomic imbalance and some degree of diastolic impairment. The present results suggest that a cardiac investigation of these patients is warranted.

Keywords: Cerebral palsy, echocardiography, autonomic nervous system, heart rate

Introduction

Cerebral palsy (CP) describes a group of chronic disorders that affects movement and posture development. It is the most common cause of severe physical disability in childhood, with an estimated prevalence of 2.4 per 1000 children. [1]

Some studies have suggested that an autonomic abnormality is associated with CP. The modulation effects on autonomic function might be disturbed resulting in unbalanced sympathovagal activity, with decreased sympathetic response after stress in CP patients.[2] Disturbances in homeostatic functions, which possibly result from autonomic dysfunction, were also observed. Another potential risk factor for autonomic alterations among CP children is sleep disturbances, such as obstructive sleep apnea or snoring. [3]

Echocardiography and heart rate variability are noninvasive diagnostic tests for the accurate evaluation of cardiac structure, function and autonomic tone to the heart. They are both sensitive and accurate tools for evaluating the impact of systemic conditions on cardiac performance. [4-5]

To the best of our knowledge, there are no studies that used echocardiography in individuals with CP to analyze cardiac performance in this population. Thus, the aim of this study was to investigate the autonomic tone and any possible structural or functional cardiac abnormalities related to CP.

Methods

Thirty-three individuals who were diagnosed with CP and were referred to our specialized rehabilitation center in Sao Paulo, Brazil, were consecutively included in this study. The inclusion criteria included a clinical diagnosis of CP, age 5-14 years-old, lack of seizures for at least 30 days prior to inclusion in the study and informed consent provided by parents/caregivers. The exclusion criteria included a previous history of cardiac disease, the presence of fever and the use of medications that might affect heart rate or cardiac function.

The presence of frequent snoring and body mass index (BMI) were also investigated in both groups.

The control group was comprised of 22 individuals who were healthy sibling volunteers of similar ages. The siblings were chosen as controls because they share similar age, cultural, genetic, and socioeconomic conditions.

Ethics approval was provided by the Universidade Federal Sao Paulo.

Echocardiogram

The blood pressure of the CP and control individuals was measured with the children comfortably seated after 10 minutes of rest. Following this, both groups underwent a 2-dimensional echocardiographic study according to standard guidelines [4], using the Sequoia 512 system (Acuson, Mountain View-CA). Continuous and pulse Doppler flows were recorded from a four-chamber view. The echocardiographic variables were assessed using the modified biplane Simpson rule. The stroke volume obtained was used to calculate the cardiac output according to the following formula: Stroke volume (L) x cardiac rate (bpm). Pulse Doppler diastolic mitral flow analysis was used to calculate the E/A ratio. The left ventricular mass index was obtained based on 2-dimensional echocardiography linear measurements [4]. Relative wall thickness (RWT) was measured with the following equation: 2 X left ventricular posterior wall in diastole/left ventricular diastolic diameter.

Heart Rate Variability

All individuals were monitored using a 3-channel ECG Holter monitor (SEER® Light, GE Medical Systems, Milwaukee, WI-USA). The twenty-four-hour HRV was calculated [5]. Subsequently, the data were processed and analyzed with a 250 Hz sampling frequency. Frequency domain indices were used. Power spectral analysis of the HRV was calculated within 3 frequency bands: very low-frequency (0.0033-0.04 Hertz), which may reflect the activity of the renin-angiotensin-aldosterone system, although its role remains unclear; low-frequency (0.04-0.15 Hz), which is related to modulation in the sympathetic and parasympathetic tone by baroreflex activity; and high-frequency (0.15-0.40 Hz), which indicates the respiratory modulation of R-R intervals, with the efferent impulses on the cardiac vagus nerve. The total power (0-0.40Hz) and the ratio of low-frequency to high-frequency power were also calculated as an indicator of sympathovagal balance.

Results

The CP group was composed of 33 patients, and the control group was composed of 22 children. The groups did not differ significantly regarding sex and age, but the CP group presented significantly lower BMI (Table 1). Significant differences between the CP and control groups were observed in terms of snoring, heart rate, E/A mitral inflow ratio, left ventricular mass index and blood pressure. A tendency towards statistical significance for the difference between the groups regarding cardiac output was found (Table 1).

When logistic regression analysis was performed, snoring was not significantly associated with E/A mitral inflow or left ventricular mass (p=0.19).

Higher values for high-frequency and low-frequency and lower values for the low-frequency/high-frequency ratio were observed for CP group (Table 2).

Table 1. Descriptive characteristics and mean (±SD) values for echocardiographic parameters of the cerebral palsy and control groups

Variables	CPG (n=33)	CG (n=22)	p value*
Sex, n(%)			
Female	12 (36.4)	8 (36.3)	0.48[a]
Male	21 (63.2)	14 (63.7)	
Age, mean [±SD]	10.1 ± 2.6	9.2 ± 22	0.20[b]
BMI	14.9 ± 1.8	16.6 ± 2.4	0.02*[b]
Snoring, n(%)			
Presence	26 (78.8)	0 (0)	<0.001*[a]
Absence	7 (21.2)	22 (100)	
Echocardiographic parameters			
LVDD (mm)	32.7 ± 5.9	35.2 ± 7.3	0.35
LVSD (mm)	19.1 ± 3.8	20.7± 5.8	0.46
SEPTUM (mm)	5.8 ± 1.1	6.2 ± 1.5	0.59
PW (mm)	5.7 ± 0.9	6.4 ± 1.3	0.10
Cardiac output (L/min)	3.0 ±0.9	2.8±0.5	0.05
SPP	22.6±3.4	21.7±4.7	0.3
HR (bpm)	96.8 ± 18.2	79.4 ± 12.5	0.01*[b]
EF (%)	72.7 ± 6.0	70.3 ± 1.1	0.56
E/A Mitral inflow	1.5±0.5	2.2 ±0.3	0.01*[b]
RWT	0.34±1.3	0.37±0.6	0.07
LV mass/height (g/m)	37.3±12.3	45.8±13.4	0.03*[b]
SBP	123.2±7.6	115.0±4.1	0.01*[b]
DBP	80.5±3.9	72.3±3.7	0.01*[b]

Cerebral palsy group (CPG) and control group (CG); BMI: Body Mass index; LVDD: Left ventricular diastolic diameter; LVSD: Left ventricular systolic diameter; PW: LV posterior wall; SPP: Systolic pulmonary pressure; HR: Heart rate; EF: Ejection fraction; RWT: Relative wall thickness; LV mass: left ventricular mass calculated from American Society of Echocardiography measurements; SBP: Systolic blood pressure; DBP: Diastolic blood pressure. The data were compared with a. the Chi squared test and b. Student's t-test, *p<0.05.

Table 2. Mean (±SD) values for HRV parameters of 24 h recording from the cerebral palsy (CPG) and control (CG) groups

Parameters	CPG (n=33)	CG (n=22)	p value*
VLF (ms^2)	32.8±8.9	29.2±7.1	0.24
HF (ms^2)	23.9 ± 9.5	17.6 ± 6.8	0.04*
LF (ms^2)	29.0 ± 11.3	24.2 ± 6.8	0.04*
LF/HF	1.2 ± 0.2	1.5 ± 0.3	0.04*
Total power	81.8 ± 28.4	73.5±19.8	0.08

HF: High frequency; VLF: Very Low frequency; LF: Low frequency; LF/HF: ratio of LF component to HF component. * Student's t-test comparing cerebral palsy group (CPG) and control group (CG), p<0.05.

Discussion

The main findings of this study were reduced left ventricular mass index and a decreased E/A ratio in the CP group that could be related to diastolic impairment in this population. In addition, a hyperdynamic status and an imbalance in the sympathovagal activity, represented by low modulation were found. To the best of our knowledge, this is the first study to demonstrate cardiac alterations and autonomic dysfunction among CP children compared to sibling controls, using echocardiogram and electrocardiographic recordings.

Some of the differences between the groups could be related to the hyperdynamic status in the CP group. In this particular case, the highest heart rate observed in the CP group could diminish ventricular filling and consequently cause changes in the E/A ratio. [4] These findings could be related to higher levels of adrenergic activation in CP individuals that could lead to unrecognized changes in diastolic function. Eidem et al. [6] stated that the limit for the mitral inflow E/A ratio is 1.6, below which the ratio is abnormal, and impairment of relaxation might be considered. No studies that evaluated the ventricular mass index in CP individuals were found, indicating that future studies on this topic are required.

Twenty-four-hour electrocardiographic recordings are particularly useful for risk stratification regarding a variety of pathological conditions, but can also be useful for quantifying autonomic dysfunction[5], although previous studies seem to have rarely focused on autonomic nervous system function of the CP individuals. Considering the HRV results, the findings suggest that an autonomic nervous system imbalance exists toward a sympathetic predominance.

HRV has been evaluated in CP individuals [7] but only during the tilt test. In the present study we obtained results with the 24-hour HRV monitoring.

Isolated HRV values obtained either at rest or under stress revealed no significant differences; however, a difference occurred in the response to stress in CP individuals presenting a small increase in the LF/HF ratio, which could indicate the existence of an autonomic response deficit in these patients [2] that is most likely due to a ceiling effect because patients are at the upper limit of sympathetic activity.

The presence of pathological oral reflexes in CP patients [8] make the ingestion of food more difficult, and this factor could have contributed to the reduced BMI in these patients. Another potential confounding factor is the presence of sleep-disordered breathing, which is common in this population [3]. Obstructive sleep apnea has been linked to high sympathetic tone and diastolic dysfunction in children [9]. Polysomnography was not performed, but the presence of snoring was assessed, which is a major sign of obstructive sleep apnea. However, the presence of snoring did not explain the echocardiographic alterations observed in this sample based on a regression analysis. Interestingly, we did not find any report of snoring among the controls. A potential explanation for the higher incidence of snoring is that parents may have paid more attention to the CP patients snore.

There are physiopathological explanations for the occurrence of cardiac problems among CP patients; these include altered autonomic tonus and neurological damage. The routine two-dimensional echocardiogram is a simple non-invasive method that allows the assessment of early cardiac consequences in this population. The present results suggest that the investigation of these patients with echocardiogram is warranted.

In conclusion, the chronic autonomic imbalance may have ultimately led to some degree of diastolic impairment in CP patients. Future studies that include tissue Doppler analysis may contribute to the understanding of the cardiovascular pathophysiology of this complex condition and may impact possible pharmacological interventions.

Acknowledgments

This study was supported by FAPESP grants 08/00960-6.

References

[1] Rosenbaum, P; Paneth, N; Leviton, A; et al. A report: the definition and classification of cerebral palsy April 2006. *Dev Med Child Neurol Suppl.*, 2007, 109, 8-14.

[2] Hirtz, D; Thurman, DJ; Gwinn-Hardy, K; Mohamed, M; Chaudhuri, AR; Zalutsky, R. How common are the "common" neurologic disorders? *Neurology*, 2007, 68(5), 326-337.

[3] Bjelakovic, B; Ilic, S; Dimitrijevic, L; et al. Heart rate variability in infants with central coordination disturbance. *Early Hum Dev.*, 2010, 86(2), 77-81.

[4] Felderhoff-Mueser, U; Bührer, C. Clinical measures to preserve cerebral integrity in preterm infants. *Early Hum Dev.*, 2005, 81(3), 237-44.

[5] MacCulloch, MJ; Williams, C; Davies, P. Heart-rate variability in a group of cerebral palsied children. *Dev Med Child Neurol.*, 1971, 13(5), 645-650.

[6] Park, ES; Park, CI; Cho, SR; Lee, JW; Kim, EJ. Assessment of autonomic nervous system with analysis of heart rate variability in children with spastic cerebral palsy. *Yonsei Med J.*, 2002, 43(1), 65-72.

[7] Yang, TF; Chan, RC; Kao, CL; et al. Power spectrum analysis of heart rate variability for cerebral palsy patients. *Am J Phys Med Rehabil.*, 2002, 81(5), 350-354.

[8] Veugelers, R; Benninga, MA; Calis, EA; et al. Prevalence and clinical presentation of constipation in children with severe generalized cerebral palsy. *Dev Med Child Neurol.*, 2010, 52(9), e216-221.

[9] O'Driscoll, DM; Foster, AM; Ng, ML; et al. Acute cardiovascular changes with obstructive events in children with sleep disordered breathing. *Sleep*, 2009, 32(10), 1265-1271.

[10] TTE/TEE Appropriateness Criteria Writing Group; Douglas, PS; Khandheria, B; et al. *J Am Soc Echocardiogr*, 2007, 20 (7), 787-805.

[11] Heart rate variability. Standards of measurement, physiological interpretation, and clinical use. Task Force of the European Society of Cardiology and the North American Society of Pacing and Electrophysiology. *Eur Heart J.*, 1996, 17(3), 354-381.

[12] Kuban, KC; Allred, EN; O'Shea, M; et al. An algorithm for identifying and classifying cerebral palsy in young children. *J Pediatr.*, 2008, 153(4), 466-472.

[13] Paulus, WJ; Tschöpe, C; Sanderson, JE; et al. How to diagnose diastolic heart failure: a consensus statement on the diagnosis of heart failure with normal left ventricular

ejection fraction by the Heart Failure and Echocardiography Associations of the European Society of Cardiology. *Eur Heart J.*, 2007, 28(20), 2539-2550.

[14] Lang, RM; Bierig, M; Devereux, RB; et al. Recommendations for chamber quantification. *Eur J Echocardiogr.*, 2006, 7(2), 79-108.

[15] Bonaduce, D; Marciano, F; Petretta, M; et al. Effects of converting enzyme inhibition on heart period variability in patients with acute myocardial infarction. *Circulation.* 1994, 90(1), 108-113.

[16] Bloomfield, DM; Kaufman, ES; Bigger, JT; Jr. Fleiss, J; Rolnitzky, L; Steinman, R. Passive head-up tilt and actively standing up produce similar overall changes in autonomic balance. *Am Heart J.*, 1997, 134(2 Pt 1), 316-320.

[17] Bloomfield, DM; Magnano, A; Bigger, JT; Jr. Rivadeneira, H; Parides, M; Steinman, RC. Comparison of spontaneous vs. metronome-guided breathing on assessment of vagal modulation using RR variability. *Am J Physiol Heart Circ Physiol.*, 2001, 280(3), H1145-1150.

[18] Eidem, BW; McMahon, CJ; Cohen, RR; et al. Impact of cardiac growth on Doppler tissue imaging velocities: a study in healthy children. *J Am Soc Echocardiogr*, 2004, 17(3), 212-221.

[19] Heart rate variability. Standards of measurement, physiological interpretation, and clinical use. Task Force of the European Society of Cardiology and the North American Society of Pacing and Electrophysiology. *Eur Heart J*, 1996, 17(3), 354-381.

[20] Dos Santos, MT; Nogueira, ML. Infantile reflexes and their effects on dental caries and oral hygiene in cerebral palsy individuals. *J Oral Rehabil.*, 2005, 32, 880-885.

[21] Villa, MP; Ianniello, F; Tocci, G; et al. Early cardiac abnormalities and increased C-reactive protein levels in a cohort of children with sleep disordered breathing. *Sleep Breath.*, 2012, 16(1), 101-110.

In: Handbook on Cerebral Palsy
Editor: Harold Yates

ISBN: 978-1-63321-852-9
© 2014 Nova Science Publishers, Inc.

Chapter 12

Cerebral Palsy, Which Risk Factors Could Be Important: Are They the Same for All Populations?

María de la Luz Arenas-Sordo, M.D., Ph.D.*
Instituto Nacional de Rehabilitación, Mexico

Abstract

The concept of cerebral palsy (CP) has been created to include different neurological sequels that affect our motor sphere. In 1958, the first accepted definition was published by Mac-Keith and Polani: ''CP is a persistent motor disorder appearing before the age of 3 due to a non-progressive interference in the development of the brain taking place before the growth of the central nervous system is complete''

Cerebral palsy has remained unchanged over the past 50 years; its incidence is approximately 2.5 per 1000 live births, almost the same in different countries.

Usually and in the classical form, CP has its origin in three important moments:

Prenatal, perinatal and postnatal. In all of these, one same situation: hypoxic events, could appear. Of course there are other many possibilities in each one, for example, infections, malformations and accidents.

The prenatal and perinatal causes are responsible for 70 to 80% of the cases; the rest corresponds to postnatal ones.

There are many risk factors that cause CP in pre, peri or postnatal stages; they depend on the type of country, genetic characteristics of the populations and environment, all of which we know are different.

To conclude, up to date, it is a fact that the important risk factors are preterm birth, pre or perinatal infections, hypoxia in the partum and thrombophilia and they can be more important or not, depending on the population.

It is important to remember that the predisposition or protection afforded by our genes may allow or not that a determined condition presents itself depending on the rest of the genome and the environment that interacts with it.

---

* Email: mlarenassordo@htmail.com; marenas@inr.gob.mx; asgk@unam.mx.

Introduction

The concept of cerebral palsy (CP) has been created to include different neurological sequels that affect our motor sphere. In 1958, the first accepted definition was published by Mac-Keith and Polani: "CP is a persistent motor disorder appearing before the age of 3 due to a non-progressive interference in the development of the brain taking place before the growth of the central nervous system is complete" [1,2].

In 2004, the meeting that defined and classified CP, which took place in Bethesda, defined it as "A group of movement development and posture disorders limiting activity due to non-progressive alterations occurring in the developing brain of the fetus or the small child. The motor disorder is frequently accompanied by alterations in sensitivity, cognition, communication, perception, behavior and/or epileptic crises" [1,3].

CP is the most frequent and important cause of motor disability in children [4]. For this reason we must focus all our efforts to understand its causes and try to avoid them.

Incidence

Cerebral palsy has remained unchanged over the past 50 years, its incidence is approximately 2.5 per 1000 live births, almost the same in different countries [5,6]. In premature children it is up to 4.5 per 1000. No differences between developing and developed countries were found. It was a surprise for the great majority of people who study these patients, that incidence was not less because of the advances in perinatal care through the years. However cases increased especially because of the survival of critically ill newborns. This means the etiology of many of our cases is prenatal in its origin and not postnatal as we thought [7].

Classification

CP has many classification schemes. It depends on topography, physiology, etiology, neuroanatomic features, severity, etc.

The physiologic and topographic ones are as follows:

1. Spastic: with different involvement: unilateral (hemiplegia), lower extremity involvement (diplegia) and total body involvement (quadriplegia).
2. Dykinetic: choreoathetoid and dystonic.
3. Hypotonic
4. Mixed

This classification is not at all useful because it does not consider the functional abilities of the patients, each one must be evaluated in other areas such vision, behavior, learning, cognition, etc. However it is one of the most used [6].

The etiologic classification is very difficult because we do not know all the different causes and we do not always have the certitude of the etiology. There are also many still unknown causes. The importance of this classification was to diminish the CP cases, and this has not been possible up to this moment [7].

The neuropathology does not yet have the accuracy to correlate the image with the function. It is probable that in the future the new imaging techniques will help us with more precision. Until this time just two situations are related with the hypoxia: the leukomalacia periventricular and injury of the basal ganglia.

However there is a classification that includes other problems not only those which depend on hypoxia: Focal arterial Infarct, cerebral malformation, periventricular abnormalities of the white substance, generalized cerebral atrophy, intracranial hemorrhage, delayed myelination and other abnormalities.

At present the functional classification has taken importance because it allows us to determine treatment according to the severity of the disease. The therapeutic classification divides cases into 4 categories: nontreatment, modest interventions, need for a cerebral palsy treatment team, and pervasive support [7].

There is another classification which gives us more precision and has been used; this is the "Gross Motor Functional Classification System". It is considered very useful to determine treatment and the follow up of patients [8].

Etiology/Risk Factors

Usually and in the classical form, CP has its origin in causes of three important moments:

Prenatal, perinatal and postnatal. In all of these, one same situation could appear, the hypoxic events [9]. Of course there are other many possibilities in each one, for example, infections, malformations and accidents. See table 1.

The prenatal and perinatal causes are responsible for 70 to 80% of the cases, the rest corresponds to postnatal ones [10,11].

Prenatally there are many risk factors, especially infections such as cytomegalovirus, toxoplasmosis, vaginal and urinary and intrinsically maternal diseases as diabetes, hypertension, etc. [9,12].

Besides there are maternal diseases that cause preterm birth such as chorioamnionitis and pre-eclampsia [9,13].

The preterm birth has now been considered a very important risk and it is one of the most recently studied risk factors. [14, 15]. We know that exposure to the extrauterine environment before the brain is completely formed, disrupts the genetically programmed brain genesis [16]. However it is also true that a preterm birth could be caused by an intrinsical problem of the fetus, then the neurological lesion is caused before and not after. The causes of a preterm birth are not well known, but many of them, as is clear, are secondary to genetic problems not well known and understood.

Recently special attention is given to stroke, caused by trombophilic diseases. The inherited and acquired thrombophilias of the mother and/or the fetus may be responsible for thrombosis in the maternal and/or fetal circulation, resulting in adverse pregnancy outcome such as CP [9, 17].

Table 1. Causes of CP in the different stages

Prenatal	Central Nervous system malformations, Infections, Strokes
Perinatal	Hypoxic ischemic encephalopathy, infections
Postnatal	Head trauma, strokes, infections, hypoxia.

There are many genetic traits that may predispose to thrombophilia. A much studied one is the polymorphism called Leiden Factor V [18, 19]. It is especially important to recognize that these polymorphic changes do not occur with equal frequency in all populations, so that means it is a common cause of trombophilic diseases in some populations, but not important in others.

Derived from studies that have been conducted in Mexico, including our own in which we were looking for the association of CP spastic hemiparesis type with Leiden factor V, it was determined that this polymorphism is rare in our population and our patients did not present association [20,21]. There are other polymorphism studied associated to thrombophilia; Prothrombin G20210A, MTHFR C677T, MTHFR A1298C, FVII -323 10 bp del/ins, FVII arg353gln, FGB -455, PAI1 -675, PAI1 -11053, Endothelial Protein Receptor C A4600G, TFPI -33 T?C, CBS I278T, ANX5 1C?T, THBD A43T, PAI2 N120D, N404 K, S413C, PLAT-33C/T [22,23]. Each one needs to be studied in different populations to know if they are prevalent and could cause CP. In Mexican mestizo people we also found that the Cambridge mutation is not frequent, but other polymorphisms need to be studied [21].

Although perinatal causes received the most attention in the past, they actually represent a small minority of cases; there are many factors poorly studied; for example those related to maternal illnesses that cause inflammation [9,24,25].

In our investigation many variables were studied: age, sex, jaundice, hypoxia, weight at birth, Apgar score, alcoholism, smoking, gestational weeks and infections during pregnancy, but really important to generate CP were hypoxia, tabaquism, infections, maternal age and as a protection factor, the gestational weeks [20].

We have to consider that CP is a multifactorial disease in which there are genes that predispose in different ways and enviromental action that precipitates the illness [26]. The first and the second can act as risk factors. It is important to know them to drive our efforts to reduce cases of CP, modifying those which are possible.

Conclusion

There are many risk factors that cause CP in pre, peri or postnatal stages; they depend on the type of country, genetic characteristics of the populations and environmental that we know are different. Hypoxia is still important and it could be caused by many situations, such as infections, trauma, thrombosis, preterm birth, etc. It is probably not just one of the risk factors but the sum of many of them that is responsible for CP.

In our population (Mexican mestizo), Factor V Leiden thrombophilia does not show any relevance but other risk factors to develop CP are still relevant.

We found that one of the most important risks is to have had a degree of perinatal hypoxia for problems at the time of birth. This has always shown a significant difference as has also been mentioned by several authors [27, 28,29]. In general this risk is practically not present in developed countries but it is in developing ones.

Other risk factors that were found were vaginal and urinary infections of the mothers, some authors have documented association [24]. We think this is related to inflammation. This means there is a role for inflammatory mediators either causing damage or affecting brain development at critical periods. For this reason it is important to think about studying other polymorphisms in some genes, for example the eNOS [30].

Regarding the gestational weeks, it was very evident that the more gestation weeks the more protection [9,14].

To conclude, up to date, it is a fact that the important risk factors are preterm birth, infections pre or perinatal, hypoxia in the partum and thrombophilia and they can be more important or not depending on the population.

It is important to remember that the predisposition or protection afforded by our genes may allow or not that a determined condition presents itself depending on the rest of the genome and the environment that interacts with it.

References

[1] Bax M, Goldstein M, Rosenbaum P, et al. (2005) Executive Committee for the Definition of Cerebral Palsy. Proposed definition and classification of cerebral palsy, April 2005. *Dev. Med. Child Neurol.* 47:571–576.).

[2] Morris C. Definition and classification of cerebral palsy: a historical perspective. *Dev. Med. Child Neurol.* 2007; 109(Suppl):3–7.

[3] Pakula AT, Van Naarden K, Yeargin-Allsopp M. Cerebral palsy: classification and epidemiology. *Phys. Med. Rehabil. Clin. N. Am.* 20, 2009; 425-452.

[4] Camacho-Salas A, Pallás-Alonso CR, la Cruz-Bértolo J, Simón-de las Heras R, Mateos-Beato F. Parálisis cerebral: concepto y bases de registro poblacional. *Rev. Neurol.* 2007;45: 503-8.

[5] Paneth N, Hong T, Korzeniewski S. The descriptive epidemiology of cerebral palsy. *Clin. Perinatol.* 2006;33(2):251–67.

[6] Robaina-Castellanos GR, Riesgo-Rodríguez S, Robaina-Castellanos M.S. Definición y clasificación de la parálisis cerebral: ¿un problema ya resuelto? *Rev. Neurol.* 2007; 45: 110-7

[7] Pakula AT, Van Naarden K, Yeargin-Allsopp M. Cerebral palsy: classification and epidemiology. *Phys. Med. Rehabil. Clin. N. Am.* 20, 2009; 425-452.

[8] Palisano R, Rosenbaum P, Walter S, Russell D, Wood E, Galuppi B. Gross Motor Function Classification System for Cerebral Palsy. *Dev. Med. Child Neurol.* 1997;39:214-223.

[9] Blair E, Watson L. Epidemiology of cerebral palsy. *Seminars in Fetal and Neonatal Medicine* 2006; 11: 117–125.

[10] Robaina-Castellanos GR, Riesgo-Rodríguez S, Robaina-Castellanos M.S. Definición y clasificación de la parálisis cerebral: ¿un problema ya resuelto? *Rev. Neurol.* 2007; 45: 110-7.

[11] Wu T, Fan XP, Wang WY, Yuan TM Enterovirus infections are associated with white matter damage in neonates. *J. Paediatr. Child Health.* 2014 Jun 9. doi: 10.1111/jpc.12656.

[12] Miller JE, Pedersen LH, Streja E, Bech BH, Yeargin-Allsopp M, Van Naarden Braun K, Schendel DE, Christensen D, Uldall P, Olsen J. Maternal infections during pregnancy and cerebral palsy: a population-based cohort study. *Paediatr Perinat Epidemiol.* 2013; 27(6):542-52. doi: 10.1111/ppe.12082.

[13] Wu YW, Colford JM Jr. Chorioamnionitis as a risk factor for cerebral palsy: a meta-analysis. *JAMA* 2000; 284: 1417-24.

[14] Tronnes H, Wilcox AJ, Lie RT, Markestad T, Moster D. Risk of cerebral palsy in relation to pregnancy disorders and preterm birth: a national cohort study. *Dev. Med. Child Neurol.* 2014; Mar 13. doi: 10.1111/dmcn.12430.

[15] Moster D, Lie RT, Markestad T. Long-term medical and social consequences of preterm birth. *N. Engl. J. Med.* 2008; 359: 262-73.

[16] Spittle AJ, Orton J. Cerebral plasy and developmental coordination disorder in children born preterm. *Semin. Fetal. Neonatal. Med.* 2014 Apr;19(2):84-9. doi: 10.1016.

[17] Gibson CS, MacLennan AH, Hague WM, Haan EA, Priest K, Chan A, Dekker GA; South Australian Cerebral Palsy Research Group. Associations between inherited thrombophilias, gestational age, and cerebral palsy. *Am. J. Obstet. Gynecol.* 2005;193(4):1437.

[18] Senbil N, Yüksel D, Yilmaz D, Gürer YK. Prothrombotic risk factors in children with hemiplegic cerebral palsy. *Pediatr Int.* 2007 Oct;49(5):600-602.

[19] Reid S, Halliday J, Ditchfield M, Ekert H, Byron K, Glynn A, Petrou V, Reddihough D. Factor V Leiden mutation: a contributory factor for cerebral palsy? *Dev. Med. Child Neurol.* 2006;48(1):14-19.

[20] Arenas-Sordo MD, Zavala-Hernández C, Casiano-Rosas C, Reyes-Maldonado E, Ríos C, Hernández-Zamora E, Del Valle-Cabrera MG, Yamamoto-Furusho JK. Leiden V Factor and Spastic Cerebral Palsy in Mexican Children. *Genet Test Mol. Biomarkers.* 2012;16(8):978-80. Epub 2012 May 15. ISSN 1945-0265

[21] Zavala-Hernández C, Hernández Zamora E, Martinez Murillo C, Arenas Sordo ML, González Orozco AE, Reyes-Maldonado E. Association of resistance to activated protein with the presence of Leiden and Cambridge Factor V mutations in Mexican patients with primary thrombophilia. *Cir. Cir. 2010;78:127-132* ISSN 0009-7411

[22] Wu YW, Croen LA, Vanderwerf A, Gelfand AA, Torres AR. Candidate genes and risk for cerebral palsy: a population-based study. *Pediatr Res* 2011; 70:642-646.

[23] Nelson KB, Dambrosia JM, Iovannisci DM, Cheng S, Grether JK, Lammer E. Genetic polymorphism and cerebral palsy in very preterm infants. *Pediatr Res.* 2005 Apr;57(4):494-499.

[24] Mann JR, McDermott S, Bao H, Bersabe A. Maternal genitourinary infection and risk of cerebral palsy. *Dev. Med. Child Neurol.* 2009;51(4):281-288.

[25] Nelson KB. Infection in pregnancy and cerebral palsy. *Dev. Med. Child Neurol.* 2009; 51: 253-254.

[26] Hemminki K, Li X, Sundquist K, Sundquist J. High familial risks for cerebral palsy implicate partial heritable aetiology. *Paediatr Perinat Epidemiol.* 2007; 21: 235-41.

[27] Back SA, Rosenberg PA. Pathophysiology of glia in perinatal white matter injury. *Glia.* 2014 Mar 31. doi: 10.1002/glia.22658.

[28] Khan RH, Islam MS, Haque SA, Hossain MA, Islam MN, Khaleque MA, Chowdhury B, Chowdhury MA. Correlation between grades of intraventricular hemorrhage and severity of hypoxic ischemic encephalopathy in perinatal asphyxia. *Mymensingh Med. J.* 2014;23(1):7-12.

[29] Kichev A, Rousset CI, Baburamani AA, Levison SW, Wood TL, Gressens P, Thornton C, Hagberg H. Tumor necrosis factor-related apoptosis-inducing ligand (TRAIL) signaling and cell death in the immature central nervous system after hypoxia-ischemia and inflammation. *J. Biol. Chem.* 2014;289(13):9430-9. doi: 10.1074/jbc.M113.512350.

[30] O'Callaghan ME, MacLennan AH, Haan EA, Dekker G. The genomic basis of cerebral palsy: a Huge systematic literature review. *Hum. Genet.* 2009; 126:149–172.

[31] Kichev A, Rousset CI, Baburamani AA, Levison SW, Wood TL, Gressens P, Thornton C, Hagberg H. Tumor necrosis factor-related apoptosis-inducing ligand (TRAIL) signaling and cell death in the immature central nervous system after hypoxia-ischemia and inflammation. *J. Biol. Chem.* 2014;289(13):9430-9. doi: 10.1074/jbc.M113.512350.

In: Handbook on Cerebral Palsy
Editor: Harold Yates

ISBN: 978-1-63321-852-9
© 2014 Nova Science Publishers, Inc.

Chapter 13

Management of Postural Abnormalities in Children with Cerebral Palsy

Michiyuki Kawakami, M.D., Ph.D. and Meigen Liu, M.D., Ph.D.*
Department of Rehabilitation Medicine,
Keio University School of Medicine, Tokyo, Japan

Abstract

Postural problems play a central role in the motor dysfunction of children with cerebral palsy. The performance of everyday activities is noticeably influenced by such postural deficits. In this chapter, we will review the epidemiology of postural deformities such as scoliosis, pelvic obliquity and hip subluxation/dislocation in these children. We then relate these deformities with secondary problems like pain, loss of ability, increased care burden, pressure problems, cardio-pulmonary dysfunctions, swallowing difficulties and sleep disturbance, which can all adversely affect the quality of life of the children as well as that of their caregivers. Many factors are involved in the development and aggravation of postural deformities, such as tone abnormalities, persistent primary reflexes, handedness, habitual posture, pain and inappropriate postural management. Among these factors, recent studies suggest that asymmetrical skull deformity (ASD) is frequently observed in cerebral palsy and closely related with asymmetric postural deformities. ASD is thought to be brought about by a predominantly one-sided facial direction during early childhood when the skull is softer, and once ASD becomes established, it aggravates the asymmetrical posture further. An asymmetrical tonic neck reflex caused by a one-sided face direction could contribute to the development and aggravation of postural abnormalities and limb and spinal deformities. A recent consensus statement by an expert multidisciplinary group defined a postural management program for children with cerebral palsy as "a planned approach encompassing all activities and interventions which impact on an individual's posture and function". In this comprehensive approach, postural management focused on ASD and facial direction appears to be necessary to prevent deformities in children with cerebral palsy.

---

* Correspondence address: Meigen Liu, Department of Rehabilitation Medicine, Keio University School of Medicine, 35, Shinanomachi, Shinjuku, Tokyo 160-8582, Japan. E-mail: meigenliukeio@mac.com.

1. Epidemiology of Postural Deformities: Scoliosis, Pelvic Obliquity and Hip Subluxation/Dislocation

Introduction

Postural problems play a central role in the motor dysfunction of children with cerebral palsy (CP). The performance of everyday activities is noticeably influenced by such postural deficits; the extent however, varies with the degree of the disability. [1]

Loss of supraspinal inhibition on spinal stretch reflexes results in increased reflex activity. This leads to spasticity, motor weakness, impaired sensory perception, and muscle and joint contractures. [2] Spasticity typically develops between 6 and 18 months of age and alters the previously normal skeletal anatomy. [3] The most commonly affected muscles are the paraspinal muscles, hip flexors, hip adductors, hamstrings, gastrocnemius, and soleus.

In this chapter, we will review the incidence and/or prevalence of scoliosis, pelvic obliquity and hip subluxation/dislocation in children with CP.

Scoliosis

The reported incidence of scoliosis in CP varies greatly, but the generally accepted incidence in the overall CP population is 20% to 25%.4-8) The rate varies depending on the particular study, the type of CP, the severity of neurologic involvement, and ambulatory status. The incidence is highest in patients with spastic CP (about 70%) and lowest in those with athetoid type (from 6%-50%). [5, 9] Madigan and Wallace, [5] in their survey of institutionalized patients with CP published in 1981, found that 64% of the 272 patients studied had scoliosis greater than 10 degrees on screening radiographs and that its incidence was related to the severity of neurologic involvement. In support of this conclusion, they pointed to the inverse relationship of ambulatory status and scoliosis (44% of independent ambulators, 54% of dependent ambulators, 61% of independent sitters, and 75% of dependent sitters or bedridden residents had scoliosis). Its incidence increased with age and diminished ambulatory capacity. Males were more commonly affected. [10] Progression of scoliosis was greatest during the growth spurt and might continue after skeletal maturity, especially when associated with pelvic obliquity. [11] One study noted curve progression of 0.8° per year when the largest curve was less than or equal to 50° at skeletal maturity and curve progression of 1.4° per year when the largest curve was greater than 50° at skeletal maturity. [4]

The cause of scoliosis in CP is not entirely clear, but is thought to be due to some combination of muscle weakness, truncal imbalance, and asymmetric tone in paraspinous and intercostal muscles. Whether the development of scoliosis is due to the primary cerebral insult or due to its secondary consequences is also unclear. [12]

Table I. Summary of the reports on incidence and/or prevalence of scoliosis, pelvic obliquity and hip subluxation/dislocation in children with cerebral palsy

Author	Year	Main findings
Gu et al.	2011	The participants were a total of 110 children and adolescents 18 years of age, with scoliosis. Age was found to be the most significant predictor of Cobb angle. If the Cobb angle was 40°by age 12 years, scoliosis was more likely to progress than if the Cobb angle was 40°.
Saito et al.	1998	The participants were 79 patients with severe spastic cerebral palsy and scoliosis. Of these 79 patients, 54 (68%) had scoliosis with a curve of at least 10° as analysed by the Cobb method on radiographs. In 11 (85%) of 13 patients who had a spinal curve of more than 40° before age 15 years, the scoliosis progressed to more than 60° by the time of the final examination. Meanwhile, in only three (13%) of 24 patients who had a curve of less than 40° at age 15 years, did the scoliosis progress to more than 60°.
Majd et al.	1997	The participants were 56 patients with cerebral palsy and scoliosis. 10 patients (18%) declined during the course of the study. In these 10 patients, the average initial curve was 41.1°, the average final curve was 80.6°, and the average progression rate was 4.4° per year. For the stable patients, the average initial curve was 33.9°, the average final curve was 56.5°, and the average progression rate was 3.0° per year.
Madigan and Wallace	1981	64% of the 272 patients studied had scoliosis greater than 10 degrees on screening radiographs and that the incidence of scoliosis was related to severity of neurologic involvement.
Balmer et al.	1970	A radiological review of 100 consecutive cases of children with cerebral palsy attending the out-patient clinic, revealed twenty-one with structural scoliosis of more than 10 degrees. These children were all over the age of four: seven were under ten years and fourteen were ten or over. Fifteen of the curves measured less than 30 degrees, four between 30 and 60 degrees, and two more than 60 degrees.

Table I. (Continued)

Author	Year	Main findings
Scrutton et al.	2001	Of 323 children, 117 (36.2%) had 196 hips (30.3%) needing treatment. 52% of children with quadriplegic CP and 21% of children with diplegic CP needed treatment by 5 years of age (p < 0.01).
Cooke et al.	1989	Risk of hip dislocation virtually confined to quadriplegic CP (n = 235) where prevalence was 16%.
Terjesen	2006	76 children, 42 with spastic quadriplegia and 34 with diplegia, were included in the study. The mean migration percentage of the side with the largest displacement was 25% (-18–66) at the initial radiographic examination and 51% (9–100) at the last follow-up. The mean increase in migration percentage was 7% (-2–33) per year. Linear multiple regression revealed that gait function and age were the most important variables that influenced the rate of migration percentage progression.
Miller and Bagg	1995	38 of 61 hips with low migration percentage (migration percentage < 30%) remain unchanged, 28 of 33 hips with migration percentage between 30% and 60% remain unchanged. Both hips with migration percentage > 60% progressed to dislocation. Spontaneous improvement in migration percentage in 6 patients but related to contralateral dislocation in 3 patients.
Samilson et al.	1972	Of 1013 hospitalized patients with cerebral palsy, 274 patients with dislocated or subluxated hips have been studied, a prevalence of 28 percent. The mean age at which dislocation occurred in 139 of these patients was seven years.
Lonstein and Beck	1986	464 patients were reviewed. They were placed to four function groups: independent ambulators, dependent ambulators, independent sitters, and dependent sitters. The percetage of subluxated or dislocated hips increased from 7% for independent ambulators to 60% for dependent sitters.
Connelly et al.	2009	Two hundred and eighteen children had been involved in the hip surveillance programme. Fifteen cases of dislocation were recorded. The percetage of subluxated hips (MP > 30%) increased from 3% for GMFCS I level to 76% for GMFCS V level.

Hip Subluxation/Dislocation and Pelvic Obliquity

Hip subluxation and dislocation are the second most common deformities in patients with spastic CP. Children with quadriplegic CP who cannot walk have the greatest risk of hip displacement. Samilson et al. [13] reported that 274 patients with dislocated or subluxated hips were found among the 1013 hospitalized patients with CP, a prevalence of 28 %. Cooke et al. [14] noted a prevalence of hip dislocation of 16% in a series from a tertiary centre. In a district population in the United Kingdom, 52% of children with quadriplegic CP required treatment for a hip problem by the age of five years compared with 21% of those with diplegia. [15]

Scrutton et al. [15] provided a detailed information regarding locomotor development and progressive hip problems. No child who had walked ten steps alone by 30 months needed treatment of their hips by five years of age. Children who could walk ten steps unaided at 5 years had a markedly reduced need for treatment (4.1% vs 46% for those unable to walk). The severity of motor disability at 18 months of age was not predictive of hip displacement, but by 24 to 30 months of age, it became predictive. A greater proportion of the females than males had hips needing treatment (38.8% compared to 32.8%) and slightly more of the females had bilateral hip problems than males (23.9% and 20.6%, respectively), but this could be explained by a larger proportion of boys who could walk (34.3% of female vs 48.7% of male patients). Females had a significantly higher early migration percentage and acetabular index scores, perhaps because of oestrogen-influenced joint laxity or anatomical differences in the pelvis which affected the direction of forces of the local spastic muscles.

Radiological measurement of the migration percentage can monitor hips at risk of subluxation. The migration percentage is the percentage of the femoral head lateral to the acetabulum (lateral to Perkins' line), measured parallel to Hilgenreiner's line. In the series of Miller and Bagg, [16] 16 of 21 hips in children between the age of two and six years remained unchanged over a period of eight years, whereas hips with a migration percentage of between 30% and 60% had a risk of further subluxation of 25%. Hips with a migration percentage of over 60% went on to dislocate. However, this study was restricted to patients who had been followed up for at least eight years. It did not consider all children with dislocated hips and thereby excluded those at the highest risk. Vidal et al. [17] noted an increase in the migration percentage from as early as 12 months of age. This did not reach a clinically significant level of 40% until a few years later in most children. The annual rate of progression of the migration percentage without surgery was 7.7% in children who were unable to walk.

In the study of Hagglund et al., [18] 54 of 78 hips (50 children) with a migration percentage greater than 33% required surgery, but in 18 hips it corrected to less than 33% without operation. No hip with a migration percentage greater than 42% became normal without operation.

Windswept hips deformity is also often experienced where there is an abduction contracture of one hip and an adduction contracture of the opposite hip. The spastic adductors and iliopsoas muscles overpower the weaker hip abductors and extensors. [19] This may result in scissor gait (bilateral adduction hip contracture) or windswept deformity. Samilson et al. [20] noted that windswept deformity occurred in up to 23% of their patients. Lonstein and Beck [21] found 53 patients with windswept hips deformity among the 464 patients studied (11%). Among them, the hips were windswept to the right (right hip abducted, left hip adducted) in 29 patients and to the left in 24 patients. There was a correlation between the windswept direction and the side of hip dislocation or subluxation. The hip was more commonly out on the adducted side. This side was opposite to the direction of the leg.

Pelvic obliquity is also often experienced, its formation is considered to be caused by retention of neonatal reflexes and a prolonged period of patterned spasticity, asymmetrical positioning of hips and spasticity. Lonstein and Beck [21] reported that the percentage of children with pelvic obliquity and the angle of obliquity formed by the horizontal and intercrest line was very similar for the four groups (independent ambulators, dependent ambulators, independent sitters and dependent sitter). For dependent sitters, pelvic obliquity occurred in 58% of the children and ranged from 0 to 92°. There was no correlation between the high side of pelvic obliquity and the dislocated or subluxated hip. The percentage of hips not become located did not increase as the pelvic obliquity increased.

References

[1] Carlberg EB, Hadders-Algra M. Postural Dysfunction in Children with Cerebral Palsy: Some Implications Therapeutic Guidance. *Neural Plast* 2005;12:221-8.

[2] Park TS, Owen JH. Surgical management of spastic diplegia in cerebral palsy. *N Engl J Med* 1992; 326:745–749.

[3] Beals RK. Developmental changes in the femur and acetabulum in spastic paraplegia and diplegia. *Dev Med Child Neurol* 1969; 11:303–313

[4] Balmer GA, MacEwen GD. The incidence and treatment of scoliosis in cerebral palsy. *J Bone Joint Surg Br* 1970;52(1):134-7.

[5] Madigan RR, Wallace SL. Scoliosis in the institutionalized cerebral palsy population. *Spine* 1981; 6(6):583-90.

[6] Saito N, Ebara S, Ohotsuka K. Natural history of scoliosis in spastic cerebral palsy. *Lancet* 1998; 351(9117):1687-92.

[7] Thometz JG, Simon SR. Progression of scoliosis after skeletal maturity in institutionalized adults who have cerebral palsy. *J Bone Joint Surg Am* 1988;70(9):1290-6.

[8] McCarthy JJ, D'Andrea LP, Betz RR, et al. Scoliosis in the child with cerebral palsy. *J Am Acad Orthop Surg* 2006;14(6):367-75.

[9] Majd M, Muldowny D, Holt R. Natural history of scoliosis in the institutionalized adult cerebral palsy population. *Spine* 1997;22(13):1461-6

[10] Rosenthal RK, Levine DB, McCarver CL. The occurrence of scoliosis in cerebral palsy. *Dev Med Child Neurol* 1974; 16: 664-667.

[11] 11 Ferguson RL, Allen BL. Considerations in the treatment of cerebral palsy patients with spinal deformities. *Orthop Clin North Am* 1988; 19: 419–425.

[12] Imrie MN, Yaszay B. Management of Spinal Deformity in Cerebral Palsy. *Orthop Clin N Am* 41 (2010) 531–547

[13] Samilson RL, Tsou P, Aamoth G, Green WM. Dislocation and subluxation of the hip in cerebral palsy: pathogenesis, natural history and management. *J Bone Joint Surg* [Am] 1972;54-A:863-73.

Management of Postural Abnormalities in Children with Cerebral Palsy — 183

[14] Cooke PH, Cole WG, Carey RP. Dislocation of the hip in cerebral palsy: natural history and predictability. *J Bone Joint Surg* [Br] 1989;71-B:441-6.

[15] Scrutton D, Baird G, Smeeton N. Hip dysplasia in bilateral cerebral palsy: incidence and natural history in children aged 18 months to 5 years. *Dev Med Child Neurol* 2001;43:586-600

[16] Miller F, Bagg MR. Age and migration percentage as risk factors for progression in spastic hip disease. *Dev Med Child Neurol* 1995;37:449-55.

[17] Vidal J, Deguillaume P. Vidal M. The anatomy of the dysplastic hip in cerebral palsy related to prognosis and treatment. *Int Orthop* 1985;9:105-10.

[18] Hagglund G, Andersson S, Duppe H, et al. Prevention of dislocation of the hip in children with cerebral palsy: the first ten years of a population-based prevention programme. *J Bone Joint Surg* [Br] 2005;87-B:95-101.

[19] Lamb DW, Pollock GA. Hip deformities in cerebral palsy and their treatment. *Dev Med Child Neurol* 1962; 4:488–498.

[20] Samilson RL, Bechard R. Scoliosis in cerebral palsy: incidence, distribution of curve patterns, natural history, and thoughts on etiology. *Curr Pract Orthop Surg* 1973; 5:183–205.

[21] Lonstein JE, Beck K. Hip dislocation and subluxation in cerebral palsy. *J Pediatr Orthop* 1986;6:521-6.

2. Problems Caused by Postural Deformities: Functional Outcomes of Adaptive Seating Interventions

Cerebral palsy (CP) is a broad term describing a group of nonprogressive disorders of posture and movement. The cause of CP is multifactorial, usually attributed to events during early brain development, and producing life-long lesions and abnormalities. The brain lesions manifest as secondary motor impairments, ranging from mild to severe, and may also affect sensation, cognition, communication, and/or behavior.

The motor disorders in children with CP are complex. The primary deficits include: muscle tone abnormalities, which are influenced by position, posture and movement; impairment of balance and coordination; decreased strength; loss of selective motor control. The secondary musculoskeletal problems are muscle contractures and bony deformities. [1]

Because of the motor impairments of the trunk and limbs, there is an inability to generate enough force to maintain antigravity postural control, thus leading to abnormal postures. [2] Posture refers to the position of the limbs or body as a whole whereas postural control is the ability to control the body's position in space to obtain stability and orientation. [3, 4] Postural control affects not only sitting and standing but also the ability to sequence movement appropriately. [3]

It's noted that associations exist between poor seated postures and negative functional outcomes including back and neck pain, heightened muscle tension, [5] compromised fine motor skills, [6] and reduced academic performance in children. [7]

A common intervention for addressing postural control in children with CP is adaptive seating, defined as modifications to seating devices to improve sitting posture and/or postural control in mobility-impaired individuals. [8]

Previous research has supported adaptive seating in improving postural control in children with CP. [9, 10, 11] Furthermore, researchers have suggested that improved postural control can increase functional abilities, such as upper extremity (UE) function, occupational performance and satisfaction, and performance of activities of daily living (ADL). [2, 13] These improvements were sustained even after the intervention was removed, suggesting that adaptive seating can facilitate physical functions. [14]

This chapter provides an overview and assessment of original articles that considered functional outcomes of adaptive seating interventions for children with CP.

Postural Control in Sitting

The features of adaptive seating that have a positive impact on postural control are stabilization of the pelvis in a slightly anterior-tilted position and increasing the sitting base by supporting the thighs in flexion and abduction. This strategy likely optimizes the starting conditions for movement by increasing the base of support and providing a stable origin for the trunk and lower extremity muscles. [10]

Myhr and Wendt [15] reported that postural control was best when the child was sitting in a forward-tipped seat, with a firm backrest supporting the pelvis, arms supported against a table and feet permitted to move backward.

Reid et al. [12] conducted a repeated-measures experimental cross-over study with school-aged children with spastic CP to compare the effects of flat-bench versus saddle-bench seating on postural control. The saddle bench allowed significantly better postural control as measured by a clinical rating scale Sitting Assessment for Children with Neuromotor Dysfunction [16].

Thus, improved postural control in sitting was evident during the short-duration intervention, and persisted into the third-year after the intervention. Pope and coworkers [17] reported that using Seating and Mobility system (SAM) with a mechanical base, molded seat support which positions a child in a straddle position with trunk leaning forward for a period of three years improved the child's sitting ability.

Upper Extremity Functions

In clinical practice, postural control of the trunk is purported to be an important contributor to voluntary UE functions, including motor control and dexterity. Researchers have suggested that improved postural control of children with CP will affect UE ability. [18] UE function is a critical determinant of the ability to perform daily activities and to participate in the surrounding environment.

Two studies [12, 17] found that saddle seating had no significant impact on improving fine motor, dexterity, and UE functions in children with CP. McClenaghan et al. [19] found a significant increase in thumb-press performance when the seat was 5° anteriorly tilted; conversely, a 5° posteriorly tilted seat was significantly related to a decrease in linear tapping test performance. No clear effects of contoured foam seating (CFS) on UE ability were determined in the study by Washington et al. [20] The contradictory findings in these studies may have resulted from the differences in seating interventions or outcome measures. None of the studies used the same measure of UE functions.

Stavness [11] reviewed studies published since 1980 investigating the effects of adaptive seating on UE functions in children with CP. Of the 16 studies reviewed, 3 reported postural control outcomes in addition to UE function outcomes. He concluded that the available evidence indicates that an upright sitting position improves UE functioning in children with CP. They should be fitted with wheelchairs that place them in a functional seating position, including an orientation in space of 0° to 15°, a hip belt, an abduction orthosis, footrests, a cutout tray and a forward sloping seat of 0° to 15°.

Social Interaction and Performance of Daily Activities

Some studies included parents' and/or teachers' subjective reports of children's social skills and ADL performance. Washington et al. [20] noted that parents perceived improvement in their children's social interactions and in the parents' ease of performing caregiving tasks, such as feeding, when using the CFS. Reid et al. [21] reported that a wheelchair mounted rigid pelvic stabilizer (RPS) had a facilitating effect for increasing physical functioning. The RPS allowed significantly better occupational performance and satisfaction with performance as measured by the Canadian Occupational Performance Measure [22]. There is a similar type of report to evaluate the short-term impact of adaptive seating device on the activity performance and satisfaction with performance of children with CP, as observed by their parents. [23] Parents reported that their young children with CP were more able to engage in self-care and play activities when using specific adaptive seating devices at home. Parents indicated that their child's activity performance decreased after the seating devices were removed from their homes.

Burden of Care

The effects of assistive technology devices, for example adaptive seating devices, may extend beyond young technology users to their parents and other family members. Ryan et al. [24] reported the parent-perceived effect of adaptive seating devices on the lives of young children with CP (aged 2–7 years) and their families. The introduction of adaptive seating devices had a significant positive effect on the lives of families who have children with CP, whose Gross Motor Function Classification System (GMFCS) level was III or IV, as measured by the Family Impact of Assistive Technology Scale.

Pulmonary Function

Several studies suggest the importance of supporting the trunk in an upright and aligned position to improve pulmonary function in children with CP. Reid [25] reported that children with CP exhibited a significantly higher tidal volume and minute ventilation (MV) than normal children in the tipped seat condition. Barks and Davenport [26] noted that total airway resistance and MV varied with wheelchair conditions. Especially, upper extremity support and lateral trunk support may be important for improving pulmonary function in children with CP.

Swallowing Function

Feeding a child with CP is a substantial problem both for the child and caretakers. Many of these children are hypotonic in the trunk. In an upright sitting position, therefore, the thoracic column becomes kyphotic and the cervical spine lordotic. Also the children usually have poor lip control and inadequate posterior transport of the bolus in the oral cavity. This leads to the oral contents leaking out of the mouth anteriorly. Therefore, trunk and neck positioning influences oral and pharyngeal swallow. In the reclined position with the neck flexed, aspiration decreases, oral leak and retention improves in children with CP. [27]

References

[1] Papavasiliou AS. Management of motor problems in cerebral palsy: A critical update for the clinician. *Eur J Paediatr Neurol.* 2009;13(5):387-96.

[2] Pin TW. Effectiveness of static weight-bearing exercises in children with cerebral palsy. *Pediatr Phys Ther.* 2007;19:62–73.

[3] Massion J. Postural control systems in developmental perspective. *Neurosci Biobehav Rev. 1998*;22:465– 472.

[4] *Stedman's Medical Dictionary.* 27th ed. Baltimore, Maryland: Lippincott Williams & Wilkins; 2000.

[5] Koskelo R, Vuorikari K, Hänninen O. Sitting and standing postures are corrected by adjustable furniture with lowered muscle tension in high-school students. *Ergonomics* 2007;50:1643–1656.

[6] Smith-Zuzovsky N, Exner CE. The effect of seated positioning quality on typical 6- and 7-year-old children's object manipulation skills. *Am J Occup Ther* 2004;58:380–388.

[7] Sents BE, Marks HE. Changes in preschool children's IQ scores as a function of positioning. *Am J Occup Ther* 1989;43:685–687.

[8] Chung J, Evans J, Lee C, Lee J, Rabbani Y, Roxborough L, Harris SR. Effectiveness of adaptive seating on sitting posture and postural control in children with cerebral palsy. *Pediatr Phys Ther.* 2008;20(4):303-17

[9] Roxborough L. Review of the efficacy and effectiveness of adaptive seating for children with cerebral palsy. *Assist Technol.* 1995;7: 17–25.

[10] Harris SR, Roxborough L. Efficacy and effectiveness of physical therapy in enhancing postural control in children with cerebral palsy. *Neural Plast.* 2005;12:229 -224; discussion 263–272.

[11] Stavness C. The effect of positioning for children with cerebral palsy on upper-extremity function: a review of the evidence. *Phys Occup Ther Pediatr.* 2006;26:39 – 53.

[12] Reid DT. The effects of the saddle seat on seated postural control and upper-extremity movement in children with cerebral palsy. *Dev Med Child Neurol.* 1996; 38:805– 815.

[13] Reid D, Rigby P, Ryan S. Functional impact of a rigid pelvic stabilizer on children with cerebral palsy who use wheelchairs: users' and caregivers' perceptions. *Pediatr Rehabil.* 1999;3:101–118.

[14] Rosenbaum P, Stewart D. The World Health Organization International Classification of Functioning, Disability, and Health: a model to guide clinical thinking, practice and research in the field of cerebral palsy. *Semin Pediatr Neurol,* 2004;11:5–10.

[15] Myhr U, von Wendt L. Improvement of functional sitting position for children with cerebral palsy. Dev Med Child Neurol. 1991;33(3):246-56.

[16] Reid D. Correlation of the Pediatric Volitional Questionnaire with the Test of Playfulness in a virtual environment: The power of engagement. *Early Child Dev Care.* 2005;175:153–164.

[17] Pope PM, Bowes CE, Booth E. Postural control in sitting the SAM system: evaluation of use over three years. *Dev Med Child Neurol.* 1994;36(3):241-52..

[18] Noronha J, Bundy A, Groll J. The effect of positioning on the hand function of boys with cerebral palsy. *Am J Occup Ther.* 1989;43:507–512.

[19] McClenaghan BA, Thombs L, Milner M. Effects of seat-surface inclination on postural stability and function of the upper extremities of children with cerebral palsy. *Dev Med Child Neurol.* 1992;34:40–48.

[20] Washington K, Deitz JC, White OR, et al. The effects of a contoured foam seat on postural alignment and upper-extremity function in infants with neuromotor impairments. *Phys Ther.* 2002;82:1064–1076.

[21] Reid D, Rigby P, Ryan S. Functional impact of a rigid pelvic stabilizer on children with cerebral palsy who use wheelchairs: users' and caregivers' perceptions. *Pediatr Rehabil.* 1999;3:101-18

[22] Canadian Association of Occupational Therapists: Occupational Therapy Guidelines for Cllient-Centred Practice (Toronto, ON: CAOT Publications), 1991.

[23] Rigby PJ, Ryan SE, Campbell KA. Effect of adaptive seating devices on the activity performance of children with cerebral palsy. *Arch Phys Med Rehabil.* 2009 ;90:1389-95.

[24] Ryan SE, Campbell KA, Rigby P, Germon B, Hubley D, Chan B. The impact of adaptive seating devices on the lives of young children with cerebral palsy and their families. *Arch Phys Med Rehabil* 2009; 90: 27-33.

[25] Reid D, Sochaniwskyj A. Effects of anterior-tipped seating on respiratory function of normal children and children with cerebral palsy. *Int J Rehabil Res* 1991; 14: 203-212.

[26] Barks L, Davenport P. Wheelchair components and pulmonary function in children with cerebral palsy. *Assistive Technology* 2012; 24:78–86.

[27] Larnert G, Ekberg 0. Positioning improves the oral and pharyngeal swallowing function in children with cerebral palsy. *Acta Padiatr* 1995;84:689-92.

3. Patterns of Postural Deformities

People with cerebral palsy (CP) who are non-ambulant are particularly vulnerable to development of contractures and postural deformities, which are often progressive despite the fact that the underlying pathology is static. [1, 2] The asymmetrical postural deformities that can arise include scoliosis, pelvic obliquity and hip subluxation/dislocation. Windswept hips deformity, one of the representative asymmetrical postural deformities, is also often experienced where there is an abduction contracture of one hip and an adduction contracture of the opposite hip. [3, 4]

Individual components of asymmetrical postural deformity tend to be considered and studied separately, however, a clear understanding of the relationships among them is essential if patterns of deformity are to be predicted and early postural management strategies implemented. Porter et al. [5] reported that a significant association was found between the direction of scoliosis and the direction of the windswept hip deformity ($P < 0.001$) such that the convexity of the lateral spinal curve was more likely to be opposite to the direction of wind sweeping. Significantly more windswept deformities to the right ($P=0.02$), hips subluxated/dislocated on the left ($P =0.02$) and lateral lumbar/lower thoracic spinal curves convex to the left ($P=0.01$) were also observed. The pattern cannot be easily explained by asymmetrical muscle activities. Although asymmetrical muscle activities have been observed with windsweeping, [6, 7] it is not clear in these studies whether the muscle activities were causes or effects.

To test the association between asymmetrical positioning in the first 12 months of life and the subsequent direction of postural deformities in non-ambulant people with CP, Porter et al. [8] performed a retrospective cohort study.

It was reported that most participants did have a preferred lying posture in the first year of life. Analysis of the participants who as infants preferred lying consistently on one side and went on to develop a scoliosis in later life, suggested that the convexity of the lateral spinal curve was more likely to be towards the side that had been unsupported during lying ($P = 0.031$). Participants were also more likely to experience a problem later in life with the hip on the unsupported side ($P = 0.003$). Analysis of participants who preferred supine lying as an infant with their head rotated consistently to one side, suggested that the convexity of the subsequent spinal curve was more likely to be away from the direction of head rotation i.e., towards the occipital side ($P < 0.001$).

Statistically significant associations were also found between the direction of head rotation during supine lying and the other three asymmetrical postural problems experienced later in life: direction of pelvic obliquity; direction of windsweeping; and side of hip subluxation/dislocation. These relationships were such that the pelvis was more likely to be lower on what was originally the occipital side ($P = 0.006$), the windswept pattern was more likely to be towards the facial side ($P = 0.03$) and the hip on the occipital side was more likely to subluxate/dislocate ($n = 29$, $P = 0.001$). The study provided evidence of an association between asymmetrical lying posture adopted in the first year of life and the direction of the subsequent pattern of postural deformities.

Recently, Kawakami et al. [9] reported that asymmetrical skull deformity is frequent in CP and closely related to asymmetrical posture and deformities. One hundred ten participants aged 1–18 years (mean age 9.3 years) were assessed using a checklist for asymmetrical skull deformity, postural abnormalities, and deformities. (Appendix I) Asymmetrical skull deformity was observed in 44 children (40%), 24 showing right and 20 showing left flat occipital deformity. Its frequency was significantly related to Gross Motor Function Classification System (GMFCS) 10) grades and with the patterns of asymmetrical posture and deformities (p < 0.05). (Table 1).Children with right flat occipital asymmetrical skull deformity showed predominantly rightward facial direction and right-side-dominant asymmetrical tonic neck reflex, left convex scoliosis, right-side-elevated pelvic obliquity, and left-sided hip dislocation. Those with left flat occipital asymmetrical skull deformity demonstrated the reverse tendency. Therefore, asymmetrical skull deformity is frequent in CP and closely related to asymmetrical posture and deformities. (Figure 1)

This information will be useful to manage the postural deformities in children with CP. Clinicians should be aware of positioning for children with severe disabilities, particularly those who prefer supine lying with their head rotated to one side and those who prefer consistent side lying.

References

[1] Saito N, Ebara S, Ohotsuka K, Kumeta H, Takaoka K. Natural history of scoliosis in spastic cerebral palsy. *Lancet* 1998; 351: 1687–92.

[2] Scrutton D, Baird G, Smeeton N. Hip dysplasia in bilateral cerebral palsy: incidence and natural history in children aged 18 months to 5 years. *Dev Med Child Neurol* 2001; 43: 586–600.

[3] Letts M, Shapiro L, Mulder K, Klassen O. The windblown hip syndrome in total body cerebral palsy. *J Pediatr Orthop* 1984; 4: 55–62.

[4] Young NL, Wright JG, Lam TP, Rajaratnam K, Stephens D, Wedge JH. Windswept hip deformity in spastic quadriplegic cerebral palsy. *Pediatr PhysTher* 1998; 10: 94–100.

[5] Porter D, Kirkwood C, Michael S. Patterns of postural deformity in non ambulant people with cerebral palsy: what is the relationship between, the direction of scoliosis, direction of pelvic obliquity, direction of windswept hip deformity and side of hip dislocation? *Clinical Rehabilitation. 2007*; 21, 1063–1074.

[6] Nwaobi, OM, Sussman MD. Electromyographic and force patterns of cerebral palsy patients with windblown hip deformity. *Journal of Pediatric Orthopedics.* 1990; 10, 382–388.

[7] Young NL, Wright JG, Lam TP, Rajaratnam K, Stephens D, Wedge JH. Windswept hip deformity in spastic cerebral palsy. *Pediatric Physical Therapy.* 1998; 10, 94–100

[8] Porter D, Michael S, Kirkwood C. Is there a relationship between preferred posture and positioning in early life and the direction of subsequent asymmetrical postural deformity in non ambulant people with cerebral palsy? *Child care health and development.* 2008; 34, 635–641

[9] Kawakami M, Liu M, Otsuka T, Wada A, Uchikawa K, Aoki A, Otaka Y. Asymmetric skull deformity in children with cerebral palsy: frequency and correlation with postural abnormalities and deformities. *J Rehabil Med* 2013; 45: 149–153

[10] Palisano R, Rosenbaum P, Walter S, Russell D, Wood E, Galuppi B. Development and reliability of a system to classify gross motor function in children with cerebral palsy. *Dev Med Child Neurol* 1997; 39: 214–223

Appendix I. A 10-Item Checklist for Asymmetric Skull Deformity, Postural Abnormalities and Deformities

Name (	)	Age ( )	Sex (male·female)
CP type		(athetoid· spastic· ataxic· rigid· mixed)	
GMFCS		(Level I · II · III · IV · V)	

	Item			
①	Asymmetric skull deformity	symmetrical	asymmetry apparent with palpation	asymmetry apparent with inspection
②	Side of deformity	flattened right occiput	flattened left occiput	others
③	Which direction is the child's face directed?	front side · right side · left side · either side · no apparent pattern		
④	How long does the child keep his/her face turned toward that direction?	always or most of the time	over half of the time	less than half of the time
⑤	Type of spinal deformity	none		
		scoliosis (right / left / double curve)·lordosis·kyphosis·other		
⑥	Pelvic obliquity	distance between lowest rib cage and ASIS	rt cm	lt cm
		spinomalleolar distance	rt cm	lt cm
		wind-swept deformity	none	(rt · lt)
		hip dislocation	none	(rt·lt·bilateral)
⑦	Limb position		rt	lt
		upper extremity	extensor pattern· flexor pattern· indefinite·hypotonic· normal	extensor pattern· flexor pattern· indefinite·hypotonic· normal
		lower extremity	extensor pattern· flexor pattern· indefinite·hypotonic· normal	extensor pattern· flexor pattern· indefinite·hypotonic· normal
⑧	ATNR	none	obligatory·non-obligatory	
			rt · lt · bilateral	
⑨	Facial asymmetry	none	present	
⑩	Head control	absent	present	

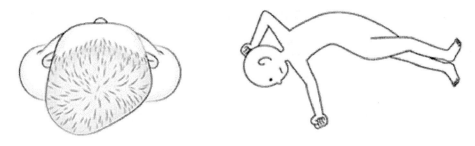

Figure 1. The illustration on the left shows asymmetric skull deformity (flattened right occiput). The illustration on the right demonstrates typical postural abnormalities and limb and spinal deformities of a child with ASD. The child shows a right-side-dominant asymmetric tonic neck reflex, left convex scoliosis, and wind-swept hip deformity.

Table 1. Frequency of asymmetrical skull deformity (ASD) and its relationship with Gross Motor Function Classification System (GMFCS), postural abnormalities and deformities. Statistical analyses were carried out with the χ^2 for independence test, setting the significance level at less than 0.05

GMFCS	I	II	III	IV	V	
ASD(+)	0	0	0	6	38	
ASD(-)	4	7	2	11	42	($X^{2=}$, $p<0.05$)

Direction of face	Rt-sided flattened occiput	Lt-sided flattened occiput	Total
($\chi 2=$, $P<0.01$)			
rt	15	3	18
rt≒lt	9	6	15
lt	0	11	11
total	24	20	44
ATNR	Rt-sided flattened occiput	Lt-sided flattened occiput	Total
($\chi 2=$, $P<0.01$)			
rt	12	1	13
rt≒lt	1	2	3
lt	0	5	5
none	11	12	23
total	24	20	44
Scoliosis	Rt-sided flattened occiput	Lt-sided flattened occiput	Total
($\chi 2=$, $P<0.05$)			
rt	6	8	14
rt≒lt	1	3	4
lt	15	3	18
none	2	6	8
total	24	20	44

Table 1. (Continued)

Inclination of pelvis	Rt-sided flattened occiput	Lt-sided flattened occiput	Total
($\chi2=$, P>0.05)			
rt	9	3	12
rt≒lt	13	14	27
lt	2	3	5
total	24	20	44
Hip dislocation	Rt-sided flattened occiput	Lt-sided flattened occiput	Total
($\chi2=$, P>0.05)			
rt	5	3	8
rt≒lt	5	2	7
lt	1	1	2
none	13	14	27
total	24	20	44

4. Future Prospects and Suggestions

As previously mentioned, Postural management, for example adaptive seating is important for children with CP. It is suggested that children in the GMFCS groups IV-V should start 24-hour postural management programmes in lying as soon as appropriate after birth, in sitting from 6 months, and in standing from 12 months. However, there is yet no report on postural management that focused on asymmetrical skull deformity and facial direction for children with CP. Clinicians should be aware of positioning for children with severe disabilities, particularly those who prefer supine lying with their head rotated to one side and those who prefer consistent side lying. In the future, a prospective intervention study focused on asymmetrical skull deformity and facial direction is desired. In addition, a prospective cohort study from early infancy is necessary to demonstrate the time course and causal relationships between asymmetrical skull deformity (including facial direction) and postural abnormalities and deformities.

In: Handbook on Cerebral Palsy
Editor: Harold Yates

ISBN: 978-1-63321-852-9
© 2014 Nova Science Publishers, Inc.

Chapter 14

Shock Wave Therapy for Reduction of Muscle Spasticity in Children with Cerebral Palsy

Elena Milkova Ilieva, M.D., Ph.D. and Maria Ilieva Gonkova, M.D.
Department of Physical and Rehabilitation Medicine,
Medical University of Plovdiv, Bulgaria

Abstract

Extracorporeal shock wave therapy has been used for the treatment of chronic musculo-skeletal disorders in the last decades. Recently a new field of its application has been studied - for reduction of muscle spasticity as a result of central motor neuron disease. The authors present the knowledge about extracorporeal shock wave therapy: physical characteristics, types, evidence based mechanisms of its effect and indications for its use.

The results of the studies about the efficacy of SWT in the treatment of muscle spasticity in adults after stroke and in children with cerebral palsy are presented and discussed.

The authors discuss also the results of their original study about the effect of radial shock wave therapy for reduction of muscle hypertonus of plantar flexor muscles of children with spastic diplegia and hemiplegia. One placebo session was applied followed four weeks later by one active treatment session. We used passive range of motion, Modified Aschworth Scale and pedobarometric measurements (static and dynamic) for outcome assessment. After RSWT, a significant increase in passive range of motion and decrease of the score of the Modified Ashworth Scale were observed, which persisted at fourth week follow-up. Pedobarometric measurement showed a significant increase in the contact plantar surface area and in heel pressure.

Conclusion: Shock wave therapy could be considered as a treatment of choice for reduction of muscle spasticity in children with cerebral palsy.

Introduction

Cerebral palsy (CP) is one of the most common chronic disabilities of childhood. It occurs worldwide and its incidence is about 1.5 to 3 per 1000 births in developed countries. As a definition, CP is "a group of permanent disorders of the development of movement and posture, causing activity limitation, that are attributed to non-progressive disturbances that occurred in the developing fetal or infant brain" [1]. The group for Surveillance of Cerebral Palsy in Europe (SCPE) published standardized procedures for describing children with CP [2]. This definition included 5 points: (1) an umbrella term (2) permanent but not unchanging (3) involves a disorder of movement and posture (4) is due to a non-progressive lesion (5) the lesion is in immature brain. Treatment is initiated in early childhood, and continues throughout life, even in adulthood.

The most common clinical feature in patients with CP is spasticity. It is a common symptom, seen in many neurological conditions - stroke, spinal cord injuries, multiple sclerosis. The good management of spasticity depends on the understanding of its underlying physiology, natural history and impact on the patient [3]. Poorly managed spasticity can be responsible for muscle shortening, development of soft tissue and tendon contractures. It is important to approach spasticity according to the level of severity, including consideration about the prevention of secondary complications.

In medical practice there are many treatment options to decrease spasticity, including oral medications, different physical agents, physiotherapy, botulinum toxin and surgery. The choice of the treatment is always complex and depends on the muscle tone and its effect on the musculoskeletal system [4]. Regardless of the level of severity, it is always very important to consider the advantages and disadvantages of the treatment method and to determine whether the spasticity is predominantly local or generalized [3].

Extracorporeal shock wave therapy (ESWT) has been widely used in the last decades in orthopedic practice for the treatment of chronic tendinopathies and enthesiopathies. Shock waves are acustic waves with high peak pressure and short pulse duration. They are disseminating in the space and have the ability to transfer a large amount of energy from one place to another. They were first applied in medicine in 1970 for disintegration of kidney stones in urology and later in gastroenterology in case of gallstones.

In 1986 new devices were invented, which allowed the use of shock waves in the treatment of musculoskeletal disorders. First studies about their effect in revision arthroplasty of the hip [5], in the treatment of bone non-unions after fractures [6], and calcific tendonitis of the shoulder [7,8] were published.

Definition of shock wave therapy: Shock waves are a sequence of single sonic pulses with steep pressure rise (0.01 µsec), high peak pressure (up to 120 MPa, over 500 Bar), followed by a low tensile amplitude (10 MPa); short duration (0.3 µsec); broad frequency spectrum (16-20 MHz) and therapeutic effect - up to 12 cm in the body [9,10,11]. The shock wave field has the shape of a mountain with a peak in the centre and steeply falling slopes. Shock waves propagate in three dimensions. The above mentioned characteristics are typical for the focused shock waves.

There are two more types of shock waves - planar and radial shock waves. Planar shock waves have peak pressure up to 3 MPa, energy flux density up to 0.14 mJ/mm^2 on skin surface and penetration depth of 5 cm.

Radial shock waves were used in medical practice for the first time in 1999. They have lower peak pressure (up to 0.10 MPa), longer wave length (200-2000 μsec) and therapeutic effect up to 3 cm in the body. In focused shock waves the energy is focused on the target zone inside the tissues, while in radial shock waves the focal point of energy is centered on the tip of the applicator and spreads radially in the tissues.

The main physical parameters of shock waves are: pressure, focal zone, energy flux density (the energy at the focal point of the shock wave per impulse), frequency, total acoustic energy and number of received shocks. According to the energy flux density (EFD), shock waves are divided into 3 groups: low-energy shock waves (0.08-0.27 mJ/mm²), medium (0.28-0.6 mJ/mm²) and high (> 0.6 mJ/mm²) [12]. Radial shock waves are in the group of low up to medium energy shock waves. Additional parameters are the number of shocks, number of treatments, intervals between treatments [13].

Generators: Three types of focused shock wave generators are used in daily medical practice: electrohydraulic, electromagnetic and piezoelectric. Planar waves are generated on the same principles, but there is a special nozzle, which changes the type of the wave and its depth penetration.

Radial shock wave is electropneumatically generated through the acceleration of a projectile inside the handpiece of the device. Then the energy is transmitted from the tip of the applicator to the target tissue [11,13].

With the introduction of combined shock wave systems, it became possible to treat patients with focused and radial shock waves simultaneously. Coupling gel is used during the procedures for alignment of acoustic impedance, transmission of larger amount of energy to the body and decrease of the percentage of reflected waves.

Effects of shock waves: Experimental studies confirm three major effects of SWT: physical, chemical and biological. There are two basic effects of shock waves: primary effect, which is a result of direct generation of mechanical forces, concentrated at the target zone; and secondary effect - indirect mechanical forces caused by cavitation, which appears during the negative pressure time [9].

Shock waves differ from ultrasound that has biphasic waves and lower intensity, but are similar to them in the fact, that one part is reflected at the boundary layer and cause the so called Hopkins effect. The direct pressure of the wave in focused SW can cause mechanical destruction of the cell and cell's membrane. It also can lead to its stimulation by reverse deformity of its membrane. This results in improved blood circulation and metabolism caused by SWT.

Indirect effect – cavitation. Besides the direct dynamic effect of shock waves on interfaces, cavitation occurs in some media like water and some tissues in the phase of negative pressure. These cavitation bubbles collapse and create 'micro-jets' that contain a high amount of energy and penetration power (1000 times higher energy), in comparison to the first hit. This causes membrane perforations or micro-bleeding. Cavitation is not limited to the focal zone, but is most prominent there [10].

These physical effects cause biological reactions. The mechanisms by which an acoustic signal is converted into biological reaction are not fully understood. Most probably mechanotransduction is the basis of biological response. Mechanotransduction is the mechanism by which reactive cells respond to mechanical stimuli. Extracellular matrix proteins and the nucleus are stimulated via the cytoskeleton thus leading to tissue regeneration [14]. The following biological effects have been scientifically studied and proven: increased cell permeability; stimulation of microcirculation (blood, lymph); release of substance P; reduction of non-myelinated nerve fibres; release of nitric oxide, which causes vasodilatation, increased metabolism and angiogenesis and has anti-inflammatory effect; anti-bacterial effect; release of growth factors (blood vessels, epithelium, bones, collagen); activation of stem cells [15]. It was found, that shock waves induce expression of vascular endothelial growth factor (VEGF), promotes tendon and bone healing /cell proliferation and tissue regeneration/ by inducing the TGF-ß1 (transforming growth factor ß1) and insulin growth factor (IGF) – I; releases bone morphogenic protein (BMPs), osteogenic protein; induces neovascularization by increasing the levels of vascular endothelial growth factor (VEGF) and proliferating cell nuclear antigen (PCNA), Nitric oxide (NO), Enzyme nitric oxide synthase (eNOS) [16,17].

It is considered, that nitric oxide (NO) plays an important role is transforming the physical mechanisms into biological reactions: proliferation and differentiation of mesenchymal cells in the area of bone and tissue damage, anti-inflammatory effect, and even reduction of muscle spasticity in patients with central nervous system (CNS) disorders. It was found that NO at low physiological concentrations down-regulates the NF-kappaß activation and the NF-kappaß dependent inflammatory genes (iNOS, TNF- α, ICAM, VCAM, COX-2) thus leading to anti-inflammatory effect [18,19].

Basic research finds a release of pro-inflammatory neuropeptides (P-substance and calcitonin gene related peptide - CGRP) in the initial phase after application of extracorporeal SWT. Later chemotaxis and mitosis of the stem cells occurs and a bony/connective tissue matrix is produced. After local neo-angiognesis, this is followed by a remodeling of the fracture gap or of the soft tissue lesion. It is considered that therapeutic effect is a result from induced inflammation, which stimulates physiological healing process [15].

One of the most important physiological effects of SWT is prompt and long-lasting analgesic effect. It is considered as a result of destruction of the neuron cell membrane and increased permeability caused by 'micro-jets', created by shock waves. Damage of non-myelinated nerve roots is also under consideration. Experimental studies found degeneration of intracutaneus nerve fibres of the skin [20] and decreased level of CGRP in the dorsal root ganglia of rats [21]. It was discovered in animal experiments that the number of pain-conducting C-fibres is reduced and the ability of nociceptors to reinnervate after the application of shock waves decreases. Gate-control mechanism is also discussed: the irritation of rapidly conducting A-δ nociceptors and nerve fibres leads to segmental inhibition and blocking for the slowly conducting C-fibres [12].

The effect of shock waves is dose related, which was found by Rompe and colleagues in an experimental study in a rabbit's Achilles tendon [12]. One of the most important aspects to be considered is not the total number of impulses used but the energy level of the shock wave. In various disease cases, a different level of intensity is applied due to the above mentioned fact about the dose-dependent effect. Usually, low-energy shock waves are used in entesopathies and tendinopathies; medium-energy - for disintegration of calcium deposits in calcifying tendonitis of the shoulder; high-energy - in the treatment of non-unions and delayed unions of long bone fractures.

Indications: Indications approved and accepted by the International Society for Medical Shock Wave Treatment (ISMST) are: calcifying tendinitis of the shoulder, plantar fasciitis with or without heel spur, lateral epicondylitis of the elbow and other tendinopathies (Achilles tendinopathy, patellar tendinopathy, trochanter tendinopathy). There is high level of evidence about the effectiveness of shock wave therapy in the treatment of calcifying tendinopthy of the shoulder and Achilles tendinopathy and moderate, but growing evidence about its effectiveness in plantar fasciitis and lateral epicondylitis. In chronic tendinopathies focused shock wave therapy is recommended in the chronic stage of the disease (duration of complaints more than 6 months), in cases reluctant to other conservative treatment modalities: physical therapy, local injections, non-steroidal anti-inflammatory drugs (NSAIDs).

Other indications are bone disorders: non-unions and delayed unions of long bone fractures (success rate ranging from 50% to 85%), pseudoarthrosis, stress fractures, avascular necrosis of the femoral head [14]. Many studies prove the beneficial effects of shock waves in the treatment of chronic wounds – diabetic and others [22].

Contraindications: blood coagulation disorders, haemophilia and patients on oral anticoagulants; pregnancy - abdominal or pelvic application; on metaphyseal areas and ossification nuclei in children; acute inflammation; osteomyelitis; tumor diseases, especially malignant; patients with pacemaker; in the area of the lungs, brain, spinal cord, large vessels and nerves; application in the area of varices; local corticosteroid injections or X-ray therapy in the last 6 weeks.

Side effects: Shock wave therapy is a non-invasive method of treatment and its side effects are limited. They more often occur after application of focused SWT: pain, erythema and skin damage; damage of small capillaries with formation of hematoma and petechiae; nerve injury with numbness and tingling; migraine and syncope; damage of pulmonary alveoli after direct application of shock waves in the area of the lungs [23,24].

Effect of SWT on muscle spasticity in patients with disorders of the central nervous system: A relatively new field of application of extracorporeal shock wave therapy is its use in patients with neurological conditions.

The Italian authors Manganoti and Amelio were the first who studied the effect of SWT on muscle spasticity of the upper limb in patients after a stroke. A total of 20 patients affected by stroke associated with severe hypertonia in the upper limbs were evaluated. It was an open study, in which each patient served as his or her own control. The results from their study showed reduction in muscle tone after application of focused SWT with 0.030 mJ/mm² intensity on the flexor hypertonic muscles of the forearm (1500 shots) and on each of the interosseus muscles of the hand (800 shots). The effect after single stimulation lasted up to 12 weeks [25]. In another study, Yoo et al. applied three sessions of SWT on the elbow flexor muscles and the wrist pronator muscle - 1000 shots, 4 Hz frequency, and 0.069 mJ/mm² intensity. The authors found a reduction in muscle tone after the treatment that was preserved at the follow-up four weeks later [26]. Bae et al. stimulated the belly and musculotendinous junction tendons of the elbow flexor muscles with focused shock waves - 1200 shots, 4 Hz frequency, 0.12 mJ/mm², three sessions. Immediately after the procedure there was statistically significant reduction of muscle spasticity, but there was not any statistically significant difference in comparison with the baseline one week and four weeks later [27]. Regarding lower limb spasticity - Sohn and colleagues studied the effect of one session FSWT on the medial head of gastrocnemius in hemiplegic stroke patients. Modified Ashworth scale showed significant reduction in spasticity after the procedure [28]. In a recently published study Moon et al. applied sham stimulation and one week later 3 sessions (1 session per week) of focused shock wave therapy on the musculotendinous junctions of the medial and lateral gastrocnemius in subacute stroke patients – 1500 impulses, with frequency of 4 Hz, intensity 0.089 mJ/mm². Patients were evaluated not only clinically and, but also biomechanically: Modified Ashworth Scale (MAS), clonus score, passive range of motion of ankle, Fugl-Myer Assessment for the lower extremity, peak eccentric torque (PET), torque threshold angle (TEA). There were no significant changes after sham stimulation. MAS and some of the peak eccentric torque parameters were significantly improved immediately and one week after ESWT. These changes were not significant at four weeks after ESWT. PET (60° per sec) and torque threshold angle were significantly improved only immediately after ESWT and not at 1 week and 4 weeks follow up [29]. Most of the studies investigate the effect of focused shock wave therapy in stroke patients. In a recent study radial shock wave therapy (RSWT) was used for reduction of m. subscapularis' increased tone in patients after stroke. Results showed significant decrease in MAS and increased range of motion. The authors found that RSWT had positive effect on pain and limited ROM in the shoulder, in addition to the decrease in spasticity [30].

In conclusion, all cited studies describe a reduction of muscle spasticity in hemiplegic stroke patients, but the duration of treatment effect maintenance is different among the studies. This could be a result of different treatment protocols: number of sessions, number of shots/per session, energy flux density, duration of the disease, volume of the muscles on which SWT is applied. In our own pilot study, we observed a significant reduction of muscle spasticity in stroke patients after application of radial shock wave therapy [31].

In the available literature, there are several studies about the effect of SWT on muscle spasticity in children and adults with cerebral palsy. Amelio and Manganotti studied the effect of focused SWT on spastic plantar flexor muscles in children with cerebral palsy (one single active session, 1500 shots on gastrocnemius and soleus muscles, 0.030 mJ/mm² intensity). Clinical and instrumental examinations were performed for evaluation of the results. Significant reduction of muscle spasticity in comparison to baseline was found. The described effect was preserved at the follow-up one month after the procedure [32]. A recent randomized, placebo-controlled clinical trial assessed the benefits of RSWT in the treatment of spasticity in young adults with CP. In that study the protocol consisted of three sessions of RSWT (once per week) on different spastic muscles and on their antagonists in a small group of 15 patients, mean age 31 years. They found a statistically significant decrease in MAS and increase of pROM in the group treated with RSWT compared to the placebo group. Their positive results were preserved for 2 months after the treatment [33]. Mirea and Onose also apply RSWT on different spastic muscle groups in children with cerebral palsy and found reduction in MAS and improvement of the global functioning of the upper and lower limbs [34].

In a systematic review and network meta-analysis, comparing the effectiveness of RSWT to FSWT in patients with plantar fasciitis, the authors pointed out potential advantages of RSWT over FSWT comprise a broader treatment area, less requirements for precise focusing, no need for adjunct local anesthesia and a lower cost. At the same time the clinical effectiveness of RSWT is similar and in some cases better than FSWT [35].

We investigated the effect of radial shock wave therapy on muscle spasticity of plantar flexor muscles in children with cerebral palsy in a double-centered study: at the Department of Physical and Rehabilitation medicine, Medical University Hospital, Plovdiv and at the Specialized Hospital for Rehabilitation of Children with Cerebral Palsy "Sv. Sofia", Sofia, Bulgaria [36]. Twenty-five children (16 boys and 9 girls), mean age 4.84±3.11 years, were involved in the study. All of the children had a diagnosis of spastic CP: spastic hemiplegia (10 children) or spastic diplegia (15 children). We used a BTL-5000 RSWT unit of BTL

Industries Inc. This was an open observational, placebo controlled double-blinded study in which each child served as its own control. Before the active stimulation a placebo session was applied. The time between the placebo and active stimulation was 4 weeks, in order to avoid a crossover effect. For the assessment of the results before, after, two weeks and four weeks later, the following clinical and instrumental methods were used: passive range of motion (pROM) in the ankle joint, Modified Ashworth Scale (MAS) and static and dynamic pedobarometric measurement. There was no significant difference in the results after the placebo session. After the active stimulation of RSWT, significant changes were observed between the results and baseline: a significant increase in pROM: from 33.25 ± 2.20 to 47.00 ± 2.29 ($p<0.001$) degrees, which persisted at the 2nd (46.87 ± 2.08 degrees, $p<0.001$) and 4th week (44.12 ± 1.93 degrees, $p<0.001$) after treatment; significant change in muscle tone proved by changes in MAS: from 2.77 to 2.00 points ($p<0.001$), which persisted at the 2nd (mean 2.05 ± 0.07 points, $p<0.001$) and 4th week (2.15 ± 0.76 points, $p<0.001$) after treatment; pedobarometric measurement showed a significant increase in the contact plantar surface area of the affected foot (from 81.32 ± 6.14 cm^2 to 101.58 ± 5.41 cm^2, $p<0.001$) and in heel pressure (from 50.47 ± 6.61 N/cm^2, to 75.17 ± 3.42 N/cm^2, $p<0.001$). No side effects were observed. The procedure was well tolerated by all children, because it is non-invasive, painless and with short duration. Based on the results of this group of children we could conclude that radial shock wave therapy is a safe, non-invasive and well-tolerated treatment method in children with CP, which could be used for reduction of muscle spasticity in cerebral palsy (Figures 1, 2).

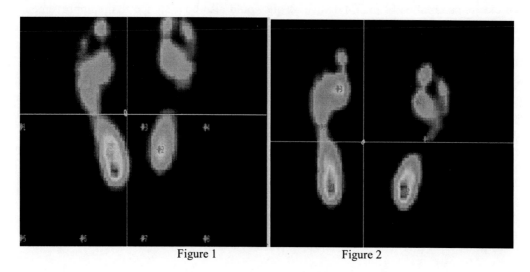

Figure 1   Figure 2

Figures 1, 2. Static pedobarometric findings of a child with right spastic hemiplegia before and after RSWT.

The depth of penetration of RSWT is lower than with FSWT but sufficient to reach the spastic muscles in children. The treatment procedure in RSWT is less painful, has wider effective regions, without the need for precise locating with image guidance and anesthesia, which reduces the patient's treatment risk and makes it suitable for children [36].

The exact mechanism underlying the positive effect of ESWT on muscle spasticity in patients with central nervous system disorders has not been clarified yet.

A number of studies have investigated the effect of shock waves and explain the mechanism of reduction of muscle spasticity: inducing enzymatic and non-enzymatic nitric oxide (NO) synthesis [19]; affecting the excitability at spinal level [37]; effect on passive stiffness of the muscles, result from expanded connective tissue; direct effect of the mechanical vibration [25]; effect on Golgi apparatus in the muscle tendon [27,29]. Most convincing is the theory about the effect of the increased levels of nitric oxide. It is known, that nitric oxide, formed by SWT, takes part in the formation of neuro-muscular junctions in peripheral nervous system and participates in neurotransmission, memory and synaptic plasticity in the central nervous system [38,39]. Recently, a study has been published about the effects of SWT in rats. The authors discuss that the effect on muscle spasticity could be a result from influence on the neuro-muscular transmission in the area of neuro-muscular synapse [40]. The reduction of muscle spasticity could not be explained as a result from any effect on spinal excitability, as there are no changes in F wave amplitude and H reflex as found by Manganotti and Sohn [25,28]. No changes in F wave minimal latency, H-reflex latency or H-M ration were detected after treatment with SWT [28]. Less convincing is the hypothesis about the effect of SWT on Golgi apparatus and decrease of the excitability of the motor nerve [27]. A direct effect of mechanical vibration on the muscle fibers can be excluded, as the clinical changes were preserved in some of the studies several weeks after the therapy.

Another very possible mechanism for reduction of muscle spasticity is the direct influence of shock waves on muscle fibrosis and on the rheological properties of the spastic muscles in cerebral palsy [32]. Positive results could also be assigned to the improvement of localized ischemia in the areas of abnormal shortening of the muscles, increased metabolism and reduced secretion of pain inducing substances [30]. In addition, possible tixotrophic effects of shock waves on tissue and vessels of the treated muscles should be considered.

Conclusion: Extracorporeal shock wave therapy is a safe and non-invasive method for reduction of muscle spasticity in patients with cerebral palsy. It is well tolerated without any serious side effects. The studies give promising and comparatively long lasting results. There are still some contradictions and ambiguities, regarding the long term effect. Further investigations are needed to clarify the mechanisms underlying its effect on muscle spasticity, the most appropriate protocol of application in CP - intensity, frequency, number of shots, number of sessions.

References

[1] Rosenbaum P, Paneth N, Leviton A, Goldstein M, Bax M, Damiano D, et al. A report: the definition and classification of cerebral palsy. *Dev Med Child Neurol* 2006;109:8-14.

[2] Surveillance of Cerebral Palsy in Europe. Surveillance of cerebral palsy in Europe (SCPE): a collaboration of cerebral palsy surveys and registers. *Dev Med and Child Neurol* 2000;42:816-24.

[3] Thompson AJ, Jarrett L, Lockley L, Marsden J, Stevenson VL. Clinical management of spasticity. *J Neurol Neurosurg Psychiatry* 2005;76:459-63.

[4] Matthews DJ, Balaban B. Management of spasticity in children with cerebral palsy. *Acta Orthop Traumatol Turc* 2009; 43:81-6.

[5] Karpman RR, Magee FR, Gruen TW, Moblev T. The lithotripter and its potential use in revision of THA. *Orthop Rev* 1987; 26-38.

[6] Valchanou VD, Michailow P. High-energy shock waves in the treatment of delayed and nonunion of fractures. *Int Orthop* 1991;151:181-4.

[7] Dahmen GP, Meiss L, Nam VC, Skruodies B. Extrakorporale Strosswallentherapies im knochennachem wechteilbereic an der schluter. *Extr Orthopedica* 1992:11-25.

[8] Loew M, Jurgowski W. Initial experiences with extracorporeal shock wave lithotripsy in treatment of tendinosis calcarea of the shoulder. *Z Orthop Ihre Grenzgeb* 1993; 131(5):470-3.

[9] Wang CJ. An overview of Shock Wave Therapy in musculoskeletal disorders. *Chang Gung Med J* 2003;26:220-30.

[10] Dreisilker U. Shock wave therapy in practice. Enthesiopathies. Leveho Buchverlag Daniela Bamberg, Heilbronn. 2010.

[11] Rompe JD. Shock wave applications in musculoskeletal disorders. Thieme Verlag, Stuttgart, 2002.

[12] Rompe JD, Kirkpatrick CJ, Kullmer K, Schwitalle M, Krischek O. Dose-related effects of shock waves on rabbit tendo Achilis. *J Bone Joint Surg Br* 1998;80B:546–52.

[13] Ogden JA, Toth-Kischakat A, Schulthesis R. Principles of shock wave therapy. *Clin Orthop* 2001;387:8-17.

[14] Ioppolo F, Rompe JD, Furia JP, Cacchio A. Clinical application of shock wave therapy (SWT) in musculoskeletal disorders. *Eur J Phys Reh Med* 2014 Mar [Epub ahead of print].

[15] Novak P. Physical basics. In Extracorporeal Shock Wave Therapy in practice, ed. U. Dresilker, 2011;28-46.

[16] Chen YJ, Wurtz T, Wang CJ, Kuo RY, Yang KD, Huang HC, Wang FS. Recruitment of mesenchymal stem cells and expression of TGF-beta 1 and VEGF in the early stage of shock wave-promoted bone regeneration of segmental defect in rats. *J Orthop Res* 2004;22(3):526–34.

[17] Wang FS, Yang KD, Chen RF, Wang CJ, Shenn-Chen SM. Extracorporeal shock wave promotes growth and differentiation of bone-marrow stromal cells towards osteoprogenitors associated with induction of TGF-beta1. *J Bone Joint Surg Br* 2002;84(3):457-61.

[18] Ciampa AR, de Prati AC, Amelio C, Cavaleri E. Nitric oxide mediates anti-inflamatory action of extracorporeal shock waves. *FEBS Lett* 2005;579(30):6839-45.

[19] Mariotto S, De Parti AC, Cavalieri E, Amelio E, Marlinghaus E, Suzuki H. Extracorporeal shock wave therapy in inflammatory diseases: molecular mechanism that triggers anti-inflammatory reaction. *Curr Med Chem* 2009;16(19):2366-72.

[20] Othori S, Inoue G, Annoji C, Saisu T, Takahashi K, Mitsuhashi S. Shock wave application to rat skin induces degeneration and reinervation of sensory nerve fibres. *Neurosci Let* 2001;315:57-60.

[21] Takahashi N, Wada Y, Othori S, Saisu T, Moroya H. Application of shock waves to rat skin decreases calcitonin gene related peptide immunoreactivity in dorsal root ganglion neurons. *Auton Neurosci* 2003;107:81-94.

[22] Mittermayr R, Antonic V, Hartinger J, Kaufmann H, Redl H, Téot L, et al. Extracorporeal shock wave therapy (ESWT) for wound healing: technology, mechanisms, and clinical efficacy. *Wound Repair Regen* 2012;20:456-65.

[23] Pettrone F. Extracorporeal shock wave therapy without local anesthesia for chronic lateral epicondylitis. *J Bone Joint Surg Ame* 2005;87(6):1297-304.

[24] Haake M, Konig IR, Decker T, Riedel C, Buch M, Muller H. ESWT in the treatment of lateral epicondylitis. A randomized multicentre trial. *J Bone Joint Surg* 2002;84:1982-90.

[25] Manganotti P, Amelio E. Long term effect of shock wave therapy on upper limb hypertonia in patients affected by stroke. *Stroke* 2005;36:1967–71.

[26] Yoo SD, Kim HS, Jung PK, The effect of shock wave therapy on upper limb spasticity in patients with stroke. *J Korean Acad Rehabil Med* 2008;32:406-10.

[27] Bae H, Lee JM, Lee KH. The effects of ESWT on spasticity in chronic stroke patients. *J Korean Acad Rehabil Med* 2010;34:663-9.

[28] Sohn MK, Cho KH, Kim YJ, Hwang SL. Spasticity and electrophysiologic changes after extracorporeal shock wave therapy on gastrocnemius. *Ann Rehabil Med* 2011;35:599-604.

[29] Moon SW, Kim JH, Jung MJ, Son S, Lee JH, Shin H, et al. The effect of ESWT on lower limb spasticity in subacute chronic patients. *Ann Rehabil Med* 2013;37(4):461-70.

[30] Kim YW, Shin JC, Yoon JG, Kim YK, Lee SC. Usefulness of radial shock wave therapy for the spasticity of the subscapularis in patients with stroke: a pilot study. *Chin Med J* 2013;126(24):4638-43.

[31] Angelova A, Ilieva E, Gonkova M. Effect of Extracorporeal Shock Wave Therapy on muscle hypertonus in patients after stroke. *Nevrorehabilitazia* 2012;6(1-2):11-14.

[32] Amelio E, Manganotti P. Effect of shock wave stimulation on hypertonic plantar flexor muscles in patients with cerebral palsy: a placebo-controlled study. *J Rehab Med* 2010; 42:339-43.

[33] Vidal X, Morral A, Costa L, Tur M. Radial extracorporeal shock wave therapy (rESWT) in the treatment of spasticity in cerebral palsy: A randomized, placebo-controlled clinical trial. *NeuroRehabilitation* 2011;29:413-19.

[34] Mirea A, Onose G, Padure L. Extracorporeal Shockwave Therapy in Spastic Children with Cerebral Palsy. 16th International Congress of Shock wave treatment. Book of abstracts. 2012;44.

[35] Chang KV, Chen SY, Chen WS, Tu YK, Chien KL. Comparative effectiveness of focused shock wave therapy of different intensity levels and radial shock wave therapy for treating plantar fasciitis: a systematic review and network meta-analysis. *Arch Phys Med Rehabil* 2012;93:1259-68.

[36] Gonkova M, Ilieva E, Ferriero G, Chavdarov I. Effect of radial shock wave therapy on muscle spasticity in children with cerebral palsy. *Int J Rehabil Res* 2013;36(3):284-90.

[37] Leone JA, Kukulka CG. Effects of tendon pressure on alpha motoneuron excitability in patients with stroke. *Phys Ther* 1998;68:475-80.

[38] Molina JA, Jiménez-Jiménez FJ, Ortí-Pareja M, Navarro JA. The role of nitric oxide in neurodegeneration. Potential for pharmacological intervention. *Drugs Aging* 1998; 12:251–9.

[39] Blottner D, Luck G. Just in time and place: NOS/NO system assembly in neuromuscular junction formation. *Microsc Res Tech* 2001;55:171-80.

[40] Kenmoku T, Ochiai N, Ohtori S, Saisu T, Sasho T, Nakagawa K, et al. Degeneration and recovery of the neuromuscular junction after application of extracorporeal shock wave therapy. *J Orthop Res* 2012;30:1660-6.

In: Handbook on Cerebral Palsy
Editor: Harold Yates

ISBN: 978-1-63321-852-9
© 2014 Nova Science Publishers, Inc.

Chapter 15

Latest Trends in Neurorehabilitation of Patients with Cerebral Palsy

Stanislava Klobucká[1,], Elena Žiaková[1,2] and Robert Klobucký[3]*
[1]Rehabilitation Centre Harmony, Bratislava, Slovakia
[2]Slovak Medical University, Faculty of Nursing and Health Professional Studies, Bratislava, Slovakia
[3]Slovak Academy of Sciences, Institute for Sociology, Bratislava, Slovakia

Abstract

Cerebral palsy (CP) still represents a live medical as well as social issue. It is one of the most common neurodevelopmental disorders in the childhood. The aim of this paper is to highlight the need for early diagnosis and adequate rehabilitation therapy of cerebral palsy. The early start of rehabilitation is the fundamental and crucial therapeutic procedure.

Ever increasing emphasis has currently been placed on active approach in the therapy, including intensive repetitive task-specific training in support of neuroplasticity. A good understanding of the maturity of gait for normal children and for each individual child with CP is decisive in planning the treatment. Locomotor functions training has become an effective means to improve walking performance in patients with gait impairment.

In the past decade there was increase in the use of robotic therapy, especially in patients with strokes, cerebrospinal trauma, and last but not least, in children with cerebral palsy. In this paper we present some of new trends in neurorehabilitation - robotic-assisted treadmill training in virtual reality environment, functional therapy of upper extremity and coordination dynamic therapy. We report here the results of robotic–assisted treadmill therapy of patient suffering from ataxic form of cerebral palsy.

Keywords: Neurorehabilitation, motor learning, gait training, robotic assisted therapy, coordination dynamic therapy

---

[*] Corresponding author: email: stanislavaklobucka@gmail.com.

Introduction

Cerebral palsy (CP) is still a current medical and social problem. It is a serious chronic neurological disorder of childhood and adulthood. It is described as non-progressive but in its manifestations, the disability of motor skills and posture to varying degrees, caused by an already occurred (and completed) damage to the developing brain in the pre-, peri- or early postnatal period (within 1 year), is not invariable. It is one of the most frequent neurodevelopmental disorders and is considered the most common cause of severe physical disability in childhood.

In foreign literature, the term "cerebral palsy" (CP) similarly as the Slovak and Czech name DMO, differs from spinal poliomyelitis (polio). The most cited definition is that of Martin Baxa, who describes it as a disorder of posture and movement caused by damage to the immature brain (Morris, 2007).

Disorder of motor function is often accompanied by impaired perception, communication, behavior, cognitive disorder, epilepsy and secondary musculoskeletal problems.

Epidemiology and Etiopathogenesis

The prevalence of CP, taking into regard the reported geographical variation, is in the range of 1.7-2.1 per 1000 live births (Andersen et al., 2008, Himmelmann et al., 2010). Information on the various forms of representation are quite different. Spastic is the most represented form, which makes up 70-75% of all cases, 10-15% of cases consist of the dyskinetic-dystonic form, while the ataxic form makes up less than 5%. From the spastic form, 30-40% of cases are diparetic, 20-30% hemiparetic and 10-15% are quadriparetic (Sankar, 2005).

The etiopathogenesis of CP is undoubtedly multifactorial and the association of individual assumptive factors of its origination is the subject of ongoing clinical epidemiological review. Despite the improvement of diagnostic possibilities, nearly 20% of cases still remain without etiological identification (Shevell, 2003).

Epidemiological analyses have defined a significant number of risk factors that can cause CP. The causes and risk factors of the occurrence of CP are classified, according to the period in which the damaging of the immature brain took place, into prenatal, perinatal and postnatal. The most important risk factors include low birth weight, intrauterine infection and multiple pregnancies (Odding, 2006).

Screening for the Risk of CP

The correct diagnosis of CP depends on knowledge of the physiological development and its variability. At this time there is no standard test for the diagnosis of CP and there is not complete agreement on how soon it is possible to specify CP. Neurological symptoms observed during the first months after birth in premature children and the development of CP do not have sensitivity or sufficient specificity to enable a reliable determining of the prognosis. Traditional and standard neurological examinations fail in predicting the risk of development and the severity of CP at an early age. For this reason, they are followed up by a developmental examination.

Postural ontogenesis, as the development of an individual to upright walking, is genetically determined. In addition to endogenously generated mobility, we focus attention on the investigation of functional, purpose-oriented and therefore motivated movement. To determine deviations from physiological development, the following ratings are used:

- Postural activity
- Postural reactivity
- Primitive reflexology (Vojta, 1972- 2007, Kolar, 2010)

Diagnostics

The suspected risk of developing CP can be pronounced in the early weeks of life, based on a detailed neurological examination and analysis of the level of psychomotor development, which is performed on all children at regular intervals in the first year of life. The second is the screening of postural development according to Vojta, that is used for the examination of children with a risk and suspicion of delays in psychomotor development (Vojta, 1972-2007).

Differential diagnosis of disorders of motor function should be made within nine months of the corrected age of the child. The identification of the central threat, however, must be determined much sooner, not later than the second month of life.

The early identification of symptoms characteristic of the possible development of CP enable the indication of early care for disabled children and means a more timely initiation of rehabilitation. This can mean a significant easing of the functional consequences and prevents the motor and cognitive complications of late diagnosis. Diagnostic procedures in children with suspected CP should, in addition to the already mentioned clinical examinations, always include basic imaging methods in infants - namely ultrasonographic examination of the brain, while in doubtful cases it is necessary to perform a CT or MRI. This should always be supplemented with examinations of eyesight and hearing. With forms poorly responsive to therapy or with mild progression or other symptomatology atypical for CP, metabolic or genetic testing is also usually required. We consider mitochondrial diseases, and many other leukodystrophies that could mimic the image of CP image as within the scope of differential diagnoses. The basis for the differential diagnosis of CP is distinguishing the progressive neurological diseases, especially those that have a specific therapy. It is always necessary to exclude a slow-growing brain or spinal cord tumor in the cervical area.

Therapy

The complex issue of children with cerebral palsy requires a multidisciplinary approach involving the cooperation of a neurologist, rehabilitation physician, physiotherapist, orthopedic surgeon, orthopedic prosthetics, psychologist, speech therapist, phoniatrist, ophthalmology and others, with links to social assistance and special needs education.

Since CP is a neurodevelopmental disorder and its manifestations in the course of development usually varies, treatment requires an adaptive approach, during which mainly reversible non-ablative therapies are applied. It is important to initiate early rehabilitation, of which physical exercise is an essential element.

Therapeutic approaches in the rehabilitation of neurological disorders were derived from the hierarchical model of the management of motor skills. Their application in physiotherapy was presented as the so-called facilitation approach (Vojta's reflex locomotion, proprioceptive neuromuscular facilitation). In connection with the development of modern neuroscience and imaging methods, the views of the management of mobility changed and were presented in various models. One of the last is the so-called system model underlying the so-called - "task oriented approach", or more generally - "the problem solving approach". This approach is represensed by, for example, Bobath's concept and program of motor learning. In these models, elements of sensorimotor learning are used.

Neurorehabilitation primarily utilizes the neurophysiological findings on sensomotor learning and adaptation.

It combines the elements:

- motor learning - conscious motion control, repetitive movements in order to improve its quality, the use of feedback and presets, the search for appropriate, existing motion sequences, optimization of motion with the appropriate combination of muscles, optimizing the timing of muscle activation and movement parameters as well.
- adaptive motor learning - modification of motor output based on sensory inputs
- conditional - associative motor learning - the use of the relationship between stimulus and motor output for conditioning response
- non-associative motor learning - use of habituation and sensitization in repeated stimuli, when using different elements of the facilitative process the stimulation of the ideal function occurs.

Therapy for children with CP is a continuous lifelong process. It should be stressed that there is currently no curative treatment for CP. It is possible to modify its manifestations but abnormalities in the child will persist.

Early rehabilitation in patients with CP is a fundamental and crucial therapeutic process. Treatment is initiated at a time when the diagnosis is not yet fully determined. The indications are serious deviations from physiological development. During the dynamic ongoing processes of the aging of the CNS (synaptogenesis, myelination, apoptosis, etc..) the neuroplastic function of brain tissue can be intensively used. A late start to physiotherapy entails a fixation of developmentally older motor patterns (symmetric, asymmetric tonic nuchal reflexes etc.), through which the child moves.

Rehabilitation options are wide and varied and physiotherapy methodologies used in the treatment of CP are numerous. This fact alone already suggests that none of them can cover all the problems of re-education of movement with this disease. Rehabilitation therapy depends on the extent of disability and medical expectations. It is important to take an individual and specific approach based on the extent of motor and mental disability. In our conditions, the most commonly used methodology is Vojta's reflex locomotion, especially in the first year of life, when it is not possible to establish cooperation with the child. The founder of this methodology was Vaclav Vojta MD, who elaborated it in the 50s of the last century. When handling a child with spastic paresis he noticed changes in spasticity on the basis of activity of muscle coordination that was the result of damage from the injury to the CNS. Therapy is also used in the treatment of motor disorders of children and adults, and does not require patient compliance. Through the starting position and the appropriate combination of excitant zones (thoracic zone, humeral medial epicondyle, medial edge of the shoulder blades, etc.) a motor response is induced at the spinal level without involving the conscious motion of the patient, which becomes an afferent stimuli to the CNS. When provoking activity, we calculate with the existence of CNS plasticity. The generated motor response is afferent to the CNS and thus enables the handling of ideal motor models. In the CNS, this motor model integrates to a higher integration circuit and is available for spontaneous mobility of the patient.

In later life, the child is usually classified under the concepts of Bobath, dynamic neuromuscular stabilization according to Kolar (Kolar, 2010), the conductive therapy of Petö, proprioceptive neuromuscular facilitation according to Kabat, Fay, Roodovej as well as others.

Currently, increasing emphasis is being placed on a pro-active approach in therapy, including intensive, repetitive, targeted training promoting neuroplasticity. The past decade has seen a rise in the significant use of robotic therapy, particularly in patients after a stroke, cerebrospinal trauma, and last but not least in children with cerebral palsy.

Training of Walking

Walking is quite challenging for children with cerebral palsy and its achievement is an important therapeutic target. Children who are able to walk are more successful in social tasks, such as participation in society and are self-sufficient in activities of daily life (daily activities) compared with children who use a wheelchair. A reduced walking speed and limited endurance during walking are two of the major functional problems. The common aim of therapy in children with cerebral palsy is to achieve upright locomotion (Mutlu, 2009) For the improvement of walking, or for its achievement in children with CP, therapy is often focused on strength and equilibrium training as well as preparation items for walking such as crawling, sitting and standing (Dodd, 2002). At present, treatment is increasingly putting emphasis on a proactive approach involving intensive, repetitive and targeted training that allows one to increase neuroplasticity (Damiano, 2006, 2009). There is growing evidence that intensive functional training is effective at improving motor skills and muscle strength in children with cerebral palsy (Meyer-Heim, 2009).

Based on the principles of *motor learning*, which describes the correlation between the repetition of activities and improvement in motor function, robot-assisted locomotor therapy was developed in the late 90s (University of Zurich, 1998) using computer controlled electronic braces. The activation of spinal and supraspinal CPG (central pattern generators) as described in animal experiments, supports the theoretical basis for this therapeutic concept.

The results of studies in animal models predict the existence of neuronal circuits in the spinal cord, responsible for locomotion, which are capable, independent of supraspinal activities, of generating a movement pattern - *central pattern generator* (Cazalets, 1995, Duysens, 1998, Mac Kay-Lyons, 2002). CPGs are activated by lower brain centers (brainstem, basal ganglia), which in turn activates the muscles performing cyclical and repetitive walking movements (Marder, 2001). Whereas higher brain centers in children with cerebral palsy are often damaged, it is assumed that the activation of the CPGs and automatic reciprocal mechanisms play an important role in stimulating walking through locomotor training (Mac Kay-Lyons, 2002). The existence of CPGs in humans could also be supported by the fact that the walking reflex mechanism is preserved even in anencephalic newborns (Borggraefe, 2008 Dietz, 2002), but conclusive evidence is still lacking. To stimulate locomotor centers in the spinal cord an optimum amount of afferent impulses is essential. This can be achieved by repeating the movements of the lower limbs in a rhythmic physiological pattern.

To stimulate locomotor centers in the spinal cord an optimum amount of afferent impulses is essential. This can be achieved by repeating the movements of the lower limbs in a rhythmic physiological pattern. In *motor learning* each new motion act takes place first through continual, voluntary conscious control. Through the repetitive movement a typical linking of the activated neurons into a pattern characteristic of the appropriate movements occurs. A sort of kinetic template on the neuronal level, the so called motor innervation pattern, is created. When the motion is sufficiently mastered, a motor innervation pattern is stored in the extrapyramidal motor system, or in the subcortical areas. In practice this means that in the process of motor learning each new movement is controlled less and less voluntarily until it is finally performed involuntarily, without the involvement of the cerebral cortex. When connecting the limbic system in the process of memory and learning, learning has an emotional shading, which can facilitate this process (biofeedback).

Locomotor training functions have become an effective way to improve walking in many not just neurological diseases and injuries.

The rehabilitation of walking, there are several basic approaches:

- walking training on the ground, conventional overground gait training (COGT)
- training with body weight strain with manual assistance, body-weight-supported treadmill therapy (BWST)
- Robot-assisted training, robotic-assisted treadmill therapy (RATT)

Robotic locomotor therapy meets the demanding criteria of the current neurorehabilitation, based on the evidence of the plasticity of the central nervous system, namely the ability of the reorganization and remodeling of the CNS activated through intense stimulation from the periphery. During development, the brain is capable of extensive anatomical and functional changes. Targeted locomotor training leads to supraspinal plasticity of the motor centers of the CNS associated with locomotor function. This is based on the latest knowledge of motor learning through repetitive movements.

Robot-assisted locomotor training builds on manually assisted gait training using the travelator. In comparison with it, we can achieve an above all constant and reproducible afferent input, precise control and the ability to regulate the main parameters of walking stereotypes and significantly facilitate the work with patients with a disorder or inability to walk. Due to this training can be longer treatment is effective and it can be expected to more quickly achieve positive results.

Several authors have demonstrated the effectiveness of robot-assisted locomotor therapy to improve walking in adults after stroke and after injuries of the brain and spinal cord SCI (Spinal Cord Injuries) (Mayr, 2007, Wirz, 2005 Hornby 2005, Mayer-Heim, 2009, Westlake, 2009, Husemann, 2007).

Preliminary studies suggest a promising effect of RATT also for patients with other neurological diseases, for example SM (Beer, 2008, Lo, 2008), Parkinson's disease (Ustinova, 2010) or TBI (Traumatic Brain Injury) (Chin, 2010).

RATT (robotic-assisted treadmill training) from 2005 began to also be used in pediatric patients with impaired motor functions of various etiologies, most commonly in children with cerebral palsy. In non-randomized studies with RATT in children with central conditional gait disorders using Lokomat, improvement was shown in motor function, speed and endurance walking and walking stereotype (Borggraefe 2008, 2010a, b, Meyer-Heim 2007 Meyer-Heim 2009).

At present there are multiple devices available enabling RATT.

Lokomat (Hocoma, AG, Volketswil, Switzerland, 1998), *GaitTrainer* (Reha-Stim, Berlin, Germany, 1997), *LokoHelp, Ambulation-assisting Robotic Tool for Human Rehabilitation, known as Arthur, Auto Ambulator, POGO* (Pneumatically Operated Gait Orthosis), *Pelvic Assist Manipulator - PAM* (commercially unavailable), a *Robotic Walking Simulator* (commercially unavailable), a *Dual Stewart Platform Mobility Simulator* (commercially unavailable), *Haptic Walker* (commercially unavailable).

Robot-Assisted Locomotor Therapy, Lokomat[®]

The Lokomat[®] is a medical - technical device that builds on manually assisted gait training using the travelator. It consists of several components: a travelator (treadmill), a specialized patented suspension system and electronically controlled orthoses. The electromechanical pressure relief system monitors and adjusts relief in real time at the desired level. The moving parts are controlled by three computers and special software. Computer-controlled drivers on each hip and knee are synchronized with the speed of the treadmill. Force sensors for these joints are connected in such a way so as to accurately measure the interaction between the patient and the Lokomat[®] System. In addition to the variable relief of body weight, we can also adjust the length of the stepping cycle, affect the quality of the swing, standing phase, as well as correct the range of motion in the hip, knee and ankle joint thanks to the software. During training, we use passive movements, where the patient tries to realize his own stereotype of walking and its quality. Training can also be active, with the possibility of using resistance or asymmetric targeting of a specific problem. An important element in the therapy is a dynamic pelvic fixation using braces and a pelvic reclining backrest, allowing the achievement of a closer status to the physiological position of the ideal walking stereotype. Dorsal flexion of the ankle joint is achieved using passive clamping of the foot (foot lifter).

Since the parameters of each workout (distance, speed, number of steps, the degree of lightening of the weight and the guidance force - the guiding force) are well defined and continuously monitored, gait training can be easily comparable interindividual as well as between individual therapeutic units. This fact offers new opportunities not only for research but also for a specific treatment plan and management of the patient (Meyer-Heim, 2009).

On monitors directed towards the patient and therapist, we can visually observe and affect the success of the exercise in real-time. For increasing incentives for pediatric patients, a program that allows training in a virtual environment has been developed. During the training, patients move though different types of virtual environments, where they solve various tasks, which increase the level of active participation of child patients in the therapeutic process.

The Virtual Environment of the Lokomat (Augmented Feedback)

The VR module for the Lokomat® system includes a flat screen placed in the front part of the Lokomat®. The VR in the Lokomat® system produces a multi-modal feedback system. The input device transforms the movements of patients into movements of a virtual character in the virtual environment. Moreover Lokomat® is able to display interaction with objects in a virtual environment. During the training, patients move in different types of virtual environments, where they solve various tasks, which increase the level of active participation of child patients in the therapeutic process. Part of the training, for example, can be to collect randomly distributed objects in a space, avoid obstacles or maintain a direction of movement. The movements of the lower limbs of children are transferred to the movement of the limbs of the virtual characters in real-time. The figure is moving in the space simultaneously with the movements of the patient. If a child can not directly control the movements of the virtual limbs by moving their own limbs, the imitation of limb movement through the device (Lokomat®) is still present, which is displayed on the screen (Figure 1).

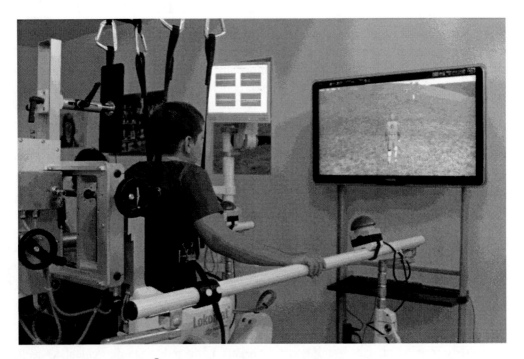

Figure 1. Training in Lokomat® system, virtual reality environment.

In this study "Lokomat® augmented feedback" was used. Training in the VR environment resembled a computer game and consists of different types of scenery, where it is possible to collect various objects randomly distributed, such as boxes of treasure, coins, snowmen, sheep, dogs, etc. In the next game, children converged on specific objects and tried to direct the limbs of virtual characters to the left and right through specific movements of the limbs. For example if they wanted to turn right, they activated the swing phase more and the right lower limb, and more of a standing phase the left lower limb. When turning left, the opposite. The important thing is that these VR tools are easy to operate and therapists are able to use them after a short period of instruction. By adjusting the intensity and level of difficulty for each task, training can be adapted to cognitive and motor skills, and where appropriate, the specific needs of each patient. All performance data is stored in the computer and the therapist may use them for control, evaluation and documentation of patient progress. The physiotherapist has an integral role in the initial setup of the software and oversees the progress and optimizes the therapy.

The pediatric Lokomat model began being clinically used in 2005. It is intended for children from 4 years of age. One of the crucial criteria is the length of the femur from 21 cm to 35 cm. Through an exchange of the orthosis for the adult module, we can broaden the spectrum of patients. The length of the femur of patients suitable for treatment with an orthosis for adults is 35-47 cm. (Figure 2)

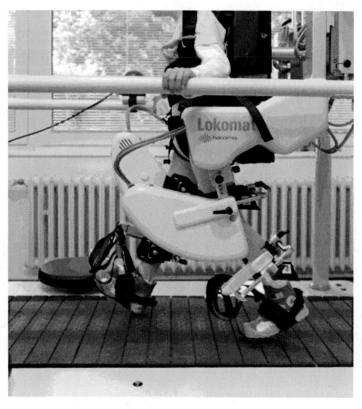

Figure 2. Robotic- assisted treadmill training in Lokomat® system.

Functional Upper Limb Therapy, Armeo

Devices with a movable orthosis arm have been used in rehabilitation for a long time, but the influence of different levels of upper-limb weight support is often difficult for adjusting and control and, moreover, do not always provide sufficient feedback regarding the return of motor recovery (Housman, 2009).

The literature mentions a number of robotic devices, for example. Massachusetts Institute of Technology (MIT) - MANUS, Mirror Image Motion Enabler (MIME), Assisted Rehabilitation and Measurement (ARM) Guide, Bi-Manu-Track, GENTLE / S and others.

However robotic devices are expensive and require high demands on security measures, which may be one of the limiting factors. In addition, the "cost to benefit" ratio has not been conclusively defined. Exclusively robotic therapy minimizes the effort spent by the patient, but also his attention, especially if the robot can perform the required movements without the participation of the patient, which on the contrary can have a negative effect on motor plasticity (Housman, 2007, 2009).

Compared with robotic, non-robotic upper-limb orthoses are potentially less expensive, safer and more suitable for semi-active training.

In order to provide actively assisted training of the upper limbs a new training system called Therapy Wilmington Robotic Exoskeleton (T-Wrex) was constructed (Housman 2007, 2009, Rahman, 2006).

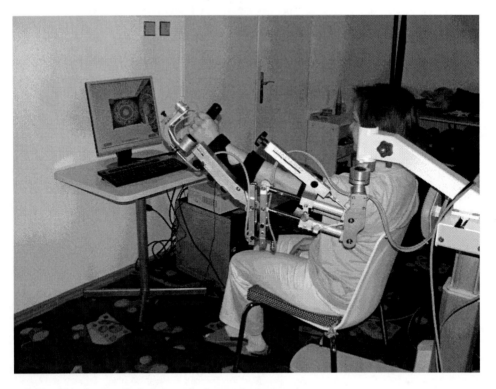

Figure 3. Functional upper limb therapy in Armeo device.

T-Wrex is a passive (non-robotic), upper-limb orthosis which is intended to relieve the weight of the upper limbs in a 3D space by using ergonomic and adjustable upper-limb rests (antigravity effect). It allows natural movement in the working space, at a size of approximately 66% of the normal working area vertically and 72% of the horizontal plane, making it easier for users with moderate to severe hemiparesis to achieve a greater range of motion than is possible without lightening the weight of the upper limbs. It also enables the use of the upper limbs, in a coordinated manner, even if only the residual possibility of movement is maintained. Since this is a non robotic device, it requires the initiation of patient motion, which requires the active participation of the patient during training.

Compared with the traditional manual upper-limb support, T-Wrex offers an easily adjustable variable level of the support of the weight of the upper limbs, customizable for different sized upper limbs. A modified version of the T-Wrex is currently distributed by the company Hocoma called ARMEO SPRING. (Figure 3)

The Armeo device is installed on a wheel chair, which can be easily and quickly placed behind the stool or wheelchair of a patient. The main structure consists of an arm exoskeleton hand with an integrated spring mechanism, consisting of two links: a single link on the forearm and a parallelogram-shaped link at the upper arm. It allows you to lighten the weight of the limbs thereby providing the opportunity to feel control of the upper limbs in all positions in the available workspace. The grip sensor detects the movement of the fingers and allows the incorporation of grip and its release into the upper-limb workout. The training takes place in a 3D workspace. Built-in electromotive motion sensors of the upper limbs and sensors recording grip strength enable the patient to interact with therapeutic computer games and provide quantitative feedback. The grip sensor enables combined training of hand and arm function and can be used as both an input device for exercise and also as a computer interface - a mouse for standard software or PC games (Hocoma). The grip sensor can be removed and the patient may, in the practice of daily activities then train the grasping of real objects (e.g., a cup, apple), while the upper limbs remain lightweight.

As part of the training the following are applied:

- Active assisted upper limb exercises (flexion, extension, abduction, adduction, extra-rotation, intra-rotation of the shoulder joint, flexion, extension of the elbow joint, forearm pronation and supination, flexion, wrist extension, grip)
- Isolated actively targeted repetitive movements
- distal and proximal exercises

After setting the therapy the patient performs the specified exercise as a separate training. All exercises are performed in the virtual reality environment where the functional role and performance of the patient are clearly represented (Klobucká, 2010).

All performance data is stored in the computer and the therapist may use them for control, evaluation and documentation of patient progress. The physiotherapist plays an integral role in the initial setup of the software and oversees the progress and optimizes the therapy.

Coordination Dynamic Therapy

Coordination Dynamic Therapy (Coordination Dynamics Therapy - CDT, Schalow) is also based on the knowledge of motor learning by repeating the motion, which describes the correlation between the repetition of activities and improvement in motor function (Hesse, 2001, 2003). CDT employs various strategies for repair. These strategies are based on the correction of the impaired auto-regulation of the CNS to compensate for the loss of mobility and reparations of damaged autonomous functions.

CDT improves the function of the CNS after injury, stroke, degenerative diseases or malformations. Patients can train movements that they want to learn - like walking, or can use rhythmic, dynamic, coordinated stereotyped movements that activate and repair the pre-motor spinal oscillating circuit (e.g., through jumping exercises on a trampoline or springboard).

Medical devices are also used for this purpose which enable cyclical, rotational movements of the upper and lower limbs with varying, alternating coordination between the upper and lower limbs.

CDT thus includes:

1. Automation training (e.g., innate movement patterns within the scope of ontogeny) such as crawling, climbing, walking and running.
2. Practice of previously learned movement patterns (e.g., learning automations with high demands on stability such as walking up the stairs).
3. Practicing dynamic rhythmic stereotyped movements such as jumping on the springboard (for repair of neuronal assemblies - spinal oscillators).
4. Training on special devices - includes implementation of integrated motion,
5. in which the upper and lower limbs are precisely coordinated. It is a practice of predefined movements in the device that will improve the synchronization and coordination of action potentials.

In the Harmony rehabilitation center we use a CDT device with distribution called Giger MD$^{®}$ (Figure 4).

Giger MD$^{®}$ is a medical device enabling kinematically related work of the upper and lower limbs in cyclic patterns. With the movements of the limbs the patient also performs three-dimensional movement of the body musculature.

This movement of the limbs - especially lying down, is often the first movement at all possible that the patient can perform alone, for example after a spinal cord injury in the cervical area. Through this, the rostral and caudal neural networks are activated across the lesion site.

Afferent and efferent inputs pass through the damaged area of the spinal cord and create coordinated communication between the cervical and lumbar intumescence. The device uses cyclical, rotational movements of the arms and legs with varying, alternating coordination between the upper and lower limbs. By adjusting the braking force of the Giger MD$^{®}$ device, we can continuously generate power more than 200W. Less braking force will warm up the muscle tendons and joints. The movement is symmetrical, harmonious and coordinated. The power is evenly distributed and the handle can be rotated forward and backward with two ways of grasping, both top and bottom.

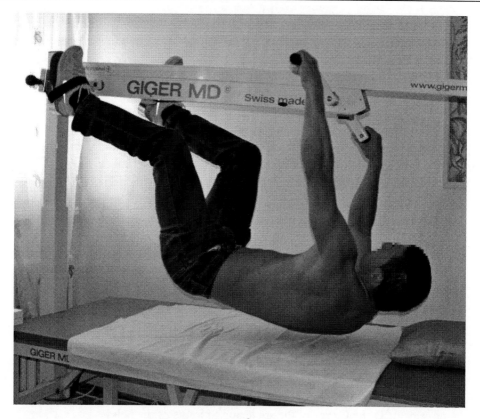

Figure 4. Coordination Dynamic Therapy, Giger MD®.

Such accuracy of coordinated movements is important for activation of the denervated neurons in and below the site of injury. The action potential is generated in the axonal processes of afferent impulses only if the total amount of potential coming from the dendrites on the nerve cell bodies exceeds the threshold of excitation. These potentials are precisely synchronized and coordinated (temporal and spatial summation of action potentials). Imprecise and uncoordinated movements generate asynchronous depolarization of afferent inputs, so sufficient potential for the spread of excitation is not reached (Schalow, 2006). Though coordination dynamic therapy we influence the rhythmically activating neural networks through the accurate to a millisecond generated exteroceptive and proprioceptive afferent impulses.

Software installed on the device allows you to view and record during therapy. The value of dynamic coordination is an integrated and determining parameter characterizing neural networks in accordance with impaired motor evaluation programs of the surface EMG (Schalow, 2006). Co-ordination of limbs expressed through "rhythmicity," analyzed through the software of the device and displayed graphically on the screen, correlated with those obtained by examination of the surface EMG (Schalow, 2006).

According to the regularity of the resulting "rhythmicity" curve, the effect of therapeutic intervention can be demonstrated and visualized which significantly contributes to the motivation of the patient (biofeedback).

The installed software allows graphical and alphanumeric data storage. It records personal data output, such as the consumption of calories, watts, number of rotations, speed, pulse.

Therapy can be carried out standing, sitting (with a modification of sitting on the ball), lying down, allowing gravity to reduce the burden to a minimum. The load pattern can also be combined together: small rotational movements, combined with a slight resistance or pressure. The location of the clamping bars and cranks and the distance between the upper and lower limbs can be variably adjusted, thereby achieving a variety of training option parameters taking into account the individual patient's needs.

As part of the training the following are applied:

- movement in the quadrupedal crossover formula requiring coordinated activity of the upper and lower limbs and torso muscles
- active exercises of the upper limbs (flexion, extension, extra-rotation, intra-rotation of the shoulder joint, flexion, extension of the elbow joint, flexion, wrist extension, grip)
- repetitive active movements
- simultaneous alternating movements
- distal and proximal exercises
- facilitation of synkinesis with the limbs on the other side
- facilitation of movement patterns
- rotational movements of the spine in 3 dimensions, extension of the spine, nutation movements in the C area of the spine and SI joints of the pelvis
- movement in open biomechanical chains (Klobucká, 2012)

Training Parameters

- Frequency: 2-5 x a week
- Duration of training: 4-12 weeks, if we detect a progressive improvement, it is appropriate to extend the therapy duration
- Time of th therapy: 30 min
- 1.5 min moving forward alternated with 1.5 min moving backward

Conclusion

The proper management of the treatment of neurological diseases is the only prevention of complications arising from structural disorders (pain, secondary musculoskeletal problems, possible malfunctions of internal organs, orthopedic, prosthetic, surgical intervention with the necessary hospitalization, or consequential spa treatment), which ultimately allows to significantly reduce the cost of subsequent health care

There are several studies positively evaluating the importance of the training of the locomotor function in patients with gait disturbances using robot-assisted locomotor training, which is also confirmed by a significant improvement in motor function, stability and walking ability compared to standard rehabilitation techniques (Borggraefe 2010, Hesse 2001, Meyer-Heim, 2009).

In recent literature there are several studies available on robotic and robot-assisted therapy of the upper limbs of children with cerebral palsy (Fasoli, 2008 Frascareli, 2009 Krebs, 2009) and adult patients after stroke (Fasoli, 2003, 2004, Housman, 2007, 2009). These studies have confirmed significant improvements in the mobility of the upper limbs in patients with moderate to severe hemiparesis, an increase in muscle strength, an increase in the range of joint mobility, improvements in neuromuscular coordination, improvements of the function of the upper limbs, an increase in patient motivation and, ultimately, improvements in self-sufficiency.

A study of foreign authors documents the beneficial effect of coordination dynamic therapy (CDT) on the motor function of patients after brain injury, spinal cord injury, stroke and cerebral palsy (Schalow, 2004-2008). As is clear from our clinical experience and the works consisting of case reports, it is possible to apply CTD in patients with juvenile and adolescent scoliosis.

Robot-assisted therapy and coordination dynamic therapy meets the criteria of the current neurorehabilitation, based on the evidence of plasticity of the central nervous system, i.e., the ability of reorganization and remodeling of the CNS activated by intense stimulation from the periphery. The results of the available studies support the current theory of motor learning by repeating motions, which describes the correlation between the repetition of activities and improvement in motor function, which is the key to stimulating motor plasticity.

A Case Report of a Patient in the Lokomat® System

Recommended training parameters during the Lokomat therapy system:

- Frequency: 2-5 x a week
- Duration of training: 4-12 weeks, if we detect a progressive improvement, it is appropriate to extend the therapy duration
- Time of walking: at first 10-30 min, and later 20-45 min
- Walking speed: 1.0-1.5 km/h, and subsequently to 2.5 km/h
- Support of patient body weight: in the beginning 50-70%, with a gradual improvement of the effort to walk without lightening
- Biofeedback: focus on the swing phase

Input Measurement, Test Range

Gross Motor Function Measure (GMFM)

GMFM is a standardized procedure for investigating children aged 5 months. It assesses changes in the gross motor skills in children with CP at the time. It was developed for clinical and research use. There are 2 versions, the 88 position (GMFM - 88) and the shortened version containing 66 positions (GMFM - 66). In this study, we use the more detailed 88 position version for the evaluation of the children's motor functions, which assess the children's motor skills in five dimensions: A - *lying and rolling,* 17 positions, B - *sitting,* 20 positions, C - *crawling and kneeling,* 14 positions, D - *standing*, 13 positions, E - *walking, running and jumping,* 24 positions.

It is expected that a 5 year old child with normal dexterity shall fulfill all 88 positions.

GMFM assesses the number of positions that the child is able to meet and does not evaluate the quality of their performance. Its use is widespread throughout the world primarily to assess the effects of the treatment of CP. The testing takes 45-60 min. (Russell, 1989, 2002, Palisano 2006, 2007).

Gross Motor Function Classification System (GMFCS)

One of the aspects that we consider in classifying cerebral palsy is also the severity of the disability. To classify gross motor function we use *The Gross Motor Function Classification System (GMFCS),* which assesses motor function taking into account the age of the affected child. It primarily monitors sitting and walking. It has separate evaluation criteria for the age groups up to 2 years, 2-4 years, 4-6 years, 6-12 years, and since 2007 also the category 12 to 18 years (Palissano,1997, 2006, 2007, Sankar, 2005, Rosenbaum, 2007, 2008).

This scale uses the distribution of gross motor function in five stages (Palissano, 1997, 2006, 2007, Sankar, 2005, Rosenbaum, 2007, 2008).

GMFCS Level I- Children walk at home, school, outdoors and the community. They can climb stairs without the use of railing. Children perform gross motor skills such as running and jumping, but speed, balance and coordination are limited.

GMFCS Level II- Children walk in most settings and climb stairs holding onto a railing. They may experience difficulty walking long distances and balancing on uneven terrain, inclines, in crowded areas or confined spaces. Children may walk with physical assistance, a hand-held mobility device or used wheeled mobility over long distances. Children have only minimal ability to perform gross motor skills such as running and jumping.

GMFCS Level III- Children walk using a hand-held mobility device in most indoor settings. They may climb stairs holding onto a railing with supervision or assistance. Children use wheeled mobility when traveling long distances and may self-propel for shorter distances.

GMFCS Level IV- Children use methods of mobility that require physical assistance or powered mobility in most settings. They may walk for short distances at home with physical assistance or use powered mobility or a body support walker when positioned. At school, outdoors and in the community children are transported in a manual wheelchair or use powered mobility.

GMFCS Level V- Children are transported in a manual wheelchair in all settings. Children are limited in their ability to maintain antigravity head and trunk postures and control leg and arm movements. (Palisano,1997)

Individual Locomotor Stages According to Vojta

- *Stage 0* - the child is apedular. It can not move forward by using the upper and lower limbs. It is not able to execute any contact (motor) by rotating or grasping objects. The supporting function is not formed. The child's head in the predilection position and its holding corresponds to the neonatal stage. Developmental age: newborn.

Latest Trends in Neurorehabilitation of Patients with Cerebral Palsy 221

- *Stage 1* - the child is apedular, it is unable to move forward, but it can turn to an object in order to touch or grasp it. In the prone position it is able to lean on its elbows.
  In the supine position it is able to lift its legs off the pad. The child has equilibrium functions. At this stage they are no longer endowed with reflexes tied to the neonatal period. Developmental age: 3-4 months.
- *Stage 2* - the child is apedular. In supination the child is able to reach for objects from the median plane. In the prone position it can use the upper limbs as a supporting and grasping organ. In the position on the abdomen it is also able to reach for objects, by using the other upper limb for support. The lower limb on the side of the grasping upper limb leans on the medial condyle of the femur and the other is in the extension phase. Muscle differentiation starts to emerge. The child tries to approach the object, but can not move forward using the arms and legs. Developmental age: the end of the 4th and beginning of the 5th month (the second half of the 5th month and 6 month is a period of transition between the 2nd and 3rd stage of locomotion).
- *Stage 3* - the child is able to crawl. This is real locomotion, the child spontaneously moves around the room on his own initiative through crawling. It is also able to turn over from its back to its belly. The child possesses the reciprocal model of stepping towards and support, in both ipsilateral and contralateral formats. In locomotor movement both oblique abdominal chains are activated. Developmental age: 7.-8. months.
- *Stage 4* - the child "bounces" (jumps on his knees and hands). It is not able to cyclically rotate the center of gravity from the axis. Support on the upper limbs is abnormal and is made up of the wrist or fist. "Bouncing" does not have a crossed pattern as we see when crawling, i.e., it is homologous. This type of locomotion does not exist in normal development. If the child is unable to reach the stage of crawling in a timely manner, it will soon completely give up locomotion.
  This model is superior to pulling oneself on the belly. The child at this stage of locomotion has no steering ability to transfer movement to an isolated segment (e.g., segmental momentum in the ankle joint). The child is able to achieve an upright kneeling position and get into an inclined sitting position. Developmental age: 9 months.
- *Stage 5* – crawling. This locomotor pattern is fully engaged when a child with central paresis can crawl throughout the apartment on its own motivation. Part of the locomotion is the crossed pattern and support is on the open palms. During crawling, the rotation of the spine and its deflection in the frontal plane is available. At a later period each crawling child can count on verticalization. Developmental age: 11months.
- *Stage 6* - the child is able to pull itself up into a standing position using the upper limbs and remain standing. It is able to move by means of the upper limbs to the side. It is a quadrupedal locomotion in the frontal plane. In the later period of this locomotion stage the onset of locomotion in the sagittal plane occurs, with the support of one upper limb. The important thing is that this locomotion must be done from one's own motivation. Developmental age: 12.-13. months.
- *Stage 7* - the child walks independently, separately, even outside the home.

- *Stage 8* - the child can stand on one leg for 3 seconds. This must be examined by a stable standing position. The flight step phase begins. Developmental age: 3 years.
- *Stage 9* - child can stand on one leg for more than 3 seconds, including on both sides. Developmental age: 4 years. (Vojta, 1972- 2007)

Walking Speed, Endurance Walking

10 meter walking test - walking speed is measured with the confirmed validity and reliability in children with confirmed neuromuscular disabilities (Pripiris, 2003 Provost, 2007), By using it we determined walking speed by measuring the time for which it takes the child to travel a distance of 10 meters at its normal pace, or with the devices usually used.

6 minute walking test - introduced under the standardized protocol of the American Thoracic Society (ATS) guidelines 6MWT (Li, 2005). It enables the assessment of walking endurance. Reliability and validity was also confirmed by this test (Paap, 2005, Li, 2005). A more meaningful value is provided by patient selected walking speed with the materials normally used when walking (Paap, 2005, Thompson, 2008). Through the test we recorded the distance the child can go in 6 minutes in a safe environment without obstacles - in our case a flat smooth sidewalk on the premises of the rehabilitation center or a corridor with a minimum length of 30 m. We used 2 warning signs (cones), which we deployed at a distance of 30 m. The patient walked between those marks. Before the test, we instructed him to undergo the greatest distance which he is able, at the same time he was allowed to vary the pace and relax as needed. The patient may be accompanied by a parent who encourages him in 30 s intervals, as recommended by the American Thoracic Society (ATS) guidelines 6MWT (Thompson, 2008). The physiotherapist followed the child at about a 1 m distance and monitored him with a stopwatch.

Case Report

The patient is a 10 year old boy with an easy-risk perinatal history (Sectio Caesarea pr. placenta praevia) with follow-up care at the neurological clinic for encephalopathy with MRI repeatedly verified by non-progressive atrophy of the cerebellum. The metabolic or genetic origin of the disease has not been confirmed.

For motor development delays and a lag in the upright mechanisms, physiotherapy intervention was initiated in the child at 12 months of age. Still in rehabilitation. During development a delayed psychomotor speed with evident mental retardation was observed. For the specific epileptic nature of the left frontal EEG activity, an antiepileptic medication is administered.

The physical examination is dominated by cerebellar ataxia, muscle tone at the border of the hypotonia, expressive phatic speech disorder with chanting is present. Oxycefalia, facial asymmetry, normal cerebral nerves, area of the cervical spine without significant disturbance of dynamics, global decreased muscle tone with tendon hyporeflexia, hypotrophic musculatur, present dysmetria as well as great asynergy are all indicated. In setting the position the upper limbs endure, lower limb instability bilaterally, in targeting easily expressed intention tremor, the right hand is preferred. Positive extension irritative pyramid phenomena are present on the lower limbs. In the standing position large-curve dextroconvex thoracic scoliosis of the spine, lumbar hyperlordosis of the spine, slanted pelvis, valgus position of the knee joints, planovalgus configuration of the feet, hyper-excursibility of the joints, as well as axial hypotonia are present. Sitting is unstable with support of the lower limbs. Standing is possible with the support of a wide base, walking a short distance with the assistance of a second person, brachybasia and ataxic. Using a mechanical wheelchair for longer distances. The sphincters control, sporadic nocturnal enuresis occurs within the secondary epileptic syndrome. At the time of the entrance examination, the patient was classified in locomotor stage 6 according to prof. Vojta. A detailed kinesiological analysis was carried out by means of the GMFM test (Russell, 2002).

The patient meets the criteria for robot-assisted locomotor therapy (central gait disturbance, femur length 21-35 cm, the ability to cooperate, indicate pain, discomfort, absence of severe contractures, fractures, absence of severe osteoporosis, intact skin cover, cardiovascular compensated).

The aim of the therapy was to improve motor function, stability of sitting, standing as well as the improvement of walking. Before therapy, the patient is normally examined as an outpatient and tested through the GMFM range (Russel, 2002). In addition to training in the LOKOMAT system other rehabilitation procedures were also ordered.

Therapy in the LOKOMAT system lasted 6 weeks with a frequency of 5 times per week, representing 30 therapeutic units. Walking speed was initially 1.1 km/h, and later increased to 1.5 km/h. The lightening of body weight was 50% at the beginning, then with a gradual reduction to almost 0. Despite the minimal lightening of body weight he was able to walk with a fixed extension of the knees. The duration of one therapeutic unit was on average 40 minutes (35-50 min, SD ± 2) with an average distance traveled of 1062 m (950 to 1,150 m, SD ± 79). The total distance covered during the 6 weeks of treatment was 31,863 m. Entry and exit tests were carried out 24 hours before treatment and 24 hours after treatment.

The obtained values indicate that the dimension of A (lying, rolling) has improved from 60.7% to 74.5%. In dimension B (sitting), we recorded a percentage increase from 70% to 80%. Crawling and kneeling (C) values improved from 61.9% to 69%. Stabilization of standing was also registered within dimension D from 25.6% to 41%. In category E (walking, running, jumping), we saw an increase in the score from 16.6% to 17.7%.

After totaling the values in each category, we can conclude an overall improvement in motor function tested using the GMFM of 9.48% (from 46.96% to 56.44%). (Figure 5)

After completing therapy in the LOKOMAT system, the stabilization of sitting and standing occurred as well as the improvement of walking stereotype. After treatment the patient was even able to walk a short distance alone (about 10 meters).

We did not observe any side effects during the therapy. After 8 years of stagnation of motor development a shift from locomotor stage 6 to stage 7 under prof. Vojta was achieved (Vojta, 1972 – 2007).

We repeated GMFM testing at intervals of 4 months. The patient continued standard kinesiotherapy during this period (Bobath concept) with a frequency of 1-2x a week. We did not record any change in the dimensions of the GMFM test. The effects of therapeutic intervention persisted.

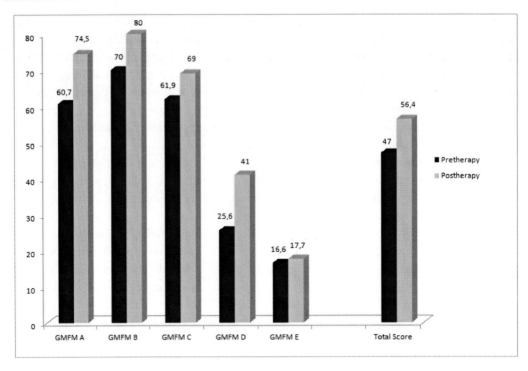

Figure 5. Improvement of motor functions evaluated by GMFM after robotic- assisted treadmill training in Lokomat.

Conclusion

A 10 year old boy with non-progressive cerebellar syndrome with the morphological correlate in the back cranial fossa underwent an objective improvement in motor and locomotor functions after 6 weeks of treatment in the Lokomat system. In accordance with the work of foreign authors we noted the effect of therapeutic intervention to stabilize the axial muscle and we observed firmed-up sitting and standing. According to the assumption of the concept of targeted locomotor training we recorded improvement in locomotor function. The achieved results correlate well with the final GMFM score. After treatment after treatment in the LOKOMAT system the patient was even able to walk a short distance alone (about 10 meters). This improvement correlated with the final score and GMFM persisted even after 4 months, which was consistent with the results of the works of foreign authors (Montinaro, 2011, Patritti 2009, Borggraefe, 2010 b-sustainability).

Acknowledgment

We are grateful to Mr. Ing. Alojz Halas - direcor of Rehabilitation Centre Harmony, for support and willingness to help in making this work.

References

Andersen, GL; et al. Cerebral palsy in Norway: prevalence, subtypes and severity. *European Journal of Pediatric Neurology*, 2008, Vol. 12, No 1, 4-13.

ATS statement: Guidelines for the six- minute walk test. *American Journal of Respiratory and Critical Care Medicine*, 2002, Vol 166, No 1, 111-117.

Bax, MCO; Flodmark, O; Tydeman, C. From syndrome toward disease. *Developmental Medicine & Child Neurology*, 2007, 49 (Suppl. 109), 39–41.

Beer, S; et. al. Robot-assisted gait training in multiple sclerosis: a pilot randomized trial. *Multiple Sclerosis*, 2008, Vol 14, No 2, 231-236.

Borggraefe, I; et al. Improved Gait Parameters After Robotic- Assisted Locomotor Treadmill Therapy in a 6-Year-Old Child with Cerebral Palsy. *Movement Disorders.*, 2008, Vol 23, No2, 280-283.

Borggraefe, I; et al. Robotic- assisted treadmill therapy improves walking and standing performance in children and adolescents with cerebral palsy. *European Journal of Pediatric Neurology*, 2010 a, Vol. 14, No 6, 496-502.

Borggraefe, I; et al. Sustainability of motor perforamnce after robotic-assisted treadmill therapy in children: an open, non randomized baseline- treatment study. *European Journal of Physical and Rehabilitation Medicine*, 2010 b, Vol 46, No2, 125-131.

Cazalets, JR; et al. Localization and Organization of the Central Pattern Generator for Hindlimb Locomotion in Newborn Rat. *The Journal of Neuroscience*, 1995, Vol 15, No 7, 4943-4951.

Damiano, DL. Activity, Activity, Activity: Rethinking Our Physical Therapy Approach to Cerebral Palsy. *Physical Therapy*, 2006, Vol 86, No 11, 1534-1540.

Damiano, DL. A Systematic Review of the Effectiveness of Treadmill raining and Body Weight Support in Pediatric Rehabilitation. *Journal of Neurologic Physical Therapy*, 2009, Vol 33, No 1, 27-44.

Dietz, V; et al. Locomotor activity in spinal man: significance of afferent input from joint and load receptors. *Brain*, 2002, Vol 125, No 12, 2626-2634.

Dodd, KJ; et al. A systematic review of the effectiveness of strength- training programs for people with cerebral palsy. *Archives of Physical Medicine and rehabilitation*, 2002,Vol 83, No 8, 1157-1164.

Duysens, J; et al. Neural control of locomotion, Part 1: The central pattern generator from cats to humans. *Gait and Posture*, 1998, Vol 7, 131-141.

Fasoli, SE; Krebs, HI; Stein, J; Frontera, WR; Hogan, N. Effects of robotic therapy on motor impairment and recovery in chronic stroke. *Archives of Physical Medicine and rehabilitation*, 2003, Vol 84, No 4, 477-482.

Fasoli, SE; Krebs, HI; Stein, J; Frontera, WR; Hughes, R; Hogan, N. Robotic therapy for chronic motor impairments after stroke: follow - up results. *Archives of Physical Medicine and rehabilitation*, 2004, Vol. 85, No 7, 1106-1111.

Fasoli, SE; Fragala- Pinkham, M; Hughes, R; Hogan, N; Krebs, HI; Stein, J. Upper limb robotic therapy for children with hemiplegia. *American Journal of Physical Medicine and Rehabilitation*, 2008, Vol 87, No 11, 929-936.

Frascareli, F; Masia, L; Di Rosa, G; Cappa, P; Petrarca, M; Castelli, E; Krebs, H. The impact of robotic rehabilitation in children with acquired or congenital movement disorders.

European Journal of Physical and Rehabilitation Medicine, 2009, Vol 45, No 1, 135-141.

Hanna, SE; Bartlett, DJ; Rivard, LM; Russell, DJ. 2008. Reference curves for the gross motor function measure: percentiles for clinical description and tracking over time among children with cerebral palsy. *Physical Therapy*, 2008,Vol 88, No 5, 596-607.

Hanna, S; et al. Stability and decline in gross motor function among children and youth with cerebral palsy aged 2-21 years. *Developmental Medicine & Child Neurology* 2009, Vol 51, No 4, 295–302.

Hesse, S. Locomotor therapy in neurorehabilitation. *NeuroRehabilitation*, 2001, Vol.16, No 3,133-139.

Hesse, S; el al. Upper and lowe extremity robotic devices for rehabilitation and for studying motor control. *Current Opinion in Neurology.*, 2003, Vol 16, No 6, 705-710.

Himmelmann, K; Hagberg, G; Uvebrant, P. The changing panorama of cerebral palsy in Sweden. X. Prevalence and origin in birth-year period 1999–2002. *Acta Paediatrica*, 2010, Vol 99, No 9, 1337- 1343.

Himmelmann, K; Hagberg, G; Beckung, E; Hagberg, B; Uvebrant, P. The changing panorama of cerebral palsy in Sweden. IX. Prevalence and origin in the birth-year period 1995-1998. *Acta Paediatrica*, 2005, Vol 94, No 3, 287-294.

Himmelmann, K; at al. Gross and fine motor function and accompanying impairments in cerebral palsy. *Developmental Medicine & Child Neurology*, 2006, Vol 48, No 6, 417–423.

Hornby, TG; et al. Robotic assisted, Body - Weight - Supported Treadmill Training in Individuals Folliving Motor Incomplete Spinal Cord Injury. *Physical Therapy,* 2005,Vol 85, No 1, 52-66.

Housman, SJ; Le, V; Rahman, T; Sanchez, RJ; Jr. Reinkensmeyer, DJ. Arm-training. *Proceedings of the 2007 IEEE 10th International Conference on Rehabilitation Robotics*, June 12-15, Noordwijk, The Netherlands, 2007.

Housman, SJ; Scott, KM; Reinkensmeyer, DJ. A randomized controlled trial *Neurorehabilitation and Neural Repair*, 2009, Vol. 23, No 5, 505-514.

Husemann, B; et al. Effects of Locomotion Training With Assistance of Robot-Driven Gait Orthosis in Hemiparetic Patients After Stroke. *Stroke*, 2007, Vol 38, No 2, 349- 354.

Chin, LF; et al. Evaluation of robotic –assisted locomotor training outcomes at a rehabilitation centre in Singapore. *Singapore Medical Journal*, 2010, Vol 51, No 9, 709-715.

Kolar, P; Kobesova, A. Postural – locomotion function in the diagnosis and treatment of movement disorders. *Clinical Chiropractic*, 2010, Vol 13, No 1, 58–68.

Klobucka, S; Kralovicova, M; Ziakova, E. Functional assisted therapy of upper extremity. *Rehabilitace a fyzikální lékařství*, 2010, Vol.17, No 4, 164-168.

Klobucka, S; Ziakova, E. Coordination Dynamic Therapy Applied in the Syndrome of Painful Shoulder. *Rehabilitace a fyzikální lékařství*, 2012, Vol 19, No3,.p. 112-116.

Krebs, H; Ladenheim, B; Hippolyte, CH; Monterroso, L; Mast, J. Robot – assisted task specific training in cerebral palsy, *Developmental Medicine & Child Neurology*, Suppl, Vol. 51, 2009, (Suppl.4).

Li, AM; et al.: The six-minute walk test in healthy children: reliability and validity. *European Respiratory Journal*, Vol 25, No 6, 1057-1060.

Lo, AC; Triche, EW. Improving gait in multiple sclerosis using robot-assisted, body weight supported treadmill training. *Neurorehabilitation and Neural Repair*, 2008, Vol 22, No 6, 661- 671.

Mac Kay-Lyons, M. Central pattern generation of locomotion: a review of evidence. *Physical Therapy*, 2002,Vol 82, No 1, 69-83.

Marder, E; Bucher, D. Central pattern generators and the control of rhytmic movements. *Current Biology*, 2001, Vol 11, No 23,986-996.

Mayr, A; et al. Prospective, Blinded, Randomized Crossover Study of Gait Rehabilitation in Stroke Patients Using the Lokomat Gait Orthosis. *Neurorehabilitation and Neural repair*, 2007, Vol 21, No 4, 307-314.

Meyer- Heim, A; et al. Feasibility of robotic assisted locomotor trainig in children with central gait impairment. *Developmental Medicine& Child Neurology*, 2007, Vol 49, No 12, 900-906.

Meyer- Heim, A; et al. Improvement of walking abilities after robotic- assisted locomotion training in children with cerebral palsy. *Archives of Disease in Childhood*, 2009, Vol 94, No 8, 615-620.

Montinaro, A; et al. Robotic- assisted locomotion training in children affected by Cerebral Palsy. *Gait and Posture*, 2011, Vol 33 Supplement 1 (2011) S55-S56. doi:10.1016/j.gaitpost.2010.10.068

Morris, Ch. Definition and classification of cerebral palsy: a historical perspective. *Developmental Medicine & Child Neurology, Suppl.s 109*, 2007, 3-7.

Mutlu, A; Krosschell, K; Spira, DG. Treadmill training with partial body –weight support in children with cerebral palsy: a systematic review. *Developmental Medicine & Child Neurology*, 2009, Vol 51, No 4, 268-275.

Odding, E. The epidemiology of cerebral palsy: Incidence, impairments and risk factors. *Disability and Rehabilitation*, 2006,Vol 28, No 4, 183-191.

Paap, E; et al., 2005. Physiologic response at the six-minute walk test in children with juvenile idiopathic arthritis. *Arthritis & Rheumatism*, 2005, Vol 53, No 3, 351-356.

Palisano, R; Rosenbaum, P; Walter, S; Russell, D; Wood, E; Galuppi, B. Development and reliability of a system to classify gross motor function in children with cerebral palsy. *Developmental Medicine & Child Neurology*,1997, Vol 39, No 4, 214–223.

Palisano, R; et al. 2006. Stability of the Gross Motor Function Classification System. *Developmental Medicine& Child Neurology*, 2006, Vol 48, No 6, 424-428.

Palisano, R; et al. 2007. Gross Motor Function Classification System (GMFCS). 2007. [cited 2008-11-11] Available from: http://www.canchild.ca/Portals/0/outcomes/pdf/GMFCS-ER.pdf

Patritti, BL; et al. 2009. Enhancement and retention of locomotor function in children with cerebral palsy after robotic gait training. *Gait and Posture*, 2011, Vol 30 Supplement 2 (2009) S9-S10. doi:10.1016/j.gaitpost.2009.08.017

Pirpiris, M; et al. 2003. Walking speed in children and young adults with neuromuscular disease: comparison between two assessment methods. *Journal of Pediatric Orthopaedics*, 2003, Vol 23, No 3, 302-307.

Provost, B; et al. 2007. Endurance and Gait in Children With Cerebral Palsy After Intensive Body Weight –Supported Treadmill Training. *Pediatric Physical Therapy*, 2007,Vol 19, No 1, 2-10.

Rahman, T; Sample, W; Jayakumar, S; King, MM; Wee, JY; Seliktar, R; Alexander, M; Scavina, M; Clarc, A. Passive exoskeleton for assisting limb movement. *Journal of Rehabilitation Research and Development*, 2006, Vol. 43, No 5, 583-590.

Rosenbaum, PL; et al. Prognosis for Gross Motor Function in Cerebral Palsy. Creation of Motor Development Curves. *JAMA*, 2002, Vol 288, No 11, 1357- 1363.

Rosenbaum, P. A report: the definition and classification of cerebral palsy April 2006. *Developmental Medicine& Child Neurology Suppl.*, 2007,s109, Vol 49, 8-14.

Rosenbaum, PL; et al. Development of the Gross Motor Function Classification System for cerebral palsy. *Developmental Medicine & Child Neurology*, 2008, Vol 50, No 4, 249-253.

Russel, D; et al. The gross motor function measure: A means to evaluate the effects of physical therapy. *Developmental Medicine& Child Neurology*,1989, Vol 31, No 3, 341-352.

Russel, D; et al. 2000. Improved Scaling of the Gross Function Measure for Children With Cerebral Palsy: Evidence of Reliability and Validity. *Physical Therapy*, 2000, Vol 80, No 9, 872- 885.

Russel, D; et al. 2002. Gross motor function measure: (GMFM-66 and GMFM-88) user's manual. 1.st edition. London: Mac Keith Press. 2002. 237.

Sankar, C; Mundkur, N. Cerebral palsy-definition, classification, etiology and early diagnosis [online]. Indian J Pediatr 2005, 72:865-868. [cited 2006 Jun 21];. Available from: http://www.ijppediatricsindia.org/article.asp?issn=0019-5456;year=2005;volume=72; issue=10;spage=865;epage=868;aulast=Sankar

Shewell, M; et al. Etiologic yield of cerebral palsy a contemporary casa series. *Pediatric Neurology*, 2003, Vol 28, No 5, 352-359.

Schalow, G; Pääsuke, M; Ereune, J; Gapeyeva, H. Improvement in Parkinson's disease patients achieved by coordination dynamics therapy, *Electromyography and clinical neurophysiology*, Vol. 44, 2004, No. 2, 67-73.

Schalow, G. Phase and frequency coordination between neuron firing as an integrative mechanism of human CNS self-organization. *Electromyography and clinical neurophysiology*, Vol. 45, 2005, No 6, 369- 383.

Schalow, G; Pääsuke, M; Jaigma, P. Integrative reorganization mechanism for reducing tremor in Parkinson's disease patients. *Electromyography and clinical neurophysiology*, Vol. 45, 2005, No 7-8, 407- 415.

Schalow, G; Jaigma, P. Cerebral palsy improvement achieved by coordination dynamics therapy. *Electromyography and clinical neurophysiolog*, 2005, Vol. 45,No 7-8, 433-445.

Schalow, G. Functional development of the CNS in pupils between 7 and 19 years. *Electromyography and clinical neurophysiology*, Vol. 46, 2006,No 3, 159-169.

Schalow, G. Hypoxic brain injury improvement induced by coordination dynamics therapy in comparison to CNS development. *Electromyography and clinical neurophysiology*, Vol. 46, 2006, No 3, 171-183.

Schalow, G.; Jaigma, P. Improvement in severe traumatic brain injury induced by coordination dynamics therapy in comparison to physiologic CNS development. *Electromyography and clinical neurophysiology*, Vol. 46, 2006, No 4, 195-209.

Schalow, G. Surface EMG- and coordination dynamics measurements-assisted cerebellar diagnosis in a patient with cerebellar injury. *Electromyography and clinical neurophysiology*, Vol. 46, 2006, No 6, 371- 384.

Schalow, G. Symmetry diagnosis and treatment in coordination dynamics therapy. *Electromyography and clinical neurophysiology*, Vol. 46, No 7-8, 2006, 421-431.

Schalow, G. Cerebellar injury improvement achieved by coordination dynamics therapy. *Electromyography and clinical neurophysiology*, Vol. 46, No 7-8, 2006, 433-439.

Schalow, G; Vaher, I; Jaigma, P. Overreaching in coordination dynamics therapy in an athlete with a spinal cord injury. *Electromyography and clinical neurophysiology*, Vol. 48. 2008, No 2, 83-95.

Thompson, P; et al. 2008. Test–retest reliability ofthe 10-metre fast walktest and 6-minute walk test in ambulatory school-aged children with cerebral palsy. *Developmental Medicine & Child Neurology*, 2008, Vol 50, No 5, 370-376.

Ustinova, K; Chernikova, L; Bilimenko, A; Telenkov, A; Epstein, N. Effect of robotic locomotor training in an individual with Parkinson's disease: a case report. *Disability and rehabilitation. Assistive technology*, 2011, Vol 6, No 1, 77-85.

Vojta, V. Die zerebralen Bewegungsstörungen im Säuglingsalter, Ferdinand Enke Verlag, Stuttgart, 1988.

Vojta, V; Peters, A; Das Vojta – Prinzip: muskelspiele in reflexfortbewegung und motorischer ontogenese. 3rd edn. Berlin: Springer; 2007.

Vojta, V. Early diagnosis and therapy of cerebral motor disorders in childhood. A. Postural reflexes in developmental kinesiology. I. Normal developmental stages. *Z Orthop Ihre Grenzgeb*, 1972, Vol 110, No 4, 450–457.

Vojta, V. Early diagnosis and therapy of cerebral motor disorders in childhood. A. Postural reflexes in developmental kinesiology. 2. Pathologic reactions. *Z Orthop Ihre Grenzgeb* 1972, Vol 110, No 4, 458–466.

Westlake, K; et al. Pilot study of Lokomat versus manual- assisted treadmill training for locomotor recovery post – stroke. *Journal of NeuroEngineering and Rehabilitation.* 2009, Vol 6, No18, doi:10.1186/1743-0003-6-18

Wirtz, M; et al. Effectiveness of Automated Locomotor Training in Patients With Chronic Incomplete Spinal Cord Injury:A Multicenter Trial. *Archives of Physical Medicine and rehabilitation*, 2005, Vol 86, No 4, 672-680.

In: Handbook on Cerebral Palsy
Editor: Harold Yates

ISBN: 978-1-63321-852-9
© 2014 Nova Science Publishers, Inc.

Chapter 16

Improvement of Gross Motor Functions in Patients with Cerebral Palsy After Robotic Assisted Treadmill Training (RATT) Depending on Age

Stanislava Klobucká[1,*], Elena Žiaková[1,2] and Robert Klobucký[3]

[1]Rehabilitation Centre Harmony, Bratislava, Slovakia
[2]Slovak Medical University, Faculty of Nursing and Health Professional Studies, Bratislava, Slovakia
[3]Slovak Academy of Sciences, Institute for Sociology, Bratislava, Slovakia

Abstract

Introduction: Robotic-assisted body-weight-supported treadmill therapy (RATT) enabled by driven gait orthosis can improve motor functions in patients with movement disorders. The aim of the study was to assess the impact of patient´s age on improvement of motor functions in patients with cerebral palsy (CP).

Methods: 78 patients (44 males) with bilateral spastic CP, aged 4 – 25 years underwent 20 therapeutic units (T.U.) of RATT using driven gait orthosis with a frequency of 3 to 5 times a week. The patients participating in the study were divided into groups according to age and severity of motor impairment determined by the Gross Motor Function Classification System (GMFCS). Outcome measures were dimension A (lying,rolling), B (sitting), C (crawling, kneeling), D (standing) and E (walking, running, jumping) of the Gross Motor Function Measure (GMFM-88).

Results: After completing 20 therapeutic units patients demonstrated highly statistically significant improvement ($p < 0,001$) in all dimensions of the GMFM. Comparing the average improvement (%) in outcome parameters in all groups after 20 T.U., we didn't recorded the difference in any of the subgroups.

---

[*] Corresponding author: email: stanislavaklobucka@gmail.com.

Conclusion: Our study indicates, that RATT can improve the gross motor functions. Effect of the age on improvement in this study has not been demonstrated. RATT can be suitable for patients with cerebral palsy of all ages. Thus, RATT is a promising treatment option in ambulatory and nonambulatory patients with CP of all ages.

Introduction

The complex issue of children with cerebral palsy requires a multidisciplinary approach involving the cooperation of a neurologist, rehabilitation physician, physiotherapist, orthopedic surgeon, orthopedic prosthetics, psychologist, speech therapist, phoniatrist, ophthalmology and others, with ties to social assistance and special needs education. Very important is the early introduction of rehabilitation, while its essential element is treatment by way of physical exercise. The goal of treatment is not a cure or achieving normality. A realistic goal of treatment is to increase functionality, improve skills and maintain health in terms of locomotion, cognitive development, social integration and independence (1). Currently, increasing emphasis is being placed on a pro-active approach in therapy, including intensive, repetitive targeted training stimulating neuroplasticity. The past decade has seen a rise in the significant use of robotic therapy, particularly in patients after a stroke, cerebrospinal trauma, and last but not least in children with cerebral palsy.

Based on the principles of motor learning, which describes the correlation between the repetition of activities and improvement in motor function a robot-assisted locomotor therapy using computer controlled electronic braces was developed in the late 90s (University of Zurich, 1998)

Several authors have demonstrated the effectiveness of robot-assisted locomotor therapy to improve walking in adults after stroke and after brain and spinal cord injury (Hornby, 2005, Husemann, 2007, Mayr, 2007, Mayer-Heim, 2009, Westlake, 2009, Wirtz, 2005). Preliminary studies suggest a promising effect of RATT (robotic-assisted treadmill training) and patients with other neurological diseases, for example multiple sclerosis or Parkinson's disease (Beer, 2008, Ustinova, 2011).

From 2005 began to also be used in pediatric patients with impaired motor functions of various etiologies, most commonly in children with cerebral palsy. In non-randomized studies with RATT, children with central conditional gait disorders using Lokomat® showed improvement in motor function, speed and endurance walking and walking stereotype (Borggraege, 2008, 2010, Mayer- Heim, 2007). In the mentioned studies, during walking training, only dimension D (standing) and E (walking, running, jumping) are evaluated in the range of GMFM (Russel, 1989, 2002). However, after completing a series of RATT therapeutic units, we also observed in our patients, among other things, a stabilization of the torso muscles, which resulted in improvement in the sitting, crawling and rolling positions. Therefore, we decided to test each patient in all dimensions in the range of GMFM-88 (A, B, C, D, E). In studies conducted in our department, we demonstrated the influence of the severity of the disability and the number of therapeutic units to improve motor function in patients with CP (Klobucka, 2013 a, 2013 c).

In a randomized clinical study, we also documented the positive impact of the virtual reality environment for training to improve motor function in patients with bilateral spastic CP. (Klobucka, 2013 b).

Development of Children with CP

The development of gross motor skills in children is described by means of achieving motor milestones such as sitting, crawling, walking. In children with CP we observe the delayed achievement of milestones in gross motor functions and also record the presence of abnormal movements and postural patterns (Beckung, 2007). The prognosis of gross motor function in children with CP is variable. Palisano et al., on the basis of gross motor functions through the GMFM-88 test, fabricated motor development curves for individuals with CP and divided them according to the severity of disability characterized by one of the five stages of GMFCS. For all five grades of motor disability, the largest increase in gross motor functions is expected during the neonatal period and early childhood; the curves begin to even out / flatten at the age 3-4 years and reach a maximum at 7 years of age, with the exception of the GMFCS E&R level 2 group, indicating that in middle childhood age in children with cerebral palsy gross motor functions do not significantly change. Other studies have shown a slow increase in the gross motor function until the age of 9-10 years (Palisano, 2000, Beckung, 2007). Hanna et al. 2008 also showed that the development of gross motor function did not differ significantly in male and female subjects. Motor development curves together with the classification of the severity of disability contributed significantly to understanding the development of individuals with CP (Palisano, 2000). Parents and therapists typically presume that the percentage of gross motor function displayed by these curves are stable, but in fact they may individually differ significantly from the average, which is necessary to keep in mind when predicting individual development and individual capacities. (Hanna, 2009). Most children with CP in GMFCS E&R levels 1 and 2 reach 90% of gross motor skills. Half of the subjects in stage 1 reach 90% of GMFM by 4 years of age, 75% by the age of 5 years. 75% of children in stage 2 reached 90% of GMFM by the age of 7 years. Most individuals in stage 3 reached a maximum of 80% of GMFM at age 7. The maximum degree of gross motor functions obtained in stage 4 can be up to 70%, but the majority of subjects reach a maximum of 30%, in the age of 4-5 years, and that remains constant; median GMFM reached by group 5 is 20% and is achieved at 7 years of age (Beckung, 2007).

Although the non-progressive nature of the underlying pathology is the principal feature of CP, the non-progessiveness does not absolutely apply to clinical manifestations, which varies over the course of a lifetime. Studies of changes in gross motor function have demonstrated that a large number of individuals experience a period of maximum gross motor skills, which decrease further with age. This drop in capabilities can be combined with the natural tendency of increased energy requirements, spasticity, developments in contractures and changes in the curvature of the spine (Hanna, 2009). As a result of increasing pain, fatigue, development of degenerative changes and a lack of physical activities, a deterioration of walking ability in ambulatory individuals can be expected. The deterioration of these abilities occurs more frequently in individuals with diparesis than hemiparesis, on average by 40-50% (Beckung, 2007, Roebroeck, 2009). Despite the fact that the functional abilities decline with age, the skills that are actively and regularly used, are developed and are maintained even in later adulthood (Roebroeck, 2009).

The aim of the present study was to evaluate the effect of age on the level of improvement on the motor function test GMFM-88 after completing 20 t.u. of RATT.

So far the effect of age on improvement in motor function after graduating RATT in patients with CP has not been demonstrated. We hypothesized that the severity of disability and patient age influences the effect of therapeutic intervention in the Lokomat® system. On this basis, we also hypothesized that greater improvement after graduating RATT would be reached by patients with CP at a younger age.

Methods

The research was conducted in the period from March 2008 to March 2014 at the Harmony rehabilitation center, Kudlákova 2, Bratislava. 78 patients (44 boys and 34 girls) with bilateral spastic cerebral palsy aged 4.3 to 25.1 years (mean age 10.4 years, SD ± 5.33) underwent 20 outpatient therapeutic units of RATT using electronically controlled orthoses in the Lokomat® system (Table 1). Patients were divided into groups according to the severity of the affliction determined through the GMFCS scale (Gross Motor Function Classification Scale) (Palisano, 2007). Patients with GMFCS level I, II (n = 23, group A 1) were assessed as a mild disability. Patients with GMFCS level III, IV were evaluated as severe disability (n = 55, group A2) (Tab. 1).

Table 1. Clinical characteristics of the 78 participants

Mean (SD) age (years)(SD)	10,4 (±5,33)
Gender	
Female	34 (43.6%)
Male	44 (56.4%)
Age group (n)	
4-11 years	51 (65.4%)
12-27 years	27 (34.6%)
GMFCS level (n)	
I	4 (5.1%)
II	19 (24.4%)
III	37 (47.4%)
IV	18 (23.1%)
Walking aids (n)	
Walker	15 (19.2%)
Crutches	22 (28.2%)
Wheelchair	15 (19.2%)
None	26 (33.4%)

Both subgroups were further divided according to the age of 11 years (A1a, A2a) and 11 years (A1b, A2b).

The A1 group consisted of 23 patients. Of which 20 were classified by age into subgroups A1a (under 11 years) and 3 patients were more than 11 years (A1b).

The A2 group consisted of 55 patients. 29 of them were classified by age into subgroups A2a (under 11 years) and 26 patients were more than 11 years (A2b).

The study included patients with bilateral spastic CP. The most common form is diparetic at which the lower limbs are more significantly disabled. With all there is also a constant disability of the upper limbs, but usually only slightly. The quadruparetic form with bilateral hemiparesis manifests in a significant disability of the upper limbs or even all four limbs being equally disabled. The diagnosis was determined by a children's neurologist in accordance with International Classification of Diseases. The femur length was at least 21 cm, which correlates with the age of approximately 4 years. Patients had to be able to reliably indicate pain, distress or possible discomfort during treatment. A prerequisite was normal, or normal, corrected vision.

Disqualifying criteria: children with fixed contracture of the lower limbs, patients after administration of botulinum toxin (BTX) into the spastic muscles, or those who have had undergone surgery (orthopedic) intervention within 3 months prior to treatment in the Lokomat ®were not included in the study. Contraindications were also severe diseases of the cardiovascular system, acute or progressive neurological diseases, uncooperative, aggressive patients, severe cognitive deficits, inability of the patient to adapt to the orthosis, serious ligamentary muscle shortening in the lower limbs, unconsolidated fractures, severe osteoporosis, arthrodesis of the hip, knee, ankle, osteomyelitis, a marked asymmetry of the limbs, extreme disproportionate growth of the lower limbs or spine.

Patients or their legal representatives were informed about the timing and circumstances of robot-assisted locomotor therapy and the use of test results for research purposes. Each patient was requested written informed consent (from parents or legal guardians).

Description of the Device

The LOKOMAT ® is a medical - technical device that builds on manually assisted gait training using the travelator. It was created through the cooperation of scientists, doctors, physiotherapists and patients in the spinal center Balgrist University Hospital in Zurich. The project was also implemented by the Swiss company HOCOMA. It consists of several components: travelator (treadmill), a specialized patented suspension system and electronically controlled orthoses (Driven Gait Orthosis, DGO). The electromechanical pressure relief system monitors and adjusts relief in real time at the desired level. The moving parts are controlled by three computers and special software. Computer-controlled drivers on each hip and knee are synchronized with the speed of the treadmill. Force sensors for these joints are connected in such a way as to accurately measure the interaction between the patient and the LOKOMAT® system. Since the parameters of each workout (distance, speed, number of steps, the degree of lightening of the weight and the guidance force - the guiding force) are well defined and continuously monitored, gait training can be easily comparable interindividual as well as between individual therapeutic units. This fact offers new opportunities not only for research but also for a specific treatment plan and management of the patient (Figure 1).

An important element in therapy is a dynamic pelvic fixation using braces and pelvic reclining backrest, allowing to achieve a closer status to the physiological position of the ideal walking stereotype. Dorsal flexion of the ankle joint is achieved using passive clamping of the foot (foot lifter). On monitors directed towards the patient and therapist, we can visually observe and subsequently influence the course of the exercise in real-time. To increase participation during RATT training in pediatric rehabilitation a special virtual reality (VR) environment was developed.

Intervention

Before the robot-assisted locomotor therapy patients underwent conventional rehabilitation (Vojta reflex locomotion method, Bobath concept, physical therapy - magnetic therapy, phototherapy, phototherapy with a biolaser and some patients also underwent complementary methods of medical rehabilitation - synergistic reflex therapy, exercise balls, hydrotherapy, acupuncture, etc. hippotherapy etc.) in various combinations depending on the type and frequency of medical equipment.

Robot-assisted locomotor therapy in the Lokomat ® system during the period of the study was based on (mainly) therapeutic intervention on the participants in this study. Other physical therapy was not part of the program. As there is no generally applicable recommendation for the RATT application in patients with CP, the duration of therapy and frequency of various therapeutic units was determined based on experience and knowledge of foreign studies and also with regard to the capacity of individual patients and their parents. Patients underwent 20 therapeutic units within 4-6 weeks, with a frequency of 3-5 times a week. One therapeutic unit lasted 55 minutes. Setting and placing the patient in the device lasts about 15 minutes in each session, walking for 30 minutes. Detaching the patient from the device after the therapeutic intervention takes about 10 minutes, so that the total duration of one therapeutic unit is limited to 55 min. Walking speed ranged from 1.1 km / h (in more severe illness) to 1.7 km / h (in moderately affected patients).

For increasing incentives for pediatric patients, a program that allows training in a virtual environment has been developed. "Lokomat ® augmented feedback" with the implementation of VR within walking training was acquired by us in 2009. Since then RATT has proceeded exclusively in the VR environment.

Tests Used

All evaluations were performed within 24 hours prior to treatment and 24 hours after the last therapy unit. Before the therapy, patients typically underwent an outpatient examination. In the study we used the more detailed 88 position version of the GMFM (Gross Motor Function Measure) which assesses the children's motor skills in five dimensions: A - *lying and rolling*, 17 positions, B - *sitting*, 20 positions, C - *crawling and kneeling*, 14 positions, D - *standing*, 13 positions, E - *walking, running and jumping*, 24 positions (Russel, 1989, 2002).

Applied Statistical Methods

The data was processed using the programs MS Office Excel 2007 and SPSS 16.0 for Windows. Datasets in our case were tested for normality by the *Kolmogorov-Smirnov test* of normality. Since the normal distribution of data was not maintained in the files, a non-parametric *Wilcoxon* test for paired values was used to compare the input and output values of GMFM in each group. For the evaluation of the intergroup differences in percentage improvement in the GMFM test, we used the *Mann-Whitney test* of two independent sets. The results are considered statistically significant at p <0.05 and highly statistically significant if p is <0.001.

Results

Evaluation of the Improvement in Motor Function and the Functional Parameters of Gait

78 patients with bilateral spastic cerebral palsy completed 20 units of therapeutic robot-assisted locomotor therapy in the Lokomat ® system over a period of 4-6 weeks at a frequency of 3-5 times a week.

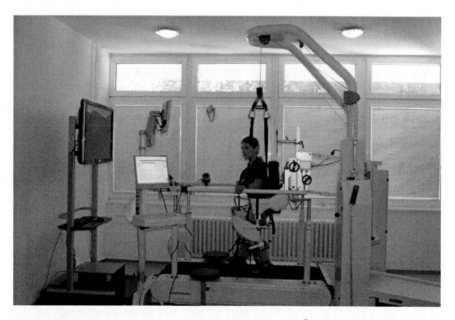

Figure 1. Robot-assisted locomotor training in the Lokomat device®.

Improvement Rate after 20 Therapy Units, Depended on the Age and the Severity of the Affliction

The groups of patients were divided according to the degree of disability. Lighter forms of CP were classified as GMFCS I, II (A1), more severe forms of GMFCS III, IV, V (A2). Both subgroups were further divided by age up to 11 years (A1a, A2a) and 11 years and older (A1b, A2b). We evaluated differences in improvements depending on the age and degree of disability.

Improvement Rate in the Group A1 after 20 Therapeutic Units Depending on the Age

Group A1 (GMFCS I, II) consisted of 23 patients. Of which 20 were classified by age into subgroups A1a (under 11 years) and 3 patients were older than 11 (A1b).

We compared the rate of improvement in subgroups A1a and A1b in the different dimensions of GMFM.

In dimension A of GMFM (lying, rolling), *the group A1 improved by an average of 6.91% (SD ± 9.45).* In the group A1a an on average improvement of 7.45% (± SD 10.00) occurred, while in group A1b it was 3.27% (SD ± 2.99). Comparing the improvement through the Mann-Whitney test, we did not find a statistically significant difference, Z = -0.184, p = 0.854. In dimension B (sitting), *group A1 improved by an average of 6.74% (SD ± 5.74).* In group A1 there was an average improvement of 7.25% (SD ± 5.93), in group A1b 3.33% (SD ± 2.88). Comparing the improvement through the Mann-Whitney test, we did not find a statistically significant difference, Z = -1.382, p = 0.167.

In dimension C (crawling, kneeling), *group A1 improved by an average of 8.69% (SD ± 13.40).* In group A1 there was an average improvement of 9.41% (± SD 14.23), in group A1b of 3.97% (SD ± 3.63). Comparing the improvement through the Mann-Whitney test, we did not find a statistically significant difference, Z = -0.185, p = 0.853.

In dimension D (standing), *group A1 improved by an average of 9.92% (SD ± 7.30).* Group A1 improved on average by 10.25% (SD ± 7.48), in group A1b by 7.69 (SD ± 6.78). Comparing the improvement through the Mann-Whitney test, we did not find a statistically significant difference, Z = -0.569, p = 0.551.

In dimension D (walking), *group A1 improved by an average of 9.78% (SD ± 5.15).* Group A1 improved on average by 9.58% (SD ± 4.98), in group A1b by 11.11% (SD ± 7.35). Comparing the improvement through the Mann-Whitney test, we did not find a statistically significant difference, Z = -0.229, p = 0.819.

In the overall evaluation *(total GMFM)* in group A1 there was an average improvement (SD) of 8.41% (SD ± 6.18). In group A1a and we recorded an average overall improvement of 8.79% (SD ± 6.43) in group A1b 5.88% (SD ± 4.00).

Comparing the improvement through the Mann-Whitney test, we did not find a statistically significant difference, Z = -0.548, p = 0.584 (Table 2, 3)

Table 2. Improvement in motor function assessed by GMFM-88 in the individual dimensions group A1 (GMFCS I, II, moderate disability) after completing 20 therapeutic units of RATT

	N	Mean improvement %	SD	Median	Min.	Max.	Z	p
GMFM A	23	6.91	± 9.45	3.92	0.00	33.33	-3.732	0.000
GMFM B	23	6.74	±5.74	5.00	0.00	21.66	-4.116	0.000
GMFM C	23	8.69	±13.40	4.77	0.00	54.76	-3.520	0.000
GMFM D	23	9.92	±7.30	7.69	0.00	28.20	-4.021	0.000
GMFM E	23	9.78	±5.15	9.72	0.00	19.44	-4.111	0.000
GMFM total	23	8.41	±6.18	7.11	2.14	25.24	-4.197	0.000

Table 3. Comparison of improvement in motor function in test GMFM-88 in the individual subgroups (A1a, A1b) after completing 20 therapeutic units of RATT depending on age and severity of disability

Group	GMFM A		GMFM B		GMFM C		GMFM D		GMFM E		GMFM TOTAL	
	A1a	A1b	A1a	A1b	A1a	A1b	A1a	A1b	A1a	A1b	A1a	A1b
Number	20	3	20	3	20	3	20	3	20	3	20	3
Mean improvement % (±SD)	7.45 (±10.00)	3.27 (±2.99)	7.25 (±5.93)	3.33 (±2.88)	9.41 (±14.23)	3.97 (±3.63)	10.25 (±7.48)	7.69 (±6.78)	9.58 (±4.98)	7.69 (±6.78)	8.79 (±6.43)	5.88 (±4.00)
Z	-0.184		-1.382		-0.185		-0.569		-0.229		-0.548	
P	p = 0.854		p = 0.167		p = 0.853		p = 0.551		p = 0.819		p = 0.584	

Legend:

A1 – mildly impaired patients of group A (GMFCS I, II)

A1a: mildly impaired patients of group A (GMFCS I, II) under 11 years

A1b: mildly impaired patients of group A (GMFCS I, II) over 11 years

Table 4. Improvement in motor function assessed by GMFM-88 in the individual dimensions group A1 (GMFCS I, II, moderate disability) after completing 20 therapeutic units of RATT

	N	Mean improvement %	SD	Median	Min.	Max.	Z	p
GMFM A	55	11.16	±8.65	9.81	0.00	29.49	-5.610	0.000
GMFM B	55	10.87	±7.84	8.33	0.00	30.00	-6.337	0.000
GMFM C	55	8.45	±7.80	7.15	0.00	30.96	-5.851	0.000
GMFM D	55	6.62	±8.67	5.10	0.00	33.34	-5.173	0.000
GMFM E	55	6.17	±6.75	4.17	0.00	30.56	-5.581	0.000
GMFM total	55	8.82	±5.21	7.39	1.45	21.55	-6.451	0.000

Improvement Rate in Group A2 after 20 Therapeutic Units Depending on Age

Group A2 (GMFCS III, IV) consisted of 55 patients. Of which 29 we classified by age into subgroups A2a (under 11 years) and 26 patients were older than 11 (A2b).

We compared the rate of improvement in subgroups A2a and A2b in the different dimensions of GMFM.

In dimension A of GMFM (lying, rolling), *group A2 improved by an average of 11.16% (SD ± 8.65).* Group A2a improved on average by 10.88% (SD ± 8.65), in group A2b by 11.46% (SD ± 8.82). Comparing the improvement through the Mann-Whitney test, we did not find a statistically significant difference, $Z = -0.127$, $p = 0.899$.

Table 5. Comparison of improvement in motor function in test GMFM-88 in the individual subgroups (A1a, A1b) after completing 20 therapeutic units of RATT depending on age and severity of disability

	GMFM A		GMFM B		GMFM C		GMFM D		GMFM E		GMFM TOTAL	
Group	A2a	A2b	A2a	A2b	A2a	A2b	A2a	A2b	A2a	A2b	A2a	A2b
Number	29	26	29	26	29	26	29	26	29	26	29	26
Mean improvement % (±SD)	10.88 (±8.65)	11.46 (±8.82)	11.76 (±7.99)	9.87 (±7.70)	8.40 (±6.31)	8.51 (±9.31)	5.31 (±7.84)	8.09 (±9.45)	4.47 (±4.65)	8.01 (±8.15)	8.42 (±4.78)	9.27 (±5.70)
Z	-0.127		-1.089		-0.611		-0.892		-1.477		-0.421	
P	p = 0.899		p = 0.276		p = 0.541		p = 0.372		p = 0.140		p = 0.673	

Legend:

A2 – moderate to severely impaired patients of group A (GMFCS I, II).

A2a: moderate to severely impaired patients of group A (GMFCS I, II) under 11 years.

A2b: moderate to severely impaired patients of group A (GMFCS I, II) over 11 years.

In dimension B (sitting), *group A2 improved by an average of 10.87% (SD ± 7.84).* Group A2 improved on average by 11.76% (SD ± 7.99), in group A2b by 9.87% (SD ± 7.70). Comparing the improvement through the Mann-Whitney test, we did not find a statistically significant difference, Z = -1.089, p = 0.276.

In dimension C (crawling, kneeling), *group A2 improved by an average of 8.45% (SD ± 7.80).* Group A2a improved on average by 8.40% (SD ± 6.31), in group A2b by 8.51% (SD ± 9.31). Comparing the improvement through the Mann-Whitney test, we did not find a statistically significant difference, Z = -0.611, p = 0.541.

In dimension D (standing), *group A2 improved by an average of 6.62% (SD ± 8.67).* Group A2a improved on average by 5.31% (SD ± 7.84), in group A2b by 8.09% (SD ± 9.45). Comparing the improvement through the Mann-Whitney test, we did not find a statistically significant difference, Z = -0.892, p = 0.372.

In dimension E (walking), *group A2 improved by an average of 6.17% (SD ± 6.75).* Group A2 improved on average by 4.47% (SD ± 4.65), in group A2b by 8.01% (SD ± 8.15). Comparing the improvement through the Mann-Whitney test, we did not find a statistically significant difference, Z = -1.477, p = 0.140. In the overall evaluation *(total GMFM)* in group A2 there was an average improvement (SD) of 8.82% (SD ± 5.21). In group A2a we recorded an average overall improvement of 8.42% (SD ± 4.78) in group A2b 9.27% (SD ± 5.70). Comparing the improvement through the Mann-Whitney test, we did not find a statistically significant difference, Z = -0.421, p = 0.673 (Table. 4, 5).

The data show that there was no statistically significant difference in the rate of improvement in motor function tested by GMFM depending on age in any of the subgroups.

Discussion

CP is a neurodevelopmental disorder and its manifestations usually change during the course of development. Treatment of CP therefore requires an adaptive approach, which places particular emphasis on reversible non-ablative therapies. The goal of the treatment of CP is not a cure or achieving normality. A realistic goal of treatment is to increase functionality, improve skills and maintain health in terms of locomotion, cognitive development, social integration and independence. The success of therapy depends on its timeliness and intensity. To stimulate locomotion in patients, especially after SCI and stroke, as well as CP, treadmill training with body weight relief in tow has been used for over 30 years. Most studies are devoted to training with body weight relief with manual assistance. It should be noted that studies dealing with the training of walking in children with CP consist mainly of case reports and open-label non-randomized studies, mostly without a control group. Groups are heterogeneous, with a small number of patients and the majority of children in the studies continued in their usual physiotherapy. BWST parameters (body-weight-supported treadmill therapy) are different in various studies, they differ in training walking velocity, degree of weight relief, as well as the frequency and duration of training.

Only few works evaluate all dimensions of the GMFM test, which does not allow for the assessment and comparison of the effects of RATT (robotic-assisted treadmill therapy) or BWST for the stabilization of torso muscles. In the last 10 years, the number of studies dealing with robotic training is growing. Robot-assisted gait training became applicable from

2005 in children with CP. It is known that cortical reorganization made possible by targeted training depends on the intensity and frequency of training (Meyer-Heim, 2009). Due to the possibility of the increased intensity and frequency of training with the maintenance of the physiological gait pattern, robot-assisted locomotor training offers almost ideal conditions for specific walking training.

The aim of this prospective clinical study was to assess the effect of age on motor function of patients with cerebral palsy after robot-assisted locomotor training in the Lokomat® system.

The Improvement Rate in Group A after 20 Therapeutic Units Based on the Age and the Severity of the Disability

Data obtained from our study indicates that there was no statistically significant difference in the rate of improvement in motor function according to the GMFM test depending on the age in any of the subgroups.

Patients in group A were divided into 2 groups according to age: 4-11 years old, over 11 years. We chose this criterion with respect to the biomechanical effect of growth acceleration in puberty and taking into account the expected maximum motor skills in children with CP.

Hanna and company (2008) and Rosenbaum (2002) processed, on the basis of a longitudinal tracking of individuals with CP in different age groups and with varying degrees of disability, motor development curves on the basis of the gross motor function test GMFM-66. According to these curves an improvement in the gross motor function occurs in individuals with CP until age10 in stage 1 of GMFCS and approximately to the age of 4 years in stage 5 of GMFCS. Gross motor functions are then constant and we usually observe observed a deterioration of motor abilities of individuals at different ages, which may occur from 10 years of age with the greatest risk in adolescence.

In children, development is not completed and an increase in the plasticity of the central nervous system is expected. During development, the brain is capable of extensive anatomical and functional changes. In children, we expect a greater impact of locomotor therapy option with the possibility of the formative influence of muscle strength on bone structure and thereby on centration joints, axial load during verticalization which will ultimately approximate the physiological positions of key joints.

Whereas in adult patients with CP growth is terminated, and hence the morphological development of the skeleton, the centration of key joints is constant and their axial adjustment under load under verticalisation is in essence unchanging. We assume greater improvement in children under 11 years. However, a statistically significant improvement was also observed in adolescents and adults, which extends the applicability of RATT in patients with CP.

In our study, there were 5 patients over age 18 years. In four of them the dimensions A, B, C, D, E, were evaluated in the GMFM test. Since they were not able to walk with crutches without the physical assistance of another person, we did not assess walking speed or endurance during walking. In one of the adults, in addition to the aforementioned parameters, walking speed and endurance while walking were also evaluated. In all five a clinically significant improvement in motor function was experienced. Improvement was associated with an improvement in movement pattern, the stereotype of movement in the joints of the lower limbs and an increase in muscle strength. In one patient, we documented an increase in walking speed after undergoing 20 T.U. (from 0.52 m / s to 0.66 m / s) and endurance during the 6-minute walk test (from 122m to 140m), which is consistent with the only previously published report on adult patients with CP who have undergone therapy in the Lokomat® system (Patritti, 2010). The patient presented in this case report was a 52 year old woman with right hemiplegic CP. The aim of this study was to evaluate whether gait training with weight relief using electronically controlled orthosis (Lokomat®) can improve locomotor function and improve the biomechanics of walking in adults with CP. The training program consisted of a 6 week RATT intervention with a frequency of 3 x a week, while one therapeutic unit lasted 30 min. During therapy she completed 18 T. J. Before therapy, after therapy and after 3 months a muscle test of the lower limbs, spasticity modified by the Ashworth scale and balance tests (Berg Balance test) were evaluated, while the functional gait parameters were evaluated by a dynamic test walk - Dynamic Gait Index, walking speed with the help of the 10 min WT and stamina the 6 min WT. The three dimensional gait analysis using a Vicon 512 was also assessed. The results showed improvement in the balance, locomotor function and biomechanics of walking of the subject. (Patritti, 2010)

In adults with CP, a functional deterioration and loss of physical activity frequently occurs, leading to a reduction in locomotor function (Andersson, 2001). Intensive training can help prevent the deconditioning process of growing older (Damiano, 2006). Robot-assisted gait training offers a means of partially fulfilling this need. It can be assumed that the activity-induced neuronal plasticity also plays a role in the functional restoration in adult patients with CP. The hypothesis is consistent with previous findings that SCI patients may be targeted with intensive training which can lead to supraspinal plasticity in the motor center related to locomotion and that an improvement of walking in the field is associated with increased activity of the cerebellum (Winchester, 2005).

Other Aspects of RATT

Several studies have also addressed the continuing achievements of robot-assisted gait training. Recent studies and published works have shown that the achieved effect of therapy persists for at least 4 months (Borggraefe, 2010, Meyer – Heim, 2007, Patritti, 2011, Montinaro, 2011). Improvement in the resulting measurements shown in our presented studies was consistent with references of patients, parents and caregivers, who generally registered more stamina, endurance, improved ability to climb stairs and an overall improvement in the mobility of children and adolescents after treatment in the Lokomat ® system in carrying out daily activities in different positions (sitting, standing, lying). They also recorded improved transfers whether with the help of crutches, walkers, with the assistance of another person, or by other means. The participants reported no adverse side effects.

Conclusion

Treatment of patients with CP should be comprehensive and requires an interdisciplinary approach. A prerequisite for effective treatment is high-quality diagnostics. An early start to rehabilitation plays a decisive role in therapy. Gait training in the Lokomat® system is safe, easily feasible and well tolerated in the studied group of patients with CP without adverse effects. In the monitored group of patients in this study there was a statistically significant improvement in motor function in the test evaluation GMFM (dimensions A, B, C, D, E, total). Both patients with severe disabilities and patients with mild disabilities improved. Data obtained from our study indicates that there was no statistically significant difference in the rate of improvement in motor function according to the GMFM test depending on the age in any of the subgroups.

Improvement concerned all ages-we observed improvement in children, adolescents and young adult patients with CP. Robot-assisted gait training using electronically controlled orthoses is a promising tool for the rehabilitation of children, adolescents and adults with central gait disorders. RATT enables almost perfect training conditions. It enables the increasing of the frequency of targeted locomotor training, training intensity within a therapeutic unit, modify walking speed and monitor the progress of treatment. It offers the possibility of more intense, prolonged gait training, which allows patients to regain or improve walking ability. This is a fundamental advantage over conventional manually-assisted gait training, which may well have the same effect, but it requires much more effort and more therapists. It would be interesting to determine the potential impact of RATT in combination with other therapeutic options such as. BTX-A. The implementation of control strategies and an adapted biofeedback system for children is an important factor in obtaining maximum participation especially for pediatric patients. Integrated technologies allowing walking in virtual reality makes this significantly easier in the Lokomat®. The stabilization of torso muscles of the previous improvements in the standing and walking parameters demonstrates the validity of the neuro-developmental concept, based on the ontogeny of the child. Improving the parameters in the evaluation of the stereotype of walking in patients with CP suggests that the paradigm of specifically targeted locomotor training can be applied in children with CP, who have not yet had the opportunity to walk with physiological stereotypes in their motor development. Proper medical management of CP is the only prophylaxis against complications resulting from structural defects (pain, secondary musculoskeletal problems, possible malfunctions of internal organs, orthopedic, prosthetic, surgical intervention with the necessary hospitalization, or consequential spa treatment), which ultimately allows to significantly reduce costs for subsequent care.

Acknowledgment

We are grateful to Mr. Ing. Alojz Halas - direcor of Rehabilitation Centre Harmony, for support and willingness to help in making this work.

References

Andersson, CH; Mattson, E. Adults with cerebral palsy: a survey describing probleme, needs, and resources, with special emphasis on locomotion. *Developmental Medicine & Child Neurology*, 2007, Vol 43, No 1, 76- 82.

Beckung, E. et al. The natural history of gross motor development in children with cerebral palsy aged 1 to 15 years. *Developmental Medicine & Child Neurology*, 2007, Vol 49, No 10, 751–756.

Beer, S; Aschbacher, B; Manoglou, D; Gamper, E; Kool, J; Kesselring, J. Robot-assisted gait training in multiple sclerosis: a pilot randomized trial. *Multiple Sclerosis*, 2008, Vol 14, No 2, 231-236.

Borggraefe, I; Schaefer, JS; Klaiber, M; Dabrowski, E; Ammann-Reiffer, C; Knecht, B; et al. Robotic-assisted treadmill therapy improves walking and standing performance in children and adolescents with cerebral palsy. *European Journal of Pediatric Neurology*, 2010, Vol 14, No 6, 496-502.

Borggraefe, I; Meyer-Heim, A; Kumar, A; Schaefer, JS; Berweck, S; Heinen, F. Improved Gait Parameters After Robotic-Assisted Locomotor Treadmill Therapy in a 6-Year-Old Child with Cerebral Palsy. *Movement Disorders*, 2008, Vol 23, No 2, 280-283.

Borggraefe, I; Kiwull, L; Schaefer, JS; Koerte, I; Blaschek, A; Meyer-Heim, A. et al. Sustainability of motor performance after robotic-assisted treadmill therapy in children: an open, non randomized baseline- treatment study. *European Journal of Physical and Rehabilitation Medicine*, 2010 b, Vol 46, No2, 125-131.

Damiano, DL. Activity, activity, activity: rethinking our physical therapy approach to cerebral palsy. *Physical Therapy*, 2006, Vol 86, No 11, 1534-1540.

Hanna, S; et al. Stability and decline in gross motor function among children and youth with cerebral palsy aged 2-21 years. *Developmental Medicine & Child Neurology*, 2009, Vol 51, No 4, 295–302.

Hanna, SE; Bartlett, DJ; Rivard, L.M; Russell, DJ. 2008. Reference curves for the gross motor function measure: percentiles for clinical description and tracking over time among children with cerebral palsy. *Physical Therapy*, 2008, Vol 88, No 5, 596-607.

Hornby, TG; Zemon, DH; Campbell, D. Robotic assisted, Body-Weight-Supported Treadmill Training in Individuals Following Motor Incomplete Spinal Cord Injury. *Physical Therapy* 2005, Vol 85, No 1, 52-66.

Husemann, B; Müller, F; Krewer, C; Heller, S; Koenig E. Effects of Locomotion Training With Assistance of Robot-Driven Gait Orthosis in Hemiparetic Patients After Stroke. *Stroke*, 2007, Vol 38, No 2, 349-354.

Klobucka, S; Kovac, M; Ziakova, E. 2013 a, Proceedings of the 9 th international congress of CP (May 15-18, 2013,Bled, Slovenia)

Improvement of Gross Motor Functions Depending on the Number of Therapeutic Units of Robotic Assisted Treadmill Training in Patients with Cerebral Palsy 19-24. ISBN 978-88-7587-685-2, printed oct. 2013 http://www.medimond.com/ebook/Q515.pdf

Klobucka, S; Ziakova, E; Klobucky, R. 2013 b The effect of Virtual Reality Environment during Robotic-Assisted Locomotor Training on Gross Motor Functions in Patients with Cerebral Palsy. *Ceska a Slovenska Neurologie a Neurochirurgie*, 2013 b, Vol 76/109, No 6, 702-711.

Klobucka, S; Kovac, M; Ziakova, E; Klobucky, R. 2013 c Effect of Robot-Assisted Treadmill Training on Motor Function Depending on Severity of Impairment in Patients with Bilateral Spastic Cerebral Palsy. *Journal of Rehabilitation Robotics*, 2013 c, 1, 71-81, E-ISSN: 2308-8354/13 © 2013 Synergy Publishers.

Mayr, A; Kofler, M; Quirbach, E; Matzak, H; Fröhlich, K; Saltuari, L. Prospective, Blinded, Randomized Crossover Study of Gait Rehabilitation in Stroke Patients Using the

Lokomat Gait Orthosis. *Neurorehabilitation and Neural repair*, 2007, Vol 21, No 4, 307-314.

Meyer- Heim, A; Ammann-Reiffer, C; Schmartz, A; Schäfer, J; Sennhauser, FH; Heinen, F. et al. Improvement of walking abilities after robotic- assisted locomotion training in children with cerebral palsy. *Archives of Disease in Childhood*, 2009, Vol 94, No 8, 615-620.

Meyer- Heim, A; et al. Feasibility of robotic assisted locomotor trainig in children with central gait impairment. *Developmental Medicine& Child Neurology*, 2007, Vol 49, No 12, 900-906.

Montinaro, A; et al. Robotic- assisted locomotion training in children affected by Cerebral Palsy. *Gait and Posture*, 2011, Vol 33 Supplement 1 (2011) S55-S56. doi:10.1016/j.gaitpost.2010.10.068

Palisano, R; et al. 2007. Gross Motor Function Classification System (GMFCS). 2007. (cited 2008-11-11) Available from: http://www.canchild.ca/Portals/0/outcomes/pdf/GMFCS-ER.pdf

Palisano, R; et al. Validation of a Model of Gross Motor Function for Children With Cerebral Palsy. *Physical Therapy*, 2000, Vol 80, No 10, 974-985.

Palisano, R; Rosenbaum, P; Walter, S; Russell, D; Wood, E; Galuppi, B. Development and reliability of a system to classify gross motor function in children with cerebral palsy. *Developmental Medicine & Child Neurology*,1997, Vol 39, No 4, 214–223.

Patritti, BL; el al. 2010. Robotic Gait Training in an Adult With Cerebral Palsy: A Case Report. *Physical Medicine and Rehabilitation*, 2010. Vol 2, No 1, 71-75.

Patritti, BL; el al. 2009. Enhancement and retention of locomotor function in children with cerebral palsy after robotic gait training. *Gait and Posture*, 2011, Vol 30 Supplement 2 (2009) S9-S10. doi:10.1016/j.gaitpost.2009.08.017

Roebroeck, ME; et al. Adult outcomes and lifespan issues for people with childhood-onset physical disability. *Developmental Medicine & Child Neurology 2009*, Vol 51, No 8, 670–678.

Rosenbaum, PL; et al. Prognosis for Gross Motor Function in Cerebral Palsy. Creation of Motor Development Curves. *JAMA*, 2002, Vol 288, No 11, 1357- 1363.

Rosenbaum, P. A report: the definition and classification of cerebral palsy April 2006. *Developmental Medicine& Child Neurology Suppl.1*, 2007,s109, Vol 49, 8-14.

Rosenbaum, PL; et al. Development of the Gross Motor Function Classification System for cerebral palsy. *Developmental Medicine& Child Neurology*, 2008, Vol 50, No 4, 249-253.

Russel, DJ; Rosenbaum, PL; Cadman, DT; Gowland, C; Hardy, S; Jarvis, S. The gross motor function measure: A means to evaluate the effects of physical therapy. *Developmental Medicine& Child Neurology*,1989, Vol 31, No 3, 341-352

Russel, DJ; Rosenbaum, PL; Avery, LM; Lane M. Gross motor function measure: (GMFM-66 and GMFM-88) User's manual. 1.st edition. London: Mac Keith Press. 2002. 237

Ustinova, K; Chernikova, L; Bilimenko, A; Telenkov, A; Epstein, N. Effect of robotic locomotor training in an individual with Parkinson's disease: a case report. *Disability and rehabilitation. Assistive technology*, 2011, Vol 6, No 1, 77-85.

Westlake, K; Patten, C. Pilot study of Lokomat versus manual- assisted treadmill training for locomotor recovery post – stroke. *Journal of NeuroEngineering and Rehabilitation.* 2009, Vol 6, No 18, doi:10.1186/1743-0003-6-18

Winchester, P; et al. Changes in Supraspinal Activation Patterns following Robotic Locomotor Therapy in Motor – Incomplete Spinal Cord Injury. *Neurorehabilitation and Neural Repair*, 2005, Vol. 19, No 4. 313-324.

Wirtz, M; Zemon, DH; Rupp, R; Scheel, A; Colombo, G; Dietz, V; et al. Effectiveness of Automated Locomotor Training in Patients With Chronic Incomplete Spinal Cord Injury: A Multicenter Trial. *Archives of Physical Medicine and rehabilitation*, 2005, Vol 86, No 4, 672-680.

www.hocoma.com

In: Handbook on Cerebral Palsy
Editor: Harold Yates

ISBN: 978-1-63321-852-9
© 2014 Nova Science Publishers, Inc.

Chapter 17

Effect of Social Support on Parenting Stress of Mothers of Children with Cerebral Palsy

Yeon-Gyu Jeong,[1], Jeong-A Bang,[1]
Yeon-Jae Jeong,[2], and Hyun-Sook Kim, Ph.D.[3]

[1]Rehabilitation Medicine, Dongguk University Ilsan Medical Center,
Goyang-si, Republic of Korea
[2]Department of Rehabilitation Medicine, Hanyang University Medical Center,
Hanyang University College of Medicine, Seongdong-gu, Seoul, Republic of Korea
[3]Department of Physical Therapy, Yeoju Institute of Technology,
Yeofu-si, Gyeonggi-do, Republic of Korea

Abstract

Background: This study investigated the effect of perceived social support on the parenting stress of mothers who have children with cerebral palsy (CP).

Method: This study was conducted using surveys, literature review, and interviews. Survey data were collected from 181 mothers of children (under 18 years of age) with CP.

Results: Level of disability, mother's health status and social support were significant predictors of the parenting stress of mothers.

Conclusion: We have to comprehend and share the psychological and physical affliction of mothers having much difficulty nurturing children with CP. Also, the government should take social responsibility for the upbringing of their children, developing back-up programs for mothers and making them comprehensively available to support the psychological and physical health of mothers of children with CP.

Keywords: Cerebral palsy, parenting stress, social support

Introduction

Cerebral palsy (CP) refers to a group of disorders in the development of movement and posture, which causes limitations of activity that are attributed to non-progressive disturbances occurring in the developing fetal or infant brain [1]. Early diagnosis and intervention is especially critical with CP, since the brain damage resulting from CP itself may be non-progressive, but it can lead to various subsequent conditions. According to the 2008 statistics compiled by the Division of Policy for Persons with Disabilities of the Ministry of Health and Welfare [2], among the age-specific brain injuries of Koreans, CP has the highest incidence between the ages 0 – 9, at 57.8%. As noted, CP is the largest category of infant brain injuries.

If the parents of children with a disability fail to cope with stress induced by the unusual challenges experienced by the family and don't develop the skills necessary for parenting, it may result in a serious family crisis. Among the family members, mothers who are primarily responsible, show the highest rate of parenting stress, which results in depression and family troubles [3].

This is due to the mother generally assuming more responsibility for the child [4], and undertaking most of the additional care necessary for a child with disability [5].

The parenting stress of mothers of children with CP can be interpreted as a composite and negative response to the physical, social, economical and psychological experience of families nurturing children with CP [6].

Moreover, stress experienced by the mothers of children with CP may be identified as physiological response stress, the level of physiological stress associated with physical fatigue, neuralgia, and convulsion, and emotional response stress, the level of response to the discomfort associated with nervousness, anxiety, distress, grief and interaction with others [7].

Therefore, adequate assistance and opportunities must be provided to help mothers cope with such stress and to accomplish excellent role performance.

Currently in Korea, the provision and standards of various supports aiding the parenting of children with CP are inconsistent, and the standards of service support or the policies pertaining to problematic situations are extremely insufficient [8].

Furthermore, there is a deficit of social welfare service policies, as well as pertinent research. In other words, until now, there has been little research into the stress of mothers parenting children with CP [9, 10, 11, 12], yet there has been little research into the correlation between social support and the parenting stress of mothers, and the proposed solutions are insubstantial.

Accordingly, this present study examined the extent and necessity of practical assistance for the reduction of the parenting stress of mothers in order to propose a basis for the establishment of effective welfare planning.

Subjects and Methods

This study surveyed 181 mothers of children under the age of 12, diagnosed with CP, who were undergoing rehabilitation therapy at university or rehabilitation hospitals located in Seoul and Gyeonggi-Do province. The scope of social support was restricted to close friends,

friends, family and medical facilities, which mothers of children with CP embraced as social support mediums. All research subjects agreed to participation in the study, and data were collected via survey. The response rate of the mothers of children with CP was 100%. The present study was supported by Dongguk University and approved by Dongguk University Institutional Review Boards, and written consent was provided by all the subjects.

The "Stress Level of Mothers with Children with CP Measurement Tool" (SMCP) was developed by Lee, Ji-won [13], who conducted an in-depth interview of 20 mothers of children with CP to evaluate their stress levels. In this study it was used as the measurement tool for measuring the stress levels of the mothers of children with CP. It has 44 questions, each of which are answered on a 5 point scale on which "strongly agree" is scored as 5 points and "strongly disagree" is scored as 1 point, with a higher score signifying greater parenting stress.

The test-retest of the SMCP shows a correlation of Pearson $r=0.97$, and a reliability of Cronbach $\alpha=0.94$.

A measuring tool for social support was developed for informal and formal support. First, in order to measure informal support, the CPSS (Carolina Parents Support Scale), developed by Bristol [14], was modified and supplemented via consultation with an associated specialist in order to correspond to Korean reality, resulting in a tool consisting of 8 questions. Each question was scored on a scale of 4 points, with "very supportive" yielding 4 points and "very unsupportive" yielding 1 point, a higher score implying greater acquisition of informal support. The reliability of the modified survey was Cronbach $\alpha=0.767$. Then, in order to measure the formal support, CPSS was modified and supplemented again to correspond to Korean reality, resulting in a survey consisting of 9 questions. Each question was scored on a scale of 4 points, with "very supportive" yielding 4 points and "very unsupportive" yielding 1 point, a higher score implying greater acquisition of formal support. The reliability of the modified survey was Cronbach $\alpha=0.838$.

Data regarding additional variables influencing parenting stress for mothers, such as the sex of children (1=Male, 2=Female), age (1=Less than 24 month, 2=Between 24 ~ 72 months, 3=More than 72 months), term of disability (1= Less than 1 year, 2= Between 1~3 years, 3=Between 3 ~ 5 years, 4= More than 5 years), severity of disability (1= Mild, 2= Average severity, 3= Very severe), age of mothers (1= Less than 30 years of age, 2= More than 30 years of age), level of education (1=High school graduate or lower, 2=University graduate or higher), family income (1= Less than 1,000,000 KRW, 2=Between 1,000,000 ~ 3,000,000 KRW, 3=Between 3,000,000 ~ 5,000,000 KRW, 4=More than 5,000,000 KRW) were collected.

Furthermore, a tool (1 question) developed by Ware, Davis, and Donald [15], scored on a scale of 4 points, with "very healthy" yielding 4 points and "very unhealthy" yielding 1 point, a higher score implying better health conditions, was utilized to examine the health conditions for mothers of children with CP.

The characteristics of the subjects are presented as frequencies and percentages. Analysis of variance (ANOVA) was conducted in order to examine the relevance between the parenting stress of mothers and the characteristics of the children. Hierarchial multiple regression analysis was employed to uncover variations ($p<0.05$) significant in the univariate analysis with respect to factors influencing the parenting stress of mothers while solution enter was utilized to identify predictable factors. The characteristics of children were entered in the first step and the characteristics of the mothers in the next. In the final step the total scores of social support were entered into the prediction model independently as formal and informal supports. Statistical analysis was performed utilizing SPSS ver. 17.0.

Result

As shown in Table 1, the correlation between factors associated with the parenting stress of mothers and the parenting stress itself, resulted in positive correlations with severity of disability, while the correlations pertaining to education levels and health conditions of mothers and family income were negative.

The results of hierarchial multiple regression analyses are presented in Tables 2 and 3. As a result of analyzing factors influencing the parenting stress of mothers of children with CP, as well as modifying the efficacy of other variables in the final step, the overall model, the severity of disability of children, health condition of mothers and social support were identified as significant predictors of parenting stress. Among others, independent examination of social support, as formal and informal support, subsequently identified informal support as a significant predictor of parenting stress.

Table 1. Correlation of Parenting Stress of Mothers

	Parenting Stress	Term of Disability	Severity of Disorder	Education Level of Mother	Family Income	Health of Mother	Social Support
Parenting Stress	1	0.090	0.302^{**}	-0.168^{*}	-0.281^{**}	-0.227^{**}	-0.260^{**}

* $p<0.05$, ** $p<0.01$.

Discussion

The present research surveyed 181 mothers of children diagnosed with CP who are currently undergoing rehabilitation treatment at university hospitals or special rehabilitation hospitals, in order to examine the factors influencing the parenting stress of mothers of children with CP with reference to social support provided to the mother.

The general characteristics of the children with CP, such as sex and age were not significantly different, though parenting stress was positively associated with the severity of the disorder of the children with CP, revealing that parenting stress increases with increased severity of the disorder ($r=0.302$, $p<0.01$). This outcome is in agreement with the results of preceding studies [3, 8, 9, 10, 16], reporting that parenting stress of the parent increases with the severity of a child's disability. Our results are analogous to those of Lena E. Svedberg [17], who concluded that parents nurturing CP children who cannot walk perceive more stress than those with CP children who can walk. Moreover, there are many circumstances of CP, in which mental retardation accompanies physiological disability, exacerbating the stress of parents [18].

Parenting stress was not dependent on age or general characteristics of mothers.

Table 2. The factors associated with Parenting Stress of Mothers

Variables			Parenting Stress
			Mean(SD)
Child	Sex	Male	146.56 (33.85)
		Female	139.49 (30.13)
	Age	Less than 24 months	143.23 (32.81)
		Between 24-72 months	139.91 (34.20)
		More than 72 months	144.96 (30.89)
	Term of disability [*]	Less than 1 year	145.00 (31.49)
		Between 1-3 years	139.39 (36.12)
		Between 3-5 years	127.20 (32.17)
		More than 5 years	148.33 (29.74)
	Severity of disability [**]	Mild	125.57 (33.05)
		Average severity	143.97 (31.57)
		Very severe	152.12 (28.01)
Mother	Age	Less than 30 years of age	131.43 (26.42)
		More than 30 years of age	142.77 (32.05)
	Level of education [*]	High school graduate or lower	149.67 (32.52)
		University graduate or higher	138.74 (31.29)
	Family income [**]	Less than 1,000,000 KRW	165.63 (18.21)
		Between 1,000,000-3,000,000 KRW	148.99 (31.67)
		Between 3,000,000-5,000,000 KRW	138.78 (28.95)
		More than 5,000,000 KRW	127.96 (38.20)
	Health conditions [**]	very unhealthy	142.71 (42.57)
		unhealthy	155.41 (33.58)
		healthy	145.46 (30.83)
		very healthy	129.78 (28.21)

* $p < 0.05$.
** $p < 0.01$.

On the other hand, parenting stress demonstrated negative correlations with the mother's level of education, level of income and health conditions, indicating that parenting stress increases with lower level of education ($r = -0.168$, $p < 0.05$), lower level of income ($r = -0.281$, $p < 0.01$) and poorer health condition ($r = -0.227$, $p < 0.01$). Haley [19] also reported lower stress levels in mothers possessing higher level of education, and Kim Soo-hyeon [12] revealed that the financial status of mothers of children diagnosed with CP influenced parenting stress in a negative correlation, concluding that the lower stress level may be due to a better ability to resolve economical difficulties experienced as a result of parenting children with disabilities.

Our results are in agreement with Lee Ji-won [13], who described the influence of the health condition of mothers on parenting, and Lena E. Svedberg [17], who identified a relationship between parent health condition and the stress they experienced in parenting children with CP, verifying that caring for children with CP has a physically negative effect.

Table 3. Hierarchial Multiple Regression Analysis I

Classification		step1	step2	step3
Child	Term of Disability	3.242	2.626	1.897
	Severity of Disability	12.974**	12.429**	12.550**
Mother	Level of Education		-3.200	-2.972
	Family Income		-6.265	-5.520
	Health Condition		-7.641*	-6.612*
Social Support	Social Support			-0.635**
R^2		0.109	0.196	0.249

* $p<0.05$, ** $p<0.01$.

Table 4. Hierarchial Multiple Regression Analysis II

Classification		step1	step2	step3
Child	Term of Disability	3.242	2.626	1.622
	Severity of Disability	12.974**	12.429**	12.497**
Mother	Level of Education		-3.200	-1.967
	Income Level		-6.265	-5.625
	Health Condition		-7.641*	-6.809*
Social Support	Formal Support			-0.268
	Informal Support			-1.117*
R^2		0.109	0.196	0.249

* $p<0.05$, ** $p<0.01$.

From this, it can be understood that, as the severity of the disability of a child with CP increases, the assistance required by the mother will increase, resulting in increased dependency and subsequent physiological stress as well as psychological burden. Inclusion of economic difficulty or problematic health condition of the mother would exacerbate the experienced burden. Therefore, intervention for parenting stress should be considered an exceptionally important issue.

The present study examined social support independently as informal support and formal support. According to research by Hong Ji-yeon [20], social support provided to the mothers of children with CP is aimed at allowing efficient coping and adaptation to stress, and proficient adjustment of social support would make successful adaptation possible. Moreover, research by Cohen and Wills [21] suggests that social support is a significant coping resource, reducing stress and improving personal adaptation levels by reducing pessimistic emotions while promoting optimistic emotions.

The present study demonstrated there is a negative correlation (r=-0.260, p<0.01) between social support and the parenting stress of mothers. This result was comparable to those of several previous studies [3, 8, 16, 22, 23] that reported a negative correlation between social support and parenting stress, and that increased social support yielded decreased parenting stress. Furthermore, in hierarchial multiple regression analysis, social support was independently examined as formal support and informal support, but of parenting stress only informal support was identified as a significant predictor (β=-1.117, p<0.01).

In other words, informal support has a perceptible influence on the parenting stress of mothers of children with disabilities, rather than formal support, indicating that emotional intervention is relatively indispensable for mothers of children with disabilities. In his research, Jeon Jae-il [24] acknowledged the significance of formal support based on an analysis of the most influential support, in affecting the quality of life of mothers of children with disabilities.

Kim Sung-su [25] revealed that an increased level of social support positively influenced childhood negligence while increased economic stress contributed to increased childhood negligence of children with developmental disorders, as well as the level of depression of mothers. Results of the in-depth survey of the present study disclosed a firm demand for lessening the physical and financial burden of caring for disabled children, indicating the significance of formal support for mothers, and the necessity of organizing a relevant welfare support system.

In summary, the present study revealed that the characteristics of children with CP and mothers, as well as social support intercorrelated, and that social support reduces the burden and stress of parenting experienced by mothers. Therefore, we must understand and ameliorate the adversity, physiological and psychological afflictions experienced through parenting of children with CP. In addition, the responsibility of parenting for children with disabilities must be administered at a national level and various support programs must be comprehensively provided for mothers to maintain their psychological and physical health.

The limitations of the present study were as follows.

First, there are difficulties in the generalization of the results of the present study. Information concerning children with CP who are enrolled in special-education schools or those who live at home, was not been incorporated. Therefore, it may be impractical to apply the results to all mothers of children with CP, and an expanded sampling region and a large number of subjects will be essential in future studies.

Second, research into social support for not only the mother of children with CP, but for the members of the family should be conducted. In particular, the brothers and sisters of children with disabilities should be carefully studied and research on understanding the difficulties and negligence felt by siblings is required.

Third, during the conduct for the present study, we perceived that there had been inadequate research into the leisure activities of mothers of children with disabilities. Various studies of leisure activities, which may improve the quality of life for mothers, must be conducted.

References

[1] Bax, M., Goldstein, M., Rosenbaum, P., Leviton, A., Paneth, N., Dan, B., Jacobsson, B., and Damiano, D. (2005). Proposed definition and classification of cerebral palsy. *Developmental Medicine and Child Neurology*, 47, 571-576.

[2] Division of Policy for Persons with Disabilities of the Ministry of Health and Welfare. (2008). Main disease labels of brain lesion [http://kostat.go.kr/]. National Statistical Office.

[3]   Ryu, H. J. (2010). The Relationship between cerebral palsy children's temperament, their Mothers' social support and maternal parenting stress. Kyeon-buk University Graduate School of Health, Masters Dissertation.

[4]   Hastings, R. P. (2003). Child behavior problems and partner mental health as correlates of stress in mothers and fathers of children with autism. *Journal of Intellectual Disability Research,* 47, 231-237.

[5]   Olsson, M. B., and Hwang, C. P. (2001). Depression in mothers and fathers of children with intellectual disability. *Journal of Intellectual Disability Research*, 45, 535-543.

[6]   Hwang, K. J. (2002). A study on the factors affecting the stress of mothers with multiple-handicapped children. Hallym University Graduate School of Social Welfare, Masters Dissertation.

[7]   Shim, Y. W. (1995). Intervention methods and comparison analysis of stress for mothers with cerebral palsy. *Korean Council of Physical, Multiple, and Health Disabilities*, 25, 67-87.

[8]   Kim, E. S., and Kim, H. S. (2009). Burden and social support of mothers with cerebral palsy. *Korean Academic Society of Rehabilitation Nursing*, 12, 39-46.

[9]   Lee, M. J., and Jeong, Y. K. (1997). Research on the correlation between stress for mothers and the level of disorder in children with cerebral palsy. *Nursing Science Research,* 1, 89-103.

[10]   Oh, S. R. (2001). Study on stress for mothers of children with disabilities. *Korean Academy of Social Welfare,* 46, 263-289.

[11]   Park, E. S. (2003). Study on coping strategies and stress for mothers of children with cerebral palsy. Daejeon University Graduate School of Health and Sports, Masters Dissertation.

[12]   Kim, S. H., and Kang, H. S. (2010). Factors influencing parenting stress in mothers of children with cerebral palsy. *Korean Academic Society of Rehabilitation Nursing*, 13, 123-131.

[13]   Lee, J. W., and Lee, H. Z. (1997). A study on the stress and coping patterns of mothers with cerebral palsy children. *Child Health Nursing Research*, 3, 190-202.

[14]   Bristol, M. M. (1979). Carolina parent support scale. University of North Carolina at Chapel Hill: Unpublished assessment instrument. (Revised 1981).

[15]   Ware, J. E., Davis-Avery, A., and Donald, C. A. (1978). Conceptualization and measurement of health for adults in the health insurance study. 5. General Health Perceptions, Santa Monica, The Rand Corporation.

[16]   Yoo, J. H. (1989). A study on the stress and coping behaviors of the mothers of the children with cerebral palsy due to the latter's abnormal and social support. Ewha Womans University Graduate School of Education, Masters Dissertation.

[17]   Svedberg, L. E, Englund, E., Malker, H., and Stener-Victorin, E. (2010). Comparison of impact on mood, health, and daily living experiences of primary caregivers of walking and non-walking children with cerebral palsy and provided community services support. *European Journal of Paediatric Neurology,* 14, 239-246.

[18]   Parkes, J., McCullough, N., Madden, A., and McCahey, E. (2009). The health of children with cerebral palsy and stress in their parents. *Journal of Advanced Nursing,* 65, 2311-2323.

[19]   Haley, A. R., (1993). Maternal distress in families with a mentally retarded child. Fordham University, Unpublished Doctoral Dissertation.

[20] Hong, J. Y. (2006). Study on the influence of family functioning perceived by mothers with developmentally disabled children on their parenting stress: focused on the moderating effect of social support. Yonsei University Graduate School of Social Welfare, Masters Dissertation.

[21] Cohen, S., and Wills, T. A. (1985). Stress, social support, and the buffering hypothesis. *Psychological Bulletin*, 98, 310-357.

[22] Kim, S. H. (2010). Study on the factors affecting parenting stress on mothers of children with cerebral palsy. Kyunghee University Graduate School of Nursing, Masters Dissertation.

[23] Voorman, J. M., Dallmeijer, A. J., Van Eck, M., Schuengel, C., and Becher, J. G. (2010). Social functioning and communication in children with cerebral palsy: association with disease characteristics and personal and environmental factors. *Developmental Medicine and Child Neurology*, 52, 441-447.

[24] Jeon, J. I., and Park, Y. G. (2006). The impact of social support for mother with mental retarded children on their quality of life. *Journal of Social Welfare Development*, 12, 381-404.

[25] Kim, S. S., and Jung, H. J. (2010). Study of effect that economic stress and depression have on child neglect in developmental disability children's mothers: The moderating effects of social support. *Korea Society for the Emotional and Behavioral Disorders*, 26(3): 257-275.

Index

A

academic performance, 183
acetabulum, 181, 182
acetylcholine, 75
acquisitions, 103
acromion, 154
action potential, 216, 217
active exercises, vii, 25, 218
Activities of Daily Living, x, 97, 108
acupuncture, 236
adaptability, 102
adaptation(s), viii, xi, 6, 42, 99, 101, 105, 110, 112,
    116, 127, 128, 130, 132, 133, 134, 135, 137, 149,
    208, 254
adduction, 154, 181, 188, 215
adductor, 74
ADHD, 67
adjunctive therapy, 122
adjustment, 5, 69, 102, 103, 104, 128, 154, 242, 254
adolescents, ix, x, 46, 53, 54, 61, 67, 88, 89, 90, 91,
    97, 110, 116, 117, 120, 124, 125, 150, 225, 242,
    243, 244, 245
adulthood, 68, 80, 194, 206, 233
adults, vii, x, xiii, 2, 44, 45, 67, 68, 76, 79, 85, 102,
    116, 136, 153, 158, 159, 182, 193, 198, 209, 211,
    213, 232, 242, 243, 244, 256
adverse conditions, 98
adverse effects, 26, 38, 75, 87, 123, 244
adverse event, 70, 100
aerobic capacity, 28
aerobic exercise, 28
aetiology, 2, 8, 9, 11, 16, 18, 84, 174
agglutination, 148
agonist, 99, 118, 119, 120
alcoholism, 172
aldosterone, 163

alters, 178
alveoli, 197
amblyopia, 72
AMF, 110
amplitude, 104, 105, 109, 152, 155, 194, 200
analgesic, 196
anatomy, 123, 178, 183
angiogenesis, 196
ANOVA, 251
antigen, 196
antiphospholipid antibodies, 43
anxiety, 71, 250
APA, 102, 103, 104, 105, 107
aphasia, 67
apoptosis, 175, 208
ARM, 214
artery, 42
arthritis, 68, 227
arthrodesis, 235
arthroplasty, 194
articulation, 54
asphyxia, viii, 11, 42, 64, 175
aspiration, 12, 64, 186
assessment, x, xiii, 17, 49, 51, 61, 71, 78, 80, 97,
    106, 107, 108, 109, 110, 113, 160, 165, 167, 184,
    193, 199, 222, 227, 241, 256
assessment tools, 80, 106, 109
assistive technology, 99, 128, 138, 139, 185
asymmetry, 106, 116, 235
ataxia, 16, 86, 120, 143, 159, 222
athetosis, 99, 152
athletes, 61
atrophy, 68, 75, 171, 222
atypical muscle tone, ix, 63, 64
autism, 256
autonomic nervous system, 165, 166
avascular necrosis, 197
axons, 44

260 Index

B

barriers, 28
basal ganglia, 44, 45, 47, 99, 152, 171, 210
base, 14, 68, 103, 108, 120, 155, 184, 223
behavior, ix, 42, 63, 67, 77, 80, 98, 101, 102, 103, 111, 126, 134, 147, 148, 170, 183, 206, 256
behavioral disorders, x, 97, 109
behavioral problems, 16
behaviors, 101, 147, 256
Belgium, 25
bending, ix, 53, 54, 59
beneficial effect, 197, 219
benefits, x, 13, 27, 31, 79, 81, 92, 116, 119, 120, 121, 133, 147, 153, 158, 198
benzodiazepine, 26
bicuspid, 144
bilateral, 61, 245
bimanual performance, viii, 42, 45, 46, 48, 82, 83
biofeedback, 73, 210, 217, 244
biomarkers, 7
biomechanics, 108, 118, 243
birth weight, viii, 4, 8, 10, 17, 19, 20, 41, 43, 47, 110, 206
births, viii, x, xii, 2, 3, 8, 10, 19, 20, 41, 42, 43, 47, 64, 65, 97, 98, 169, 170, 194, 206
birthweight, 22, 49, 65, 67, 86
bleeding, 143, 147, 195
blindness, 4
blood, xii, 75, 92, 93, 161, 163, 164, 195, 196, 197
blood circulation, 195
blood pressure, xii, 161, 163, 164
blood transfusion, 92
blood vessels, 196
body mass index (BMI), xi, 161, 162, 163, 164, 165
body weight, x, 116, 118, 121, 126, 210, 211, 219, 223, 227, 241
bone(s), 22, 27, 32, 33, 34, 38, 53, 54, 60, 71, 194, 196, 197, 201, 242
boredom, 36
bottom-up, 102
brain abnormalities, 67
brain activity, 77
brain damage, vii, ix, 12, 63, 64, 67, 75, 93, 250
brain structure, 86
brainstem, 72, 210
Brazil, x, 97, 98, 115, 127, 141, 143, 151, 153, 161, 162
breathing, 165, 166, 167
breech delivery, 12
bronchopulmonary dysplasia, 3, 5, 7
Bulgaria, 193, 198

C

caesarean section, 12, 43, 64
calcitonin, 196, 201
calcium, 70, 196
calculus, 143, 155, 156
cancer, 13
capsule, 44, 47
carbamazepine, 70
carbohydrates, 142
cardiac arrest, 93
cardiac output, xii, 161, 163
cardiac structure, 162
cardiovascular system, 235
caregivers, xi, xii, 80, 141, 142, 143, 144, 145, 146, 147, 148, 149, 153, 162, 177, 187, 243
caregiving, 90, 185
caries, 147, 149
case study(s), 38, 45, 74, 77, 80
casting, 72, 73, 76, 81, 82
catheter, 74
causal relationship, 192
CBS, 172
cell death, 175
central nervous system (CNS), x, xii, 48, 80, 100, 115, 116, 123, 169, 170, 175, 196, 197, 199, 200, 208, 209, 210, 216, 219, 228, 242
cerebellum, 99, 152, 222, 243
cerebral blood flow, 43
cerebral cortex, 210
challenges, vii, 2, 4, 9, 13, 15, 19, 28, 83, 126, 250
channel blocker, 70
chemical, 98, 195
chemotaxis, 196
Chicago, 1
childhood, vii, ix, x, xii, xiii, 19, 22, 23, 43, 63, 65, 83, 84, 88, 97, 98, 109, 113, 142, 160, 162, 177, 194, 205, 206, 229, 233, 246, 255
China, 65, 85
chorea, 99
choreoathetoid movements, 136
choreoathetosis, 98, 158
chromosomal abnormalities, 7
chromosome, 100
circulation, 171
classification, 4, 17, 22, 48, 83, 84, 85, 98, 99, 100, 113, 116, 148, 150, 166, 170, 171, 173, 200, 227, 228, 233, 246, 255
clinical diagnosis, 162
clinical examination, 207
clinical neurophysiology, 228, 229
clinical presentation, viii, 35, 37, 42, 44, 47, 104, 166

clinical symptoms, 61
clinical trials, 13, 14, 18, 35, 76
clonus, 99, 198
clothing, 69
cochlear implant, 72, 89
cognition, ix, 16, 17, 42, 63, 68, 98, 142, 170, 183
cognitive abilities, 17, 67, 80
cognitive deficit(s), 235
cognitive development, 17, 232, 241
cognitive impairment, 66, 67
cognitive level, 33
collaboration, 13, 14, 19, 85, 110, 200
collagen, 196
communication, vii, ix, x, 2, 11, 16, 22, 42, 63, 68, 71, 85, 88, 97, 109, 142, 170, 183, 206, 216, 257
communication skills, 71, 88
communication systems, 71
community, vii, 2, 17, 21, 22, 69, 149, 220, 256
community networks, vii, 2
community service, 256
compensation, 78, 82
complement, 29, 31
complexity, 33, 37, 101, 102, 104, 111, 120, 146
compliance, 40, 209
complications, 3, 8, 20, 27, 69, 90, 100, 194, 207, 218, 244
computer, vii, 25, 29, 30, 34, 39, 71, 88, 129, 138, 153, 209, 213, 215, 232
conditioning, 208
configuration, 33, 110, 130, 223
congenital heart disease, 43
connective tissue, 196, 200
connectivity, 47
consciousness, 43
constipation, 166
constraint induced movement therapy, ix, x, 42, 64, 69, 77, 82, 89, 94, 96
construction, 133
consumption, 142, 218
contracture, 55, 60, 181, 188, 235
control group, 6, 31, 32, 34, 74, 79, 81, 152, 153, 162, 163, 164, 241
controlled trials, 69, 76, 81, 117, 118, 124
convulsion, 250
cooling, 2, 12, 21
coordination, viii, ix, xiii, 4, 26, 30, 64, 65, 70, 82, 85, 96, 99, 103, 112, 121, 128, 133, 134, 135, 136, 137, 158, 166, 174, 183, 205, 209, 216, 217, 219, 220, 228, 229
coping strategies, 256
copper, 131
correlation(s), ix, 44, 45, 47, 53, 86, 108, 182, 189, 209, 216, 219, 232, 250, 251, 252, 253, 254, 256

cortex, ix, x, 34, 44, 46, 48, 54, 57, 58, 59, 63, 64, 99, 115, 116, 123, 124
cortical re-organization, viii, 41
corticosteroids, 5
cost, 15, 121, 147, 158, 198, 214, 218
cost saving, 15
covering, 143
crises, 170
critical analysis, 117
critical period, 173
cross-sectional study, 123, 147
crouch gait, ix, 53, 54, 59, 60, 61
CST, 47, 48, 79
cure, 14, 232, 241
currency, 13
cycles, 75
cycling, 31, 32, 38
cytokines, 6
cytomegalovirus, 10, 21, 171
cytoskeleton, 195

D

daily living, 32, 74, 76, 89, 184, 256
data analysis, 129
data collection, 129, 131
data set, 2
database, 17, 85
DBP, 164
deaths, 5, 10
defects, 6, 10, 64
deficit, 43, 67, 165, 250
degradation, 27
deltoid, 102
dendrites, 217
Denmark, 66
dental care, 144
dental caries, 142, 148, 149, 150, 167
dental plaque, 148
dependent variable, 24, 147
depolarization, 48, 217
deposits, 196
depression, 28, 250, 255, 257
deprivation, 48
depth, 194, 195, 199, 251, 255
desensitization, 144
destruction, 195, 196
detectable, 6, 143
detection, 6
developed countries, x, 20, 65, 83, 97, 98, 170, 173, 194
developing brain, 48, 98, 170, 206
developing countries, 65

developmental disorder, 111, 255
developmental disuse, ix, 64, 65
developmental functioning, vii, 2
dexterity, ix, 31, 32, 64, 65, 81, 184, 220
diabetes, 171
diastole, 163
diet, 142, 146, 147
differential diagnosis, 207
diffusion, 44, 45, 51, 86, 93
Diffusion Tensor Imaging (DTI), viii, 42, 5, 46, 49
diplegia, xiii, 182, 193, 198
disabled patients, vii, 25
discomfort, 69, 70, 120, 223, 235, 250
discrimination, 67
diseases, 87, 144, 148, 171, 172, 197, 207, 216, 235
dislocation, xii, 16, 18, 22, 58, 59, 68, 177, 178, 179, 181, 182, 183, 188, 189, 192
disorder, ix, xii, 63, 67, 68, 69, 75, 98, 143, 169, 170, 174, 194, 206, 208, 210, 222, 241, 252, 256
dispersion, 131, 134, 135
displaced fractures, ix, 53, 61
displacement, 16, 22, 92, 123, 125, 156, 181
disproportionate growth, 235
distal strength, ix, 64, 65
distress, 9, 16, 235, 250, 257
distribution, 4, 19, 98, 131, 183, 216, 220
dogs, 88, 213
DOI, 23, 61
dosage, 83
dosing, 77, 81
drug treatment, 70
drugs, x, 10, 69, 70, 87, 116
dysarthria, 67, 71, 88
dysphagia, 17, 23
dysplasia, 5, 20, 42, 60, 183, 189
dystonia, 70, 91, 99, 159, 160

E

echocardiogram, 165
economic status, 10
edema, 143
EEG, 125, 222
EEG activity, 222
elbows, 221
electromagnetic, 195
eligibility criteria, 13
elongation, 59
emboli, 43
embolism, 43
embolization, 43
EMG, 44, 55, 73, 91, 104, 109, 111, 217, 228
emotional health, 17

employment, 10, 68, 87
employment status, 10
encephalopathy, xi, 2, 6, 11, 12, 15, 21, 151, 152, 153, 172, 175, 222
endocrine, 66
endurance, 209, 211, 222, 232, 242, 243
energy, 31, 32, 194, 195, 196, 198, 201, 233
energy expenditure, 31, 32
England, 19, 66, 139
enlargement, 6
enuresis, 223
environment(s), viii, xii, xiii, 26, 29, 33, 34, 39, 69, 80, 81, 86, 95, 100, 101, 105, 128, 137, 160, 169, 171, 173, 184, 187, 205, 212, 213, 215, 222, 232, 236
environmental conditions, 103
environmental factors, 150, 257
enzyme, 167
epicondylitis, 197
epidemiology, vii, xii, 1, 3, 4, 8, 84, 173, 177, 227
epilepsy, ix, 4, 11, 16, 42, 63, 66, 67, 68, 70, 88, 98, 100, 206
epithelium, 196
EPS, 137
equilibrium, 101, 103, 105, 112, 209, 221
equipment, 119, 139, 236
erythropoietin, 5
Estonia, 19
ethics, 13
etiology, viii, ix, 5, 19, 41, 42, 53, 98, 170, 171, 183, 228
Europe, 4, 19, 43, 49, 65, 66, 85, 87, 88, 100, 110, 194, 200
evidence, vii, ix, xiii, 2, 3, 4, 5, 13, 14, 15, 16, 17, 18, 19, 22, 23, 27, 33, 35, 37, 38, 39, 46, 47, 48, 64, 65, 68, 69, 70, 71, 72, 76, 79, 80, 81, 84, 86, 89, 111, 112, 120, 121, 123, 125, 138, 185, 187, 188, 193, 196, 209, 210, 219, 227
evidence based interventions, vii, 2
evolution, 27, 121
examinations, 143, 198, 207
excision, 60
excitability, x, 46, 48, 115, 116, 117, 123, 124, 200, 202
excitation, 217
exclusion, 153, 162
execution, viii, x, xi, 26, 38, 81, 102, 115, 116, 118, 121, 127, 134, 155, 156, 157, 158
executive function(s), vii, 2, 17, 87
executive functioning, 87
exercise, 28, 40, 46, 51, 60, 79, 121, 122, 126, 212, 215, 235, 236
exoskeleton, 215, 228

Index

F

exposure, 70, 98, 171
extensor, ix, 53, 54, 59, 61, 99
eye movement, 72

facial asymmetry, 222
families, 10, 16, 68, 83, 90, 149, 185, 187, 250, 257
family functioning, 257
family history, 10
family income, 251, 252
family members, 185, 250
family support, 28, 68
fat, 75
fear, 67, 102
femur, 32, 182, 213, 221, 223, 235
fetal distress, 43
fetal growth, 5, 6
fetus, vii, 170, 171
fever, 162
fiber(s), 45, 46, 49, 200
fibrosis, 200
fine motor, vii, ix, xi, 2, 17, 63, 64, 69, 73, 85, 127, 129, 132, 133, 134, 136, 137, 183, 184, 226
finger movements, ix, 63, 64
first aid, 71
first molar, 144
fitness, xi, 31, 32, 116, 122
fixation, 152, 208, 211, 235
flexibility, 27
flexor, xiii, 178, 193, 197, 198, 202
flight, 222
fluctuations, 124
fluid, 11, 148
fMRI, viii, 42, 78, 93
food, 142, 147, 165
Food and Drug Administration (FDA), 75
force, ix, xi, 53, 54, 59, 81, 109, 110, 119, 127, 137, 160, 183, 189, 211, 216, 235
formation, x, 97, 148, 182, 197, 200, 203
formula, 163, 218
fractures, ix, 53, 54, 57, 59, 60, 61, 194, 196, 197, 201, 223, 235
functional changes, 210, 242
functional imaging, 34
functional MRI, viii, 42, 47, 51, 78
funding, 14, 36, 76

G

gait, ix, x, xiii, 31, 53, 54, 55, 56, 59, 60, 61, 68, 86, 91, 105, 110, 111, 115, 116, 117, 118, 119, 120, 121, 122, 123, 124, 125, 126, 160, 181, 205, 210, 211, 218, 223, 225, 227, 231, 232, 235, 241, 243, 244, 245, 246
gait disorders, 211, 232, 244
Gait Laboratory, ix, 53, 54, 60, 61
gait orthosis, xiii, 231
gallstones, 194
gaming controllers, vii, 25, 26, 30
ganglion, 201
gastrocnemius, 178, 197, 198, 202
genes, xii, 169, 172, 173, 174, 196
genetic components, 10
genetic testing, 207
genetic traits, 172
genetics, 9
genome, xii, 169, 173
geometry, 83
Germany, 211
gestation, 3, 4, 5, 6, 7, 89, 173
gestational age, viii, 3, 4, 9, 10, 19, 20, 21, 42, 174
gestational diabetes, 43
gingival, 143, 147
glasses, 71
glaucoma, 72
glia, 174
Gross Motor Function Classification System (GMFCS), x, xiii, 4, 11, 17, 31, 32, 34, 36, 85, 99, 100, 104, 105, 106, 108, 110, 115, 116, 121, 123, 129, 153, 154, 173, 185, 189, 191, 192, 220, 227, 228, 231, 233, 234, 237, 238, 239, 240, 242, 246
goal directed treatment, ix, 42
goal setting, 83, 86, 88, 106
government policy, 14
grades, 175, 189, 233
grants, 148, 166
graph, 54, 56, 57
grasping, ix, 64, 65, 74, 81, 128, 137, 138, 139, 160, 215, 216, 220, 221
gravity, 99, 119, 153, 218, 221
gray matter, 42, 44, 45, 47
gross motor, vii, x, xiv, 2, 16, 22, 23, 39, 68, 69, 89, 99, 106, 113, 115, 116, 122, 125, 126, 138, 190, 219, 220, 226, 227, 228, 232, 233, 242, 245, 246
growth, xii, 6, 7, 9, 10, 11, 21, 68, 100, 106, 167, 169, 170, 178, 196, 201, 242
growth factor, 7, 196
growth spurt, 178
guidance, 110, 116, 147, 199, 211, 235
guidelines, xi, 4, 13, 83, 84, 85, 142, 148, 163, 222

H

habituation, 208

hand function, viii, 38, 42, 44, 45, 46, 47, 49, 74, 78, 90, 94, 96, 108, 187
hand posturing, ix, 64, 65
handedness, xii, 44, 47, 177
handwriting, 4, 133, 138
healing, 196
health, vii, xi, xiv, 2, 13, 14, 16, 17, 22, 35, 36, 38, 67, 68, 70, 85, 95, 141, 142, 144, 146, 148, 149, 189, 218, 232, 241, 249, 251, 252, 253, 254, 256, 257
health care, 13, 22, 218
health condition, 251, 252, 253, 254
health insurance, 36, 256
health services, 36
health status, xiv, 70, 149, 249
hearing impairment, 72
hearing loss, 4, 89
heart failure, 166
heart rate, xi, 161, 162, 163, 165, 166
height, 100, 106, 129, 154, 155, 164
helplessness, 28
hematoma, 197
hemiparesis, x, 51, 93, 95, 100, 105, 115, 116, 129, 139, 152, 159, 160, 172, 215, 219, 233, 235
hemiplegia, ix, xiii, 2, 6, 11, 16, 17, 23, 38, 43, 45, 50, 63, 64, 65, 67, 68, 71, 79, 80, 83, 84, 89, 90, 94, 95, 96, 104, 105, 143, 170, 193, 198, 199, 225
hemiplegic CP, viii, ix, 34, 41, 42, 44, 64, 65, 66, 67, 68, 69, 72, 77, 243
hemisphere, 45, 46, 48, 78
hemorrhage, 42, 44, 67, 100, 171, 175
hip contracture, 181
history, 9, 10, 43, 131, 162, 182, 183, 189, 194, 222, 245
homes, 185
Hong Kong, 150
hospitalization, 218, 244
House, 17, 23
human body, 53
human development, 19
human development index, 19
Hunter, 21
hydrocephalus, 7
hygiene, xi, 69, 75, 141, 142, 144, 146, 147, 148, 149, 150, 167
hyperactivity, 67
hyperbilirubinemia, 100
hypertension, 7, 11, 171
hypoglycemia, 43
hyporeflexia, 222
hypotension, 5
hypothermia, 15, 64
hypoxia, xii, 100, 169, 171, 172, 173, 175

I

ICAM, 196
idiopathic, 88, 227
iliopsoas, 181
image(s), 44, 153, 155, 171, 199, 207
imagery, 125
imbalances, 118
imitation, 212
immersion, 123
immobilization, 120
immunoreactivity, 201
impairments, vii, ix, 4, 8, 11, 13, 16, 18, 22, 23, 40, 43, 46, 47, 49, 63, 64, 65, 66, 67, 70, 71, 72, 77, 82, 84, 85, 98, 100, 103, 104, 105, 109, 125, 152, 159, 183, 187, 225, 226, 227
improvements, xi, 46, 74, 81, 82, 116, 124, 146, 184, 219, 237, 244
impulses, 163, 196, 197, 210, 217
in utero, 5
in vitro, 15
in vivo, 15
incidence, x, xi, xii, 43, 67, 84, 97, 98, 127, 165, 169, 170, 178, 179, 182, 183, 189, 194, 250
incisor(s), 143, 144
income, 253
independence, xi, 28, 71, 76, 79, 81, 108, 116, 118, 158, 191, 232, 241
independent variable, 144, 147
India, 150
indirect measure, 109
individual development, 233
individualization, 144
individuals, vii, ix, x, xi, 2, 4, 13, 16, 18, 23, 47, 48, 63, 70, 71, 78, 79, 105, 112, 113, 115, 116, 120, 125, 129, 141, 142, 143, 144, 146, 147, 148, 149, 151, 152, 153, 157, 158, 162, 163, 165, 167, 184, 233, 242
induction, 201
industry, viii, 26, 30
infancy, 43, 104, 110, 112, 147, 192
infants, 2, 3, 4, 5, 6, 7, 8, 9, 10, 11, 12, 13, 15, 16, 19, 20, 43, 44, 47, 64, 85, 88, 101, 102, 104, 110, 111, 112, 113, 137, 166, 187, 188, 207
infarction, 43, 44, 46, 47
infection, 5, 6, 10, 20, 68, 100, 174, 206
infertility, 43
inflammation, 5, 6, 7, 20, 143, 172, 173, 175, 196, 197
inflammatory disease, 201
inflammatory mediators, 173
informed consent, 13, 143, 162, 235
ingest, 147

Index

ingestion, 165
ingredients, 82
inhibition, 102, 118, 167, 178, 196
initiation, 77, 105, 113, 207, 215
injections, 46, 50, 72, 75, 89, 92, 197
injure, 152
injury(ies), 6, 7, 8, 20, 42, 43, 44, 67, 104, 105, 117,
  118, 121, 171, 152, 174, 194, 197, 209, 210, 211,
  216, 217, 219, 228, 229, 250
insulin, 7, 196
integration, 31, 69, 76, 100, 102, 123, 209
intellect, 71
intellectual disabilities, 148, 256
intensive care unit, 3, 72
intercellular adhesion molecule, 7
interface, 215
interference, xii, 134, 137, 169, 170
interleukin-8, 7
International Classification of Diseases, 235
interneuron, 47
interrogations, 49
intramuscular injection, 75
investment, 76
investors, 36
ions, 123
ipsilateral, 44, 46, 47, 48, 51, 60, 78, 93, 221
IQ scores, 186
Ireland, 53
ischemia, 100, 175, 200
Islam, 47, 49, 51, 93, 175
isolation, 71
Italy, 63

J

Japan, 177
jaundice, 12, 172
joint control, viii, 26, 30
joints, 17, 33, 153, 154, 211, 216, 218, 223, 235, 242
Jordan, 94
jumping, 106, 216

K

kidney stones, 194
kinetic data, ix, 53, 110
knee extensor disruption, ix, 53, 54, 59, 61
knees, 53, 54, 59, 68, 116, 118, 154, 221, 223
Korea, 249, 250, 257
kyphosis, 70

L

landscape, 131
latency, 102, 200
later life, 188, 209
lateral epicondylitis, 196, 202
laterality, 78
lead, vii, ix, 2, 18, 28, 45, 46, 47, 64, 65, 68, 69, 75,
  77, 95, 142, 165, 195, 243, 250
learning, 4, 48, 67, 69, 73, 77, 78, 81, 84, 93, 101,
  121, 124, 128, 132, 133, 134, 137, 138, 170, 205,
  208, 209, 210, 215, 216, 219, 232
legs, 216, 221
leisure, 71, 255
lesions, 6, 27, 42, 44, 45, 47, 49, 67, 88, 98, 99, 183
level of education, 251, 253
liability insurance, 14
life expectancy, 13
ligand, 175
light, 31, 32, 71, 82, 129
limbic system, 210
linear model, xi, 141, 144, 146
lithotripsy, 201
local anesthesia, 198, 202
localization, viii, 42
locomotor, 93, 112, 125, 181, 209, 210, 211, 218,
  221, 223, 224, 226, 227, 229, 232, 235, 236, 237,
  242, 243, 244, 246
loneliness, 71
low birthweight, 64
low risk, 16
lumbar spine, 32, 107
lying, xiii, 106, 188, 189, 192, 216, 218, 220, 223,
  231, 236, 238, 239, 243
lymph, 196

M

magnesium, 5
magnetic resonance image, 78
magnetic resonance imaging (MRI), viii, 2, 7, 20, 34,
  42, 43, 44, 47, 49, 67, 86, 207, 222
magnitude, 73, 76, 105, 109
management, vii, xii, 17, 18, 21, 37, 50, 69, 70, 72,
  73, 74, 76, 85, 87, 89, 91, 92, 177, 182, 188, 192,
  194, 200, 208, 211, 218, 235, 244
manipulation, ix, 63, 65, 77, 128, 147, 186
manual abilities, vii
mapping, 84, 102, 125
marketing, 36
marrow, 201
Maryland, 110, 186

mass, xi, 101, 109, 112, 161, 162, 163, 164, 165
maternal smoking, 5
atrix, 195, 196
matter, 6, 17, 42, 45, 47
measurement(s), xiii, 10, 17, 84, 107, 109, 143, 154, 155, 163, 164, 166, 167, 181, 193, 199, 228, 243, 251, 256
mechanical ventilation, 100
meconium, 64
medial epicondyle, 209
median, 221, 233
medical, xiii, 4, 9, 13, 14, 69, 87, 143, 145, 174, 194, 195, 205, 206, 208, 211, 216, 235, 236, 244, 251
medication, 26, 27, 69, 120, 222
medicine, 3, 18, 35, 126, 194, 198
membranes, 6, 43
memory, 4, 48, 67, 133, 200, 210
meningitis, 7, 43
mental health, 256
mental retardation, 67, 68, 71, 222, 252
mentally impaired, 67
mesenchymal stem cells, 201
messages, 22, 87
meta-analysis, 4, 16, 19, 21, 22, 42, 48, 86, 89, 120, 174, 198, 202
metabolic disorder(s), 100
metabolism, 71, 195, 196, 200
meter, 222
methodology, 13, 209
Mexico, 172
microcephaly, 7
microcirculation, 196
Microsoft, vii, 25, 29, 30, 31, 36
migration, 69, 181, 183
miscarriage(s), 10
mitosis, 196
models, 81, 208, 209
modifications, 69, 78, 184
Modified Ashworth Scale (MAS), xiii, 193, 198, 199
momentum, 221
Moon, 92, 197, 202
morbidity, 43
mortality, 8, 43, 85
motion accuracy, viii, 26
motion control, 136, 208
motivation, vii, 25, 26, 28, 30, 34, 36, 37, 38, 39, 78, 117, 126, 131, 217, 219, 221
motor activity(s), x, 97, 136
motor behavior, 89, 101, 111, 134
motor control, ix, x, 27, 34, 63, 64, 69, 81, 86, 97, 103, 112, 115, 118, 120, 121, 126, 158, 183, 184, 226
motor disabilities, x, 97, 108, 109

motor impairment, ix, x, xiii, 11, 16, 43, 44, 47, 64, 65, 67, 79, 88, 94, 98, 99, 104, 105, 108, 115, 118, 121, 125, 142, 152, 159, 183, 225, 231
motor neuron disease, xiii, 193
motor skills, 31, 69, 73, 78, 98, 128, 129, 132, 135, 147, 148, 183, 206, 208, 209, 213, 219, 220, 233, 236, 242
motor system, 103, 210
motor task, 124
movement disorders, xiii, 90, 106, 225, 226, 231
movement planning, ix, 64, 65
multiple factors, 70
multiple regression analyses, 252
multiple regression analysis, 251, 255
multiple sclerosis, 33, 194, 225, 227, 232, 245
multivariate analysis, 18, 21
muscle atrophy, 75
muscle contraction, 99, 101, 104, 105
muscle hypertonus, xiii, 193, 202
muscle relaxant, x, 116
muscle spasms, 70
muscle strength, x, 32, 69, 75, 116, 117, 118, 119, 120, 209, 219, 242
muscles, xiii, 17, 26, 27, 59, 68, 74, 75, 92, 101, 102, 103, 105, 109, 118, 119, 120, 142, 158, 178, 181, 184, 193, 197, 198, 199, 200, 202, 208, 210, 218, 232, 235, 241, 244
musculoskeletal, ix, 16, 17, 42, 63, 68, 98, 100, 104, 106, 114, 125, 183, 194, 201, 206, 218, 244
musculoskeletal system, 100, 104, 194
mutation(s), 43, 172, 174
myocardial infarction, 167
myopia, 72

N

necrosis, 175
negative consequences, 102
negative effects, 48, 121
negative experiences, 147
neonates, 5, 8, 15, 174
neovascularization, 196
nerve, 26, 70, 196, 197, 200, 201, 217
nervous system, 80, 100, 101, 162, 165, 196
nervousness, 250
Netherlands, 41, 66, 226
neural network(s), 216, 217
neural system, 98
neuralgia, 250
neurodegeneration, 202
neurodevelopmental disorders, xiii, 205, 206
neuroimaging, 43, 49, 78
neuro-imaging, viii, 41, 42, 98, 100

neurological disease, 207, 210, 211, 218, 232, 235
neurological disorders, viii, 26, 154, 208
neurological rehabilitation, 123
neurologist, 207, 232, 235
neuromotor, 2, 4, 99, 106, 108, 109, 187
neuronal circuits, 209
neuronal networks, viii, 42, 48
neurons, 48, 201, 210, 217
neuropeptides, 196
neuroprotection, vii, 1, 3, 4, 8, 16
neurorehabilitation, vii, xiii, 2, 76, 117, 126, 205, 210, 219, 226
neurorehabilitation therapies, 76
neurotransmission, 200
neurotransmitter(s), 48, 78
New England, 18, 125, 148
Nintendo Wii Fit, vii, 25, 39
nitric oxide, 5, 196, 200, 202
nitric oxide synthase, 5, 196
non-progressive disturbance, x, 97, 109
non-steroidal anti-inflammatory drugs (NSAIDs), 197
normal children, xiii, 70, 125, 186, 187, 205
normal development, 48, 98, 221
normal distribution, 237
North America, 166, 167
Norway, 66, 225
nuclei, 197
nucleus, 195
nutrition, 17

O

oblique fracture, ix, 53
obstacles, 212, 222
obstructive sleep apnea, 162, 165
occupational therapy, viii, 26, 27, 34, 46, 69, 71, 72, 73, 76, 80, 90, 129
optimization, 124, 208
oral cavity, 142, 144, 147, 148, 186
oral diseases, 146
oral health, xi, 17, 141, 142, 144, 145, 146, 147, 148, 149
organ(s), 218, 221, 244
organism, 100, 128
orthopedic surgeon, 208, 232
oscillators, 216
ossification, 54, 197
osteomyelitis, 197, 235
osteoporosis, 223, 235
osteotomy, 60
outpatient, 39, 223, 234, 236
oxygen, 4, 76

P

pain, xii, 16, 17, 28, 30, 36, 59, 60, 61, 67, 68, 69, 70, 74, 79, 177, 183, 196, 197, 198, 200, 218, 223, 233, 235, 244
Pakistan, 84
palate, 142
parallel, 154, 181
parenting, xiv, 249, 250, 251, 252, 253, 254, 255, 256, 257
parents, 17, 44, 69, 80, 143, 153, 162, 165, 185, 235, 236, 243, 250, 252, 257
paresis, 44, 128, 209, 221
Parkinson disease, vii, 25, 30
participants, xi, 78, 79, 105, 109, 129, 130, 131, 133, 134, 136, 137, 151, 153, 154, 156, 158, 188, 234, 236, 243
patella, ix, 53, 54, 55, 57, 59, 60, 61
patellar fractures, ix, 53, 54, 57, 59
patellar tendon, 53, 59
pathogenesis, 182
pathology, viii, 11, 33, 37, 42, 77, 188, 233
pathophysiological, 118
pathophysiology, 166
pathways, vii, ix, 1, 2, 3, 11, 44, 45, 47, 63, 64, 78, 83
patient care, 13, 15
patient motivation, viii, 26, 28, 219
Pedobarometric measurement, xiii, 193
pellicle, 148
pelvis, 181, 184, 188, 192, 218, 222
pen pressure, 129
peptide, 196, 201
perception, ix, 4, 28, 42, 63, 68, 98, 100, 142, 170, 178, 206
perfusion, 6, 68
perinatal, xii, 2, 5, 7, 18, 19, 20, 21, 43, 44, 49, 83, 100, 169, 170, 171, 172, 173, 174, 175, 206, 222
periodontal, xi, 141, 142, 143, 144, 147, 148, 149
periodontal disease, xi, 141, 142, 147, 148, 149
periosteum, 59
peripheral nervous system, 200
permeability, 196
PET, 198
petechiae, 197
pharmacotherapy, 72, 74
phosphate, 71
physical activity, x, 28, 31, 32, 39, 40, 97, 243
physical characteristics, xiii, 128, 193
physical exercise, 29, 208, 232
physical health, xiv, 249, 255
physical impairment, ix, 63, 64
physical mechanisms, 196

physical properties, 128
physical therapist, vii, 25
physical therapy, 28, 40, 69, 90, 117, 118, 124, 125, 126, 186, 197, 228, 236, 245, 246
physiology, 123, 159, 170, 194
physiotherapy, viii, 26, 31, 34, 39, 46, 51, 60, 72, 76, 80, 87, 117, 118, 129, 194, 208, 222, 241
pilot study, 39, 91, 154, 198, 202
placebo, xiii, 5, 73, 92, 193, 198, 199, 202
placenta, 222
plantar fasciitis, 196, 198, 202
plaque, 143, 147
plasticity, 48, 80, 86, 209, 210, 214, 219, 242, 243
play experience, vii, 25
playing, vii, 25, 30, 34, 40, 44
pneumothorax, 4
polarity, 123
policy makers, 14
polio, 206
polyhydramnios, 11
polymorphism(s), 172, 173, 174
population, xii, 2, 5, 9, 11, 12, 15, 19, 20, 21, 22, 31, 46, 67, 71, 86, 88, 91, 122, 123, 160, 162, 165, 169, 172, 173, 174, 178, 181, 182, 183
positive correlation, 252
postural adjustments, ix, 64, 65, 101, 102, 104, 109, 110, 111, 112, 113
postural control, x, 97, 100, 101, 103, 104, 105, 107, 108, 110, 111, 112, 183, 184, 185, 186, 187
postural development, x, 97, 109, 207
posture, viii, ix, xii, 30, 31, 33, 41, 42, 63, 64, 68, 69, 70, 74, 90, 98, 99, 100, 102, 104, 106, 107, 108, 112, 113, 142, 153, 162, 170, 177, 183, 184, 186, 188, 189, 194, 206, 250
potential benefits, 117
power generation, 54
predictor variables, xi, 141
preeclampsia, 6
pregnancy, 10, 18, 43, 171, 172, 174, 197
premature infant, 3
prematurity, 3, 4, 5, 7, 72, 100
preparation, 39, 209
preschool, 22, 111, 149, 186
preschool children, 149, 186
preterm infants, vii, 1, 3, 6, 7, 8, 20, 42, 43, 89, 166, 174
prevention, vii, 2, 5, 14, 16, 18, 19, 64, 68, 69, 112, 119, 144, 147, 148, 183, 194, 218
primary caregivers, 145, 146, 256
principles, 29, 69, 81, 88, 195, 209, 232
problem solving, 208
professionals, 68, 117, 118, 120, 123, 148
progestins, 3

prognosis, vii, 4, 8, 88, 104, 116, 117, 124, 183, 207, 233
programming, 91, 112
pro-inflammatory, 196
project, 35, 36, 235
prolapse, 5, 11
proliferation, 196
propagation, 57
prophylactic, 8
prophylaxis, 20, 244
protection, xii, 169, 172, 173
proteins, 195
pruning, 48
psychologist, 208, 232
puberty, 28, 242
public health, 3
P-value, 37

Q

quadriceps, 53, 54, 55, 57, 59, 61, 75, 119
quality of life, xii, 13, 70, 87, 88, 95, 116, 128, 146, 149, 177, 255, 257

R

radio, 154
radius, 154
Rasch analysis, 106
rating scale, 184
RATT, vi, xiii, 210, 211, 231, 232, 233, 234, 236, 238, 239, 240, 241, 242, 243, 244
reaction time, 33, 34
reactions, x, 115, 117, 125, 195, 196, 229
reactivity, 207
real time, 29, 123, 211, 235
reality, xiii, 38, 39, 40, 78, 93, 122, 123, 124, 126, 159, 205, 212, 215, 232, 244, 251
reasoning, 119
receptors, 225
reconstruction, 155
recovery, 84, 93, 105, 120, 126, 203, 214, 225, 229, 246
recreational, 10
recruiting, 15
rectus femoris, 55
reflexes, xii, 68, 144, 148, 149, 165, 167, 177, 178, 182, 208, 221, 229
regeneration, 48, 195, 201
registries, vii, 1
regression, xi, 103, 141, 144, 145, 147, 163, 165
regression analysis, 163, 165

regression model, xi, 141, 144, 145
rehabilitation program, 27, 81
relaxation, 165
relevance, 39, 172, 251
reliability, 23, 85, 110, 111, 113, 125, 138, 190, 222, 226, 227, 229, 246, 251
relief, 211, 235, 241, 243
renin, 163
repair, 216, 227, 246
repetitions, 30, 121, 155
reproduction, 3
requirements, 13, 198, 233
researchers, 2, 14, 15, 18, 31, 99, 117, 152, 157, 184
resilience, 98
resistance, 69, 120, 125, 155, 174, 186, 211, 218
resources, x, 68, 76, 83, 86, 98, 116, 119, 121, 124, 128, 244
respiratory distress syndrome, 7, 64
response, 10, 46, 51, 72, 80, 83, 102, 105, 162, 165, 195, 208, 209, 227, 250, 251
responsiveness, 23, 107
restoration, 78, 243
restrictions, 116
retardation, 67
retinopathy, 4, 7, 20, 72
rhythmicity, 217
rickets, 71
risk(s), vii, viii, xii, 1, 2, 3, 5, 6, 7, 8, 9, 10, 11, 12, 13, 16, 18, 19, 20, 21, 36, 41, 42, 61, 64, 70, 71, 83, 84, 89, 92, 137, 142, 144, 146, 147, 162, 165, 169, 171, 172, 173, 174, 181, 183, 199, 206, 207, 222, 227, 242
risk factors, vii, viii, xii, 1, 2, 3, 8, 9, 10, 12, 18, 19, 20, 21, 41, 64, 83, 84, 89, 144, 169, 171, 172, 173, 174, 183, 206, 227
robotics, 121
root(s), 155, 196, 201
rotations, 218

S

saliva, 150
scaling, 125
school, 17, 39, 41, 69, 72, 74, 80, 128, 129, 137, 150, 152, 157, 158, 184, 186, 220, 229, 251, 253, 255
school activities, 152, 157, 158
school performance, 129
science, 126
scoliosis, xii, 68, 70, 91, 177, 178, 179, 182, 188, 189, 191, 219, 222
scope, 207, 216, 250
secretion, 200
security, 214

seizure, 21, 38, 68, 70, 71, 88, 142
self-care activities, ix, 63, 64
self-efficacy, 28
self-esteem, 71
self-organization, 228
self-sufficiency, 219
semicircle, 154
sensation, ix, x, 16, 42, 63, 64, 68, 97, 98, 103, 142, 183
senses, 67, 102
sensitivity, 7, 129, 148, 170, 206
sensitization, 208
sensorimotor dysfunction, ix, 63, 64
sensors, 211, 215, 235
sensory systems, 103
sepsis, 6, 7
service provider, 16
services, 13, 16, 21, 36, 71, 88
sex, 21, 43, 44, 86, 143, 144, 147, 163, 172, 251, 252
shape, 128, 194
sheep, 21, 213
shock, xiii, 57, 193, 194, 195, 196, 197, 198, 200, 201, 202, 203
shock waves, 194, 195, 196, 197, 200, 201
showing, viii, 26, 34, 56, 58, 70, 99, 101, 189
sibling(s), xi, 161, 162, 165, 255
side effects, 197, 199, 200, 223, 243
significance level, 191
signs, 11, 33, 43, 74, 99, 222
silver, 131
Singapore, 226
skeleton, 242
skill acquisition, 84, 98
skin, 155, 194, 196, 197, 201, 223
sleep apnea, 165
sleep disturbance, xii, 16, 162, 177
sleep medicine, 22
sleeve fracture, ix, 53, 58, 59
Slovakia, 25, 205, 231
smoking, 3, 5, 172
smoking cessation, 3
smoothness, 158
snoring, 162, 163, 165
SNP, 5
social acceptance, 34
social activity, x, 97
social adjustment, 17
social consequences, 174
social integration, 232, 241
social interactions, 185
social responsibility, xiv, 249
social situations, 10
social skills, vii, 2, 185

social support, xiv, 249, 250, 251, 252, 254, 255, 256, 257
social welfare, 250
socialization, 71
sodium, 26, 70
software, 130, 131, 153, 155, 211, 213, 215, 217, 218, 235
soleus, 178, 198
solution, 32, 36, 109, 251
spasticity, ix, x, xiii, 17, 22, 23, 26, 27, 38, 46, 59, 61, 63, 64, 68, 69, 70, 73, 74, 75, 76, 79, 86, 87, 89, 91, 92, 97, 99, 109, 116, 117, 118, 119, 120, 143, 178, 182, 193, 194, 196, 197, 198, 199, 200, 201, 202, 209, 233, 243
special education, 4
speech, 67, 68, 71, 159, 208, 222, 232
spinal cord, 27, 44, 194, 197, 207, 209, 210, 211, 216, 219, 229, 232
spinal cord injury, 216, 219, 229, 232
spinal cord tumor, 207
spine, 68, 186, 218, 221, 222, 233, 235
splinting, 72, 73, 74, 90, 92
stability, 100, 103, 133, 135, 152, 158, 183, 187, 216, 218, 223
stabilization, 101, 105, 184, 209, 223, 232, 241, 244
standard deviation, 156
standardization, 120
standing test, 31
state(s), 16, 17, 26, 28, 39, 70, 75, 86, 107, 108, 109
status epilepticus, 43
stem cells, 196
stereotypes, 210, 244
sternum, 154
steroids, 6, 7
stimulation, x, 44, 47, 48, 51, 74, 78, 80, 90, 91, 96, 116, 118, 121, 123, 124, 126, 147, 195, 196, 197, 199, 202, 208, 210, 219
stimulus, 103, 147, 208
strabismus, 72
stratification, 165
strength training, 28, 90, 155
stress, xiv, 71, 121, 149, 162, 165, 197, 249, 250, 251, 252, 253, 254, 255, 256, 257
stress fracture, 197
stress test, 121
stretching, x, 28, 40, 69, 116, 118
stroke, vii, viii, xi, xiii, 11, 25, 30, 38, 42, 43, 44, 45, 49, 76, 79, 80, 83, 93, 94, 123, 127, 135, 137, 160, 163, 171, 193, 194, 197, 198, 202, 209, 211, 216, 219, 225, 229, 232, 241, 246
stroke volume, 163
stromal cells, 201
structural defects, 244

structure, viii, 42, 48, 215, 242
subacute, 197, 202
subgroups, xiii, 21, 231, 234, 237, 238, 239, 240, 241, 242, 244
subluxation, xii, 22, 177, 178, 179, 181, 182, 183, 188
subscapularis, 198, 202
substrates, 77
successive approximations, 77
sulfate, 5
surface area, xiii, 143, 193, 199
surgical intervention, 27, 69, 70, 218, 244
surplus, 81
surveillance, 16, 17, 18, 21, 22, 73, 85
survival, 3, 42, 170
survival rate, 3
survivors, 3, 7, 8
sustainability, 224
Sweden, 19, 66, 226
Switzerland, 211
symptoms, ix, 43, 47, 63, 64, 99, 122, 206, 207
synapse, 200
synaptic plasticity, 200
synaptogenesis, 48
synchronization, 216
syndrome, 9, 69, 75, 99, 189, 223, 224, 225
synthesis, 112, 200

T

target, viii, xi, 26, 75, 117, 119, 120, 123, 151, 152, 153, 154, 158, 195, 209
target zone, 195
task conditions, 102
Task Force, 166, 167
task performance, 100
TBI, 211
techniques, viii, ix, 22, 28, 29, 35, 36, 42, 49, 64, 65, 69, 76, 77, 78, 79, 80, 94, 122, 123, 171, 219
technology(s), 71, 185, 202, 229, 244, 246
teeth, 143, 144, 147
temperament, 256
tendinitis, 196
tendon(s), 27, 53, 194, 196, 197, 200, 202, 216, 222
tension, 60, 183, 186
testing, vii, 5, 15, 25, 31, 34, 36, 124, 220, 223
thalamus, 44, 45, 47, 67
therapeutic approaches, 106, 109
therapeutic goal, 123
therapeutic interventions, 69, 79
therapeutic process, 208, 212
therapist, 28, 38, 80, 81, 120, 121, 123, 133, 208, 212, 213, 215, 232, 235

therapy interventions, 90
threshold of excitation, 217
thrombosis, 43, 171, 172
time commitment, 76
time frame, 43
tissue, 75, 143, 166, 167, 194, 195, 196, 200, 208
TNF, 196
tobacco, 100
toddlers, 88, 92
tonic, xii, 43, 47, 177, 189, 191, 208
tooth, 143, 147, 148
toxic effect, 70
toxin, ix, x, 17, 26, 42, 46, 50, 51, 60, 69, 70, 72, 75, 87, 89, 91, 92, 95, 116, 120, 194, 235
toxoplasmosis, 171
training programs, 225
trajectory, 156
transforming growth factor (TGF), 196, 201
transition period, 101
translation, 13, 108
transmission, 195, 200
transplantation, 75
transport, 152, 186
trauma, xiii, 172, 205, 209, 232
traumatic brain injury, 22, 228
tremor, xi, 127, 133, 134, 136, 222, 228
trial, 5, 13, 14, 15, 18, 20, 23, 31, 39, 50, 81, 82, 87, 89, 90, 91, 92, 94, 95, 96, 102, 125, 126, 130, 160, 198, 202, 225, 226, 245
triceps, 91
triggers, 201
trochanter, 196
trunk control, x, 97, 104, 106, 107, 108
tumor, 7, 197
tumor necrosis factor, 7
twins, 5

U

ulna, 154
ultrasonography, 4
ultrasound, 6, 7, 20, 43, 67, 195
umbilical cord, 75, 92
Unilateral spastic CP, viii, 41, 42
unions, 194, 196, 197
United Kingdom, 181
United States (USA), 10, 13, 65, 98, 115, 163
upper extremity, ix, xiii, 23, 32, 38, 40, 45, 46, 64, 65, 73, 77, 79, 80, 81, 92, 94, 95, 110, 184, 186, 205
urine, 11
uterus, 77

V

vacuum, 12
vagus, 163
vagus nerve, 163
valgus, 222
validation, 23, 35
valorization, 35
variables, 10, 132, 144, 163, 172, 251, 252
variations, 78, 251
vascular endothelial growth factor (VEGF), 196
VCAM, 196
velocity, x, 68, 104, 105, 109, 112, 116, 121, 152, 156, 157, 158, 241
ventilation, 4, 186
Vermeer, 152, 160
vessels, 197, 200
vestibular system, 123
vibration, 200
video games, vii, 25, 26, 28, 29, 30, 31, 33, 36, 40
virtual reality (VR), 236
vision, 72, 170, 235
visual acuity, 67
visual disorders, viii, 26
vitamin D, 70
vitamin D deficiency, 70
vocational training, 68
vomiting, 144, 148
vulnerability, 6, 48, 98

W

walking, xiii, 4, 16, 31, 54, 59, 68, 69, 70, 106, 109, 114, 120, 122, 125, 126, 205, 207, 209, 210, 211, 216, 219, 220, 222, 223, 225, 227, 231, 232, 233, 235, 236, 238, 241, 242, 243, 244, 245, 246, 256
Washington, 185, 187
weakness, x, 53, 75, 99, 103, 115, 117, 119, 120, 178
well-being, 16, 17, 95, 149
Western Australia, 5, 9, 18, 20
white matter, 6, 20, 42, 44, 47, 67, 174
withdrawal, 121
World Health Organization, 3, 187
wound healing, 202

X

Xbox Kinect, vii, 25, 29, 30, 31